ADDICTIONS & SUBSTANCE ABUSE

Strategies for Advanced Practice Nursing

Madeline A. Naegle, RN, CS, PhD, FAAN
New York University

Carolyn Erickson D'Avanzo, RN, DNSc
University of Connecticut

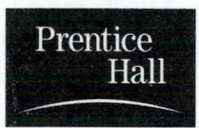

Prentice
Hall

Prentice Hall Health
Upper Saddle River, New Jersey 07458

Library of Congress Cataloging-in-Publication Data

Naegle, Madeline A.
    Addictions & substance abuse : strategies for advanced practice nursing / Madeline A. Naegle, Carolyn E. D'Avanzo.
        p. ; cm.
    Includes bibliographical references and index.
    ISBN 0-8385-8676-7 (alk. paper)
    1. Substance abuse--Nursing. 2. Substance abuse--Patients--Rehabilitation. 3. Substance abuse--Treatment. I. Title: Addictions and substance abuse. II. D'Avanzo, Carolyn E. III. Title.
    [DNLM: 1. Substance-Related Disorders--nursing. 2. Substance-Related Disorders--Nurses' Instruction. WY 160 N141a 2000]
    RC564 .N335 2000
    616.86'06--dc21

                                                                    00-029857

Publisher: Julie Alexander
Acquisitions Editor: Maura Connor
Production Editor: Barbara Barg, Navta Associates, Inc.
Production Liaison: Janet Bolton
**Director of Manufacturing
  and Production:** Bruce Johnson
Managing Editor: Patrick Walsh
Manufacturing Buyer: Ilene Sanford
Art Director: Marianne Frasco
Marketing Manager: Kristin Walton
Editorial Assistant: Beth Ann Romph
Cover Design: Jayne Conte
Composition: Barbara Barg, Navta Associates, Inc.
Printing and Binding: RR Donnelley, Harrisonburg, VA

Prentice-Hall International (UK) Limited, *London*
Prentice-Hall of Australia Pty. Limited, *Sydney*
Prentice-Hall Canada Inc., *Toronto*
Prentice-Hall Hispanoamericana, S.A., *Mexico*
Prentice-Hall of India Private Limited, *New Delhi*
Prentice-Hall of Japan, Inc., *Tokyo*
Prentice-Hall Singapore Pte. Ltd.
Editora Prentice-Hall do Brasil, Ltda., *Rio de Janeiro*

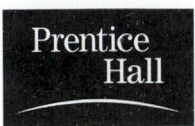

10 9 8 7 6 5 4 3 2
ISBN 0-8385-8676-7

We dedicate this book to our families, Amanda, Ben and Cara McGowan and Jonathan and Lorraine D'Avanzo, Ratha and Sita Touch, Tinh Do and Pholla Meas. Their love and encouragement have supported this project.

Contents

Preface

Addictions and Substance Abuse: Strategies for Advanced Practice Nursing is a further step in the ongoing efforts to increase practicing nurses' knowledge and skills related to addictions. Whether educators and/or direct care providers, nurses comprise the largest group of health care professionals and have great potential to decrease the prevalence of problems relating to addictions as well as the morbidity and mortality of persons with substance-related disorders. Often nurses recognize that substance use or abuse is causing problems for clients and/or their families but lack sufficient knowledge to intervene with confidence. This book is designed as a reference for several general content areas foundational to advanced practice. It holds some answers and hopefully stimulates ongoing questions about effective ways to make differences in client's lives. The development of a chapter for each specialty posed too great a task, therefore chapters provide basic knowledge for interventions in a range of settings and specialties. The book includes three chapters on addiction and substance abuse issues that influence nursing practice. Chapter 5 discusses the wide variation of substance-related problems in persons of differing ethnic backgrounds. These early chapters contribute frameworks for the specific interventions discussed later in the book.

Addictions and Substance Abuse is designed to support evidence-based practice by master's prepared nurses in advanced practice roles. The interventions and approaches described require the autonomy, knowledge, and skills that characterize the roles of nurse practitioners, clinical specialists, case managers, and consultants. The recent emergence of scientific research on substance use and its influence on major human systems makes it imperative that all nurses upgrade their knowledge of this field. This book contributes resources to meet some of these important goals. In a field where tradition has often dictated practice, new information and its configuration into prevention and treatment modalities are most welcome. Although much of the material herein is reference, learner outcomes and competencies can be developed around the case studies and critical thinking questions provided at the end of the chapers. Educators will find this book a useful resource text.

The appendices are important components of this volume. They provide direction and resources that are up-to-date, inexpensive, and easy to access. Websites are constantly emerging and under revision and the number of agencies and organizations interested in bringing treatment providers together are increasing. The best sources to find up-to-date approaches and increasing current knowledge are provided. If each reader of this volume develops interest in and the facility to further pursue knowledge about evidence-based and effective practice in relation to substance use, abuse, and dependence, then the goals of this venture will be more than realized.

Acknowledgments

We acknowledge and thank our colleagues who have helped us to understand the needs of practicing nurses as they care for clients with substance-related illnesses. We are particularly grateful to those colleagues who have contributed their efforts to enrich this volume with timely and substantive works.

We thank our students whose enthusiasm and commitment to the study of substance abuse have been sources of inspiration as well as reminders of the need to persevere with this venture.

Funding of the ATOD Faculty Development Programs by the Center for Substance Abuse Prevention, United States Department of Health and Human Services, supported acquisition of knowledge about substance-related disorders which was the origin of this project. We wish to acknowledge the mentorship and support of Olga Church who directed the FDP at the University of Connecticut and our colleagues in the AMERSA organization.

We thank the editors and production staff at Prentice Hall for their assistance in the final organization of manuscripts and a smooth transition to a new publisher. A special thank you is reserved for Sally Barhydt, formerly of Appleton and Lange, without whose support and confidence this book would have remained in the realm of ideas. We also thank the following reviewers for their insight and helpful comments:

Jeanne A. Clement, EdD, RN, CS, FAAN
Professor of Nursing
Ohio State University, Columbus, OH

Benna Cunningham, RN, MSN, FNP
Professor of Nursing
Medical College of Georgia, Athens, GA

Janice Cook Feigenbaum, RN, PhD
Professor of Nursing
D'Youville College, Buffalo, NY

Mary Jo Gorney-Moreno, PhD, RN
Professor of Nursing
San Jose State University, San Jose, CA

Nancy M. Valentine, RN, PhD, MPH, FAAN
Special Assistant to Secretary and Advisor to Under Secretary for Health
Veterans Health Administration, Washington, DC

Diane Snow, PhD
Professor of Nursing
University of Texas at Arlington, Arlington, TX

Contributors

David Duncan, DrPh
Senior Study Director
Substance Abuse Research Group
Westat Corporation
Rockville, MD

Patricia C. Dunn, EdD, LCSW, ACSW
Associate Professor
School of Social Work
Rutgers University
New Brunswick, NJ

Laina Gerace, PhD, RN
Rockford Regional Program
University of Illinois, Rockford
Rockford, IL

Robert Granfield, PhD
Department of Sociology
University of Denver
Denver, CO

Judith Haber, RN, PhD, APRN, FAAN
Professor and Director of Master's
  Programs and Advanced Certificate
  Programs
New York University
New York, NY

Carl A. Kirton, RN, MA, CS, ANP
Clinical Assistant Professor of Nursing
New York University
New York, NY

Sophronia Larig, CNM, MSN, CNP
Independent Practice, Women's Health
Forest Hills, NY

Phyllis Lisanti, RN, PhD
Clinical Associate Professor of Nursing
New York University
New York, NY

Deborah J. Mahoney, ScD, RN, CSPNP
Associate Professor
University of Massachusetts
Boston, MA

Pamela J. Maraldo, RN, PhD, FAAN
Principal
Women's Health Management Solutions
New York, NY

Jane Murdock, RN, EdD
Emeritus Associate Professor
School of Nursing
University of Connecticut
Storrs, CT

Kevin Ryan
Department of Justice Studies and
  Sociology
Norwich University
Northfield, VT

Marie Talashek, RN, PhD, FAAN
College of Nursing
University of Illinois, Chicago
Chicago, IL

1

Introduction and Overview

Carolyn E. D'Avanzo, RN, MSN, DNSc

LEARNER OUTCOMES

On completion of this chapter, the learner will be able to:

1. Identify natural substances and chemicals used historically as physical and psychological remedies.
2. Define the disease model of alcoholism and its role in reducing the stigma of addictions.
3. Synthesize information about the prevalence of alcohol, nicotine, and other drug abuse and the consequences to society as a whole.
4. Explore policy changes linked to significant changes in substance abuse prevention and treatment.

KEY TERMS

disease model of alcoholism
drug dependence

illicit/illegal drugs
licit/legal drugs

prevalence

Although drug abuse is recognized as a global problem with far-reaching consequences for industrialized as well as developing countries, societies have yet to develop effective prevention and intervention activities that decrease the enormous health and social consequences of drug dependence. Our communities need to develop better understandings about the many personal (heredity, personality characteristics) and environmental (social, economic, political, cultural) factors that contribute to drug use. Particularly important are factors that determine vulnerability to drugs, initiation of use, drug use progression, and resources used by individuals to limit or stop drug use prior to reaching psychological and/or physiologic dependence.

Historical Perspectives

Natural substances and chemicals have been used throughout history, and their use has been integral to social, economic, and medical contexts. Drugs have frequently been used to alter states of consciousness in efforts to achieve secondary goals: medicate uncomfortable psychological states, improve performance, alter mood, facilitate relaxation and socialization, or reach other highly individual goals emanating from one's culture and personality. Historically, alcohol may have been the first substance observed to produce a change in physical and psychological state when ingested, but the use of various natural plants such as poppies (opium), hemp (marijuana), and coca beans (cocaine) also dates back thousands of years. Remedies made from these plants were used to treat illness, relieve pain, and increase the capacity of individuals to tolerate long days of labor within and outside the home.

Herbalists and shaman from many cultures commonly used, and continue to use, plants, seeds, and animal products to treat physical and mental illnesses and mood disorders, as well as to enhance a sense of well-being. Native North and South American cultures, for example, incorporated the use of seeds and natural plants, such as peyote and mushrooms, in their rituals to induce euphoric states to increase their receptivity to revelation from supernatural beings. Over time, although the helpful effects of certain drugs were recognized, negative effects such as impaired work performance, antisocial behavior, crime, and violence were also observed. For these reasons, legal promulgations to control the export, trade, sale, and use of drugs were initiated and have existed for thousands of years.

The recognition that the abuse of substances could constitute forms of emotional and mental illness occurred around the middle of the twentieth century, as these conditions became evident in men and women returning from World War II. At that time, dominant public views of addiction linked excessive use of prescription drugs (e.g., morphine and cocaine), heavy alcohol consumption, and use of illicit drugs (e.g., marijuana) to emotional instability, poor character, and weak will. Conversely, in psychiatric circles, **drug dependence** was viewed as symptomatic of unresolved unconscious conflicts, fixation at an earlier level of development, and problems of personality structure. In the 1960s, Jellinek's **disease model of alcoholism** was published. It initially identified types of alcoholism differentiated by patterns of onset, loss of control, and rate of progression and described alcoholism as a chronic, relapsing disease with a genetic component (Jellinek, 1960). This major shift in definition became the cornerstone of the Alcoholics Anonymous movement. The model, along with the ground-breaking work of developing self-help models by Alcoholics Anonymous, is credited with both decreasing the stigma associated with addiction and shifting public attitudes toward defining addiction as a disease. George Vaillant's longitudinal study of men and their patterns of alcohol use revealed highly individual patterns of alcoholism, as well as recovery from alcoholism with and without professional intervention (Vaillant, 1983; Vaillant, Gale, and Milofsky, 1984). The current disease model derived from Jellinek's and Vaillant's work acknowledges a wide range of individual patterns of abuse and addiction. The widespread use of illicit drugs that emerged in the late 1960s peaked in the 1970s, bringing the attention of the government, health professions, and the public to the study of both the origins and the nature of drug problems. Due to intensified scientific research efforts, genetic factors and other constitutional characteristics were shown to support the biologic theory of addiction; psychological and sociocultural models of causation also were developed. Increasingly, the development of addictions, whether to tobacco, drugs, or alcohol, is acknowledged as derived from the same neurologic and psychological process.

Current policy on American control of narcotics stems from the Drug Abuse Prevention and Control Act of 1970, which stated that federal law supercedes state legislation. This effectively transferred authority for drug enforcement policies from the Treasury Department to the Bureau of Narcotics and Dangerous Drugs under the Department of Justice and created a schedule of drugs reflecting their potential for abuse. The National Institute of Alcohol Abuse and Alcoholism and the National Institute of Drug Abuse were both established in 1972, which facilitated more extensive research on addictions and made findings readily available to policymakers, health care providers, and the public. The establishment of the Centers for Substance Abuse Treatment and Substance Abuse Prevention within the Substance Abuse and Mental Health Services Agency (SAMHSA) further expanded studies and demonstrations in the areas of prevention, education, and treatment. Increasingly, public education and policy development have emerged from such research.

Prevalence

One source of information on drug use for health professionals in the United States is the National Household Survey on Drug Abuse (NHSDA) (SAMHSA, 1998), which randomly selects individuals from households and other residences and asks them about their patterns of use. The National Household Survey on Drug Abuse definition states that the **prevalence** of a condition is the number or rate at which individuals have a specified condition at a given point or for a period of time. Current drug use means use of a drug at least once in the past month; lifetime prevalence is the percent of people who have ever used the drug, regardless of the number of times they may have used it. The survey also reports use of substances in the previous year (past-year use). Four age groups (12–17, 18–25, 26–34, and 35 and over) and three racial/ethnic groups (Hispanic in origin, regardless of race; white non-Hispanic; and black non-Hispanic) are interviewed in National Household Surveys. The NHSDA reports frequency distributions and rates both for **licit/legal drugs** such as alcohol and nicotine (cigarettes and smokeless tobacco) and for **illicit/illegal drugs** (marijuana, cocaine, hallucinogens, and heroin). Survey participants are selected from noninstitutionalized households, college dormitories, and military installations. A major difficulty when attempting to generalize NHSDA results to the total population of the United States is that segments of the population that may contain substantial numbers of drug users have only recently been included in the survey. These include transients not residing in shelters, military personnel on active duty, and those incarcerated in jails and prisons. The value of self-report is, of course, dependent on both the memory and the honesty of subjects but has been found through research to provide valid approximate guidelines. The NHSDA measures the prevalence of alcohol, drug, and tobacco use in the estimated 216 million members of the U.S. population age 12 and older. Such data help provide a general resource to nurses and others to help them identify emerging and long-standing trends in use.

In the early 1960s, it was reported that less than 5 percent of adult Americans had tried illicit drugs; by 1988, almost 37 percent reported they had tried at least one. From 1977 to 1990, there was a decrease in use in all categories of drugs in the 18–25 age group, a trend thought to be consistent in other age groups as well (Coleman, 1993). Data from the early to mid-1990s suggested some stability of drug use in Americans age 18 and older. Despite some encouraging trends, there remain approximately "18 million alcoholics, 28 million children of alcoholics, 6 million cocaine addicts, 14.9 million people who abuse other substances, 25 million addicted to nicotine, 54 million who are at least 20% overweight, 3.5 million school-age children with attention-deficit disorder or Tourette syndrome, and about 448,000 compulsive gamblers" in the United States (Blum et al., 1996, p. 143).

Legal Drugs

Alcohol and nicotine, both licit/legal drugs, are most frequently abused in the United States. Over 51 percent of the U.S. population (about 111 million people) report current (in the previous month) alcohol use (SAMHSA, 1998), with over 4.6 million of that number between the ages of 12 and 17. Approximately 11 million Americans report heavy drinking (defined as drinking five or more drinks per occasion on 5 or more days in the previous 30 days). Another 32 million report binge drinking (defined as drinking five or more drinks on some occasion on at least 1 day in the past 30 days). Consumption of alcohol alone is the most common pattern of drug use in the United States: The Household Survey estimates that 4 percent to 33 percent of adults seeking outpatient primary care services have problems with alcohol. Over 152 million people (over 70 percent of the surveyed population) had tried a cigarette at some point in their lives; about 29 percent (64 million) were current smokers (use in the past month).

Illegal Drugs

Before using any other drugs, individuals tend to use nicotine, followed by alcohol, inhalants, and marijuana. For that reason, nicotine and alcohol have been labeled gateway drugs. These are followed by cocaine, hallucinogens, and heroin (used by progressively fewer individuals). In a governmental report (Rouse, 1995), alcohol and illegal drugs together accounted for over 11 percent of preventable deaths in the United States; smoking, however, accounted for 39 percent, the greatest portion of preventable deaths.

In the 1997 NHSDA, almost 14 million Americans (over 6 percent) reported current use of illicit drugs (in the past month). Of the illicit/illegal drugs, marijuana was the most frequently abused, with about 71 million of the over 216 million persons represented in

1997 reporting they had tried it, and over 11 million reporting current use (in the past month). The National Household Survey states that the estimates on cocaine are subject to potentially significant underreporting, although the trends are considered to be reliable. The estimated number of occasional cocaine users (use for fewer than 12 days in the previous year) was also similar to that of 1996. Cocaine use has decreased from 1985 when it was over 7 million; the use of crack cocaine has changed little since 1988. The 1997 survey reported over 4 million Americans have used crack cocaine, a highly addictive drug, at some time, and about 604,000 are current users. Crack use was highest among blacks (3.1 percent), followed by whites (1.9 percent), and Hispanics (1.6 percent). The age of initiation of use, later than for marijuana, is about 21 years of age.

At its peak, cocaine was used by about 1.5 million persons each year between 1980 and 1982. In 1992, an estimated half-million people used cocaine for the first time. Over 22 million of the 216 million people represented in the 1997 survey reported they had used cocaine at some time (10.5 percent); over 1.5 million reported current use (in the past month). Although the use of cocaine gradually diminished in the 1980s, its use is still prevalent and is associated with violent acts such as rape and armed robbery (Giannini et al., 1993).

In addition, the 1997 data indicate that there were over 1.6 million current hallucinogen users. Of this number, 369,000 reported using phencyclidine (PCP) in the previous year, and almost 2 million reported past-year lysergic acid diethylamide (LSD) use. There were 883,000 current inhalant users and 612,000 current stimulant users. About 597,000 individuals used heroin in the last year—twice as many as in the early 1990s. Noninjectable heroin is believed to be primarily responsible for this rise in incidence. Recent data indicate that heroin use is rising in 14-year-olds, an alarming trend. About 2.3 million of the over 216 million represented in the 1997 survey reported lifetime drug use with needles. Over 4 million persons reported use of prescription-type sedatives for nonmedical reasons, and 6.9 million had used tranquilizers. Overall, the drug problem in the United States affects significant numbers of persons and seriously impacts health and health care delivery. The War on Drugs and efforts to educate the public on the dangers of both licit and illicit drug use have produced inconsistent outcomes relative to decreasing the drug problem.

The Toll of Alcohol and Other Drugs on Health

In the United States, substance abuse ranks number one as the primary cause of illness, disability, and mortality in preventable health conditions (McGinnis and Foege, 1993). Tobacco use is the single most important preventable cause of death in the United States, and cirrhosis of the liver is caused by alcohol abuse about 50 percent of the time. Increasing mortality rates due to substance abuse are also attributed to acquired immunodeficiency syndrome (AIDS) (Horgan, 1993). The SAMHSA Drug Abuse Warning Network (DAWN) (1996) monitors the consequences of drug use using two indicators: drug-related hospital emergency department (ED) visits and drug-related deaths recorded by medical examiners. This institutional data collection system captures the problem end of drug abuse. The four most frequently reported drugs associated with deaths are cocaine, heroin, alcohol in combination with other drugs, and codeine.

Cardiovascular Disease

Use of alcohol and cigarettes causes serious health problems in their users, over and above the problem of dependency. Excessive alcohol use has potentially harmful effects on the cardiovascular system such as elevated blood pressure, abnormalities in heart rhythms, and congestive heart failure due to weakened heart muscle (alcoholic cardiomyopathy). These links were identified in the 1950s (Doll and Hill, 1952). Women's hearts may be even more susceptible to the adverse effects of alcohol (including cardiomyopathy) than men's; because they metabolize alcohol differently from men, women appear to become alcoholic at lower levels of consumption. Tobacco use is considered to be a major risk factor for diseases of the heart and blood vessels, and cigarette smoking is responsible for an estimated 21 percent of all coronary heart disease deaths (40 percent of those under age 65).

Emphysema and Chronic Bronchitis

As of 1997, almost 7 million people were current users of smokeless tobacco, and over 64 million were current cigarette users. Tobacco use is a major risk factor for chronic obstructive pulmonary disease (COPD), a major cause of chronic morbidity and disability. Cigarette smoking accounts for 82 percent of these deaths and causes pneumonia, bronchitis, and frequent respiratory infections.

Cancer

It is estimated that one in three cancer deaths is linked to smoking. According to 1996 estimates (American Cancer Society, 1996), tobacco use was responsible for about 170,000 deaths, and smoking cigarettes was responsible for 87 percent of all lung cancer deaths. Although lung cancer mortality in men is leveling off, the number of deaths from lung cancer in women is increasing at a steady rate worldwide. Passive or involuntary smoking causes lung cancer and other diseases in healthy nonsmokers, as well as severe respiratory problems in children. Tobacco is also associated with cancers of the bladder, head, and neck. Risk factors for esophageal cancer (with less than a 5 percent five-year survival) include smoking and alcohol consumption, frequently in combination (Goroll, May, and Mulley, 1995).

Costs of Substance Abuse and Dependence

Cost-of-illness studies evaluate both the direct and indirect costs of substance abuse and dependence. Direct costs are those for which payments are actually made and include expenditures for health care, research, training costs for physicians and nurses, insurance payments, and costs of drug-related crime. Indirect costs are those for which resources are lost, for example, morbidity and mortality costs. Morbidity costs refer to the value of lost productivity because the individual is unable to perform usual activities or cannot perform them at full effectiveness. Mortality costs refer to the value of lost productivity due to the individual's premature death. In addition, the psychosocial costs associated with substance abuse and dependence (e.g., trauma, chronic grief, and psychological disability) affect society, families, and individuals.

Analyses published in 1992–1993 indicate that fetal alcohol syndrome and AIDS cost the United States $2.1 and $6.3 billion, respectively, in 1990. Yearly crime, criminal justice, and property loss associated with crime cost $15.8 billion and $46 billion for alcohol and drugs, respectively. Lost productivity due to alcohol-related and drug-related illnesses cost $36.6 and $8.0 billion, respectively, and health care costs related to alcohol and drugs were $10.6 and $3.2 billion, respectively. Alcohol abuse and drug abuse are costly across all occupations but take on special significance in occupations in which public safety may be jeopardized, such as truck drivers, train engineers, and airline pilots. Major payers for alcohol and drug treatment include private sources, state/local government, and Medicaid, and these have decreased their amounts of support. State/local government is the primary payment source for alcohol and drug treatment. It is estimated that 19 percent of all Medicaid inpatient costs are related to substance abuse, in that the diseases or health conditions for which individuals sought treatment were directly linked to the use of alcohol, tobacco, and/or drugs (Rouse, 1995). About 8 percent of the 19 percent of total Medicaid costs go toward additional days of hospitalization required by medical/surgical clients to treat secondary diagnoses of substance dependence.

Health insurance coverage for persons treated for drug-related problems varies by income level, and health insurance is an important determinant of treatment. The higher the income of those treated, the greater is the likelihood that they will have health insurance. At more moderate levels of income ($10,000–$29,000), there are differences between those treated for alcohol and drug abuse: About 65 percent of treated alcoholics have health insurance, compared with about 80 percent of treated drug abusers. Whites, blacks, and Cuban Americans are most likely to have private health insurance; Puerto Ricans are most likely to have public health insurance (e.g., Medicare or Medicaid). Mexican Americans are most likely to be uninsured. From 1982 to 1991, employers expanded their private health insurance coverage for substance abuse detoxification. The percentage of employees covered by insurance in businesses employing 100 or more workers increased from 50 percent or less of employees to over 95 percent of employees in medium and large companies from 1982 to 1991.

Public subsidies are the most important source of funding for facilities specializing in drug abuse treatment (40 percent of revenues). Public subsidies are provided through state and local funds and federal block grants. Other public sources of funding include Medicaid, Medicare, and Tricare Allied Health Care for retired military personnel and their dependents. Together, public sources account for over 50 percent of treatment funds. Private insurance, including health maintenance organizations (HMOs), accounts for another 30 percent, and client fees for 11 percent, of the total funding received by the specialty drug abuse facilities. Studies of individuals who have received treatment for substance abuse indicate favorable economic impacts (e.g., higher rates of employment and less use of public assistance).

Implications for Nursing Practice

The most common causes of injuries seen in emergency departments are traffic accidents, falls, and violence, which often lead to traumatic brain and spinal cord injuries (the two most severe disabling conditions). Approximately 25 percent of injuries treated in the ED are alcohol-related. Nurses working in other primary care and specialty areas may not be as aware of the impact of substance abuse and dependence on these services. For example, on general medical service units, 18 percent to 25 percent of the clients may be alcoholics, have other substance abuse problems, or be dually diagnosed. Estimates for surgical services are 25 percent, psychiatric services may reach 30 percent to 40 percent, and outpatient settings range consistently between 15 percent and 25 percent (Babor, 1990; Coleman and Veach, 1990; Moore et al., 1989). The costs to society as a whole are estimated at a staggering $240 billion annually (Rice, 1993; Robert Wood Johnson Foundation, 1992) and result in psychological, social, health, and financial problems that affect the quality of life for individuals and their families.

This book provides a broad knowledge base for advanced practice nurses (APNs) treating the varied manifestations of substance use and abuse. Because drug taking is a part of this society and eradication of the problem is unlikely, intervention to decrease related health problems must be part of nursing practice. The focus on primary health care within the managed care model, the growing autonomy of APNs, and consumer awareness are increasing the need for APNs to manage substance-related problems. The physical and psychological problems that are the sequelae to drug use challenge nursing practitioners in a variety of settings.

The shift in nursing practice from acute care, in which 67 percent of registered nurses (RNs) are presently employed, to community health and ambulatory settings, where 10 percent and 8 percent of nurses (respectively) are employed, is a major paradigm shift for the profession (Klainberg, Holzemer, Leonard, and Arnold, 1998). For many nurses in this time of professional chaos and uncertainty, the knowledge and skills needed to practice in this expanded role must be examined in light of societal needs. The Chinese character that means both chaos and opportunity provides a model for progress. If APNs can expand goals to improve health services for substance-abusing clients, new opportunities will emerge. Resources to educate and support nursing practice in the areas of substance use, abuse, and dependence must be specialty-specific, although they emerge from the common knowledge base of drug use and addiction. We look to our colleagues to creatively use the information herein to shape medical practice to benefit clients, families, groups, and communities.

Case Study

John Hill is a 54-year-old accountant who has made an appointment for a routine physical. As you begin your assessment, it becomes clear that John is severely depressed. He tells you that he is in the process of a divorce and is also in danger of losing his job in a large accounting firm. He admits that he has been drinking heavily for years, but that prior to this time it has gone unnoticed by his employers. Although his drinking is generally limited to weekends, he is increasingly unable to function on Mondays and is experiencing more frequent blackouts than in the past. His employer has given him an ultimatum: either get help from the firm's employee assistance program or get out. John says he has "dried out" several times and returned to drinking; therefore, he feels it may be pointless to try again. He also states that the Alcoholics Anonymous self-help model is less than ideal for him because he doesn't believe in a higher power.

1. Using your knowledge of the disease concept of alcoholism, how would you explain the relapsing nature of John's alcoholism that is influencing his attitude toward treatment?
2. What are some positive aspects of John's confrontation with his employer?
3. How can you best intervene in this situation and aid in the coordination of substance abuse treatment and services?
4. What other self-help groups can you suggest to John that do not include acceptance of the concept of a higher power?
5. As an advanced practice nurse, what legal, ethical, and professional responsibilities should you assume for John's follow-up care?

CRITICAL THINKING QUESTIONS

1. What personal and environmental factors in your own life may put you at risk for substance abuse?
2. What are the pros and cons of the Alcoholics Anonymous self-help model?
3. Should the use of natural mood-altering substances by Native North Americans be legalized as religious ritual or be punishable as illegal drug use?
4. How do managed care models impact the prevention and treatment of substance abuse by advanced practice nurses?

REFERENCES

American Cancer Society. (1996). *Cancer Facts and Figures—1996*. Atlanta, GA: Author.

Babor, T.F. (1990). Alcohol and substance abuse in primary care settings. In J. Mayfield and M. Grady (eds.), *Primary Care Research: An Agenda for the 90s*. Washington, DC: U.S. Department of Health and Human Services.

Blum, K., Cull, J.G., Braverman, E.R., and Comings, D.E. (1996). Reward deficiency syndrome. *American Scientist 84,* 132–145.

Coleman, P. (1993). Overview of substance abuse. *Primary Care 20*(1), 1–18.

Coleman, P.R., and Veach, T. (1990). Substance abuse and the family physician: A survey of attitudes. *Substance Abuse 11,* 84–93.

Doll, R., and Hill, A.B. (1952). Study of the aetiology of carcinoma of the lung. *British Medical Journal 2,* 1271–1285.

Giannini, A.J., Miller, N.S., Loiselle, R.H., and Turner, C.E. (1993). Cocaine-associated violence and relationship to route of administration. *Journal of Substance Abuse Treatment 10*(1), 67–69.

Goroll, A.H., May, L.A., and Mulley, A.G. (1995). Management of gastrointestinal cancers. In A.H. Goroll, L.A. May, and A.G. Mulley (eds.), *Primary Care Medicine*. Philadelphia: J.B. Lippincott Co.

Horgan, C. (1993). *Substance Abuse: The Nation's Number One Health Problem, Key Indicators for Policy*. Institute for Health Policy, Brandeis University. Princeton, NJ: Robert Wood Johnson Foundation.

Jellinek, E.M. (1960). *The Disease Concept of Alcoholism*. New Brunswick, NJ: Hillhouse Press.

Klainberg, M., Holzemer, S., Leonard, M., and Arnold, J. (1998). *Community Health Nursing: An Alliance for Health*. New York: McGraw-Hill.

McGinnis, M.J., and Foege, W. (1993). Actual causes of death in the United States. *Journal of the American Medical Association 270*, 2208.

Moore, R.D., Bone, L.R., Geller, G., Mamon, J.A., Stokes, E.J., and Levine, D.M. (1989). Prevalence, detection, and treatment of alcoholism in hospitalized patients. *Journal of the American Medical Association 261*, 403–407.

Rice, D. (1993). The economic cost of alcohol abuse and alcohol dependence. *Alcohol World: Health and Research 17*, 10–12.

Robert Wood Johnson Foundation. (1992). *Substance Abuse* (annual report). Princeton, NJ: Robert Wood Johnson Foundation.

Rouse, B. (ed.). (1995). *Substance Abuse and Mental Health Statistics Sourcebook*. DHHS Publication No. (SMA) 95-3064. Washington, DC: Superintendent of Documents, U.S. Government Printing Office.

Substance Abuse and Mental Health Services Administration (SAMHSA), Office of Applied Studies. (August 1996). *Preliminary Estimates from the Drug Abuse Warning Network: 1995 Preliminary Estimates of Drug-Related Emergency Department Episodes, Advance Report Number 17*. Rockville, MD: Author.

Substance Abuse and Mental Health Services Administration (SAMHSA), Office of Applied Studies. (1998). *National Household Survey on Drug Abuse: Population Estimates 1997*. DHHS Publication No. (SMA) 98-3250. Rockville, MD: Author.

Substance Abuse and Mental Health Services Administration (SAMHSA), Office of Applied Studies. (1998). *National Household Survey on Drug Abuse: Population Estimates 1998* (http://www.health.org/pubs). Rockville, MD: Author.

Vaillant, G.E. (1983). *The Natural History of Alcoholism*. Cambridge, MA: Harvard University Press.

Vaillant, G.E., Gale, L., and Milofsky, E.S. (1984). Natural history of male alcoholism: Paths to recovery. In D.W. Goodwin, K.T. Van Dusen, and S.A. Mednick (eds.), *Longitudinal Research in Alcoholism*. Boston: Kluwer-Nijhoff.

2

The Advanced Practice Role

Pamela J. Maraldo, RN, PhD, FAAN

LEARNER OUTCOMES

On completion of this chapter, the learner will be able to:

1. Describe the relationship between nursing and managed care.
2. List nursing's most recent advances in terms of regulatory changes in the Medicare statute.
3. Discuss the rate of increase in mental health and substance abuse expenditures.
4. Explain the main barriers to independent practice for advanced practice nurses.
5. Describe the types of changes that need to occur before advanced practice nurses can function as primary care providers.

KEY TERMS

advanced practice nurse (APN)
autonomy

consumer education
integrated care

medical model

Managed care is in trouble. The once-spectacular vision of better medicine at lower costs as a result of market-driven health care has dimmed amid disappointing earnings for managed care companies and consumer dissatisfaction.

Although managed care dramatically reduced the inflation in health insurance costs for employers in the mid-1990s, this seems to have been a one-time savings because the underlying demographic and technological trends remain unchanged, and employers and benefits consultants report sharply rising premium costs ahead. With premium costs continuing to rise, more employers are dropping or reducing coverage than are expanding it (Kuttner, 1999).

We are at a critical crossroads in health care, and questions remain: Where did we go wrong? Where do we go from here? Critics charge that the cost decreases have occurred because managed care organizations (MCOs) have not cared for many sick people. They collected huge boluses of cash signing up enrollees and then imposed arbitrary rules restricting health care, such as 24-hour drive-by deliveries, denial of referrals to specialists, and bureaucratic denials of important services, that aroused the public ire.

In addition, disastrous misjudgments led to the collapse of the stock of the industry's most celebrated health maintenance organizations (HMOs). In 1997, Oxford recorded $29 million in losses, and the company realized additional losses in 1998. Other companies suffered Oxford's fate. Many health care companies in a relatively short period have gone from being Wall Street's darlings to Wall Street's outcasts. By 1997, the stock-market boom in health care companies was largely over (Kuttner, 1999).

Some of the managed care industry's problems may be the result of inventing itself based on the conventional medical model and failing to take into account that there is no entirely gentle way to alter a system that has been in place for a number of years. Yet, the legendary excesses in hospitalization rates and surgeries posed substantial economic threats under the old fee-for-service (FFS) system and were more infuriating to consumers and policymakers alike than the current wave of anger over managed care. As Governor Lamm, Chairman of the PEW Commission, recently pointed out, the number of specialists often determines how many and what types of procedures are performed in the community. The highest correlation to the number of tonsillectomies, prostatectomies, hysterectomies, and hernia repairs is not the level of health in a population, but the number of specialists in the area (Lamm, 1996).

Rates for appendectomies, which are not elective procedures, are nearly geographically uniform, but elective procedures, over which doctors have discretion, vary in disturbing proportions. Lamm (1996, pp. 220–221) concludes with the observation, "Much of what we do in health care serves the interests of the physician or a particular institution rather than the interests of the public. Well meaning people continually turn away from facing the ethical implications of this dynamic."

Regardless of financing mechanism, quality of health care is on the national agenda. Much of the interest in quality has developed in response to the dramatic transformation of the health care system in recent years. New organizational structures and reimbursement strategies have created incentives that may affect quality. Even though there is some evidence of poor quality, the concern about quality "arises more from fear and anecdote than from facts" (Schuster, McGlynn, and Brook, 1998, p. 517). There is surprisingly little systematic evidence about quality of care in the United States.

Many have been quick to conclude that managed care is responsible for much of the poor quality that has been found. Studies published in the research literature, however, have neither clearly confirmed nor refuted this conclusion. Some studies find that MCOs provide better care than FFS models, some find that FFS provides better care, and others find that the care is about the same. Results vary depending on the setting, the type of care assessed, and the methodology used to analyze the issue (Schuster, McGlynn, and Brook, 1998).

Managed care sought to correct the excesses and put financial incentives in place to encourage prevention and to keep people out of expensive hospitals and away from costly specialists and medical procedures, but managed care has failed in its execution to a large extent because physicians are not educated to practice that way. Traditional medical education trains physicians to practice in a very linear way: Germ A causes disease B, and it's treated by drugs C or surgery D. Keeping people well requires the ability to look for the emotional and psychological as well as physical patterns that precede a particular illness.

A person's psychology and social sphere have no influence over conventional medical science even though scientific evidence clearly shows that emotional and social patterns of behavior have a profound effect on health and well-being. It is well established that stress can suppress immune function, and anger (like other suppressed emotions) is bad for the heart. Further, social connection has profound consequences for health. People who suffered abuse in childhood (or who had a parent who was an alcoholic, was an addict, or was battered) were shown to be two to four times more likely to suffer serious illnesses such as heart disease, stroke, or emphysema than others (Goode, 1999). Yet, physicians are trained to take action only when they see symptoms, which may often be too late (McEwen and Stellar, 1993).

Medicine in modern society has defined its mission in terms of curing disease (the medical disorder) while overlooking illness (the client's experience of the disease). Often medical practitioners ignore clients' emotional reactions to their medical problems or dismiss their reactions as irrelevant to the cause of the problem. No matter how well intentioned medical practitioners are, that attitude is spawned by a **medical model** that entirely dismisses the notion that the mind influences the body in consequential ways. Limited emphasis on mind/body relationships results in a narrow focus that often excludes emotional and addictive illnesses. Spiegel (1999) recently stated, "We have been closet Cartesians in modern medicine—treating the mind as though it were reactive to but otherwise disconnected from disease in the body" (Spiegel, 1999, p. 1328).

But much of that is now changing. A growing number of scientists recognize that we are in the middle of a scientific revolution—a major paradigm shift—with tremendous implications for health and disease. Recent technological innovations have allowed us to examine the molecular basis of emotions and to understand how emotions are inseparable from physiology. As neuroscientist Candice Pert (1998) recently stated, "It is the emotions I have come to see that link the mind and the body."

What causes people to consume alcohol and licit and illicit substances is emotions that are inhibited, cut off, unprocessed, unintegrated, or unreleased. Trauma and stress continually lodged at the level of the receptors block nerve pathways and interrupt the smooth flow of information chemicals, a physiological condition we experience as "stuck" or "unhealed emotions: chronic sadness, fear, frustration, anger." "Reaching for that drink or joint is usually precipitated by some disturbing or unacceptable feeling that we don't know how to deal with" (Pert, 1998).

Meeting the challenge of integrating the biomedical and the psychosocial aspects of care will be increasingly vital to the provision of effective health care. This challenge can uniquely be met by the **advanced practice nurse** (APN) in a variety of roles, such as the nurse practitioner (NP), clinical nurse specialist (CNS), or case manager.

The Inexorable Trend Toward Integration

Economic pressures as well as new scientific discoveries are forcing movement toward **integrated care.** As managed care continues to face downward pressure on prices from employers, the need for new models of care becomes ever more apparent. The fragmentation of services that scrolls back to our highly specialized system calls for reintegration in many respects. The integration of psyche and soma is a major challenge; because mental health had been carved out from the premium dollar, it is now time to carve it back in. Any integration of services will be virtually ineffectual unless funding mechanisms are integrated as well.

As the Institute of Medicine's report on primary care recently expressed, mental health carve-out systems have major drawbacks and, in fact, can subvert certain core principles and values of primary care—comprehensiveness and continuity (de Gruy, 1996). Carve-out providers have no incentive to reduce general medical costs and may try to shift costs into the general medical sector. Moreover, one-third to one-half of clients referred for mental health services fail to accept the referral, and the refusals generally come from clients who are high users (de Gruy, 1996). Recent federal legislation that sought parity of mental health benefits with other medical benefits has been undermined by insurers. Companies are bypassing the federal law by changing the structure of benefits for inpatient and outpatient mental health/substance abuse care in a discriminatory manner. Although 19 states have laws that require negotiation of similar levels of coverage for mental and physical illnesses, health plans circumvent this by limiting previous spending caps (*New York Times,* 1998).

With respect to mental health and substance abuse outcomes, the most compelling evidence is related to the management of depression. It has been demonstrated that integrating mental health professionals into the primary care setting results in impressive improvements in client outcomes. The report further states, "At this moment the field is ripe for discovering who to integrate into the primary care team, how to integrate them, and to which problems the team should address itself" (de Gruy, 1996, p. 425).

There is no question that extraordinary evidence exists that failing to take psychosocial issues into account in the primary care arena is a very costly matter. Integrated primary care offers large medical cost offsets:

- Untreated depressed primary care clients use two to three times the annual medical services as their nondepressed counterparts (Simon, Ormel, von Korff, and Barlow, 1995).
- Only 15 percent to 25 percent of medical decisions made by physicians in primary care are based on health morbidity; the remaining decisions revolve around psychosocial needs, client preferences, and doctor-client relationships.
- Providing behavioral health services to medical clients may result in cost offsets in the range of 20 percent to 40 percent (Friedman et al., 1995).

Society is paying a high price for the inescapable cost and human consequences of neglecting mental health problems in primary care. Indeed, the primary care arena has been referred to as the de facto mental health arena (McDaniel, Campbell, and Seaburn, 1995). That is because the majority of problems that present themselves in primary care do not have a medical diagnosis and are, in fact, psychological in origin.

Missed mental health and substance abuse diagnoses, or misdiagnoses, turn out to have serious cost consequences. Frequently related consequences are experienced as conditions such as fatigue, migraines, gastrointestinal upset, insomnia, and organ pathology. Studies have shown that the mental health cost offset of properly diagnosing these conditions in the primary care arena is substantial. Anxiety disorders, depression, and substance abuse are among the most commonly misdiagnosed conditions—with costly consequences in primary care.

The advanced practice role is well suited to provide specialized care to the acute and the chronically ill clients in the biopsychosocial context of their lives. New scientific discoveries in the areas of mind/body research and molecular biology call for holistic approaches, especially in addressing the needs of the chronically ill. As Benson (1996, p. 52) recently stated:

> Traditionally, doctors have thought that if a symptom could not be measured, it must be fake or non-existent. We've distrusted a patient's ability to perceive authentic bodily change. But my research and that of many others [have] demonstrated that perceptions and physicality are very tightly braided in the body, so it is impossible to separate objective and subjective change.

It is in this arena—client advocacy and assistance in mobilizing clients' beliefs and emotions to produce healing—that APNs can have a profound influence. APNs are comfortable in both worlds, the biomedical and the psychosocial. Increasingly, caring for clients effectively will require professional skills in both realms.

The role of the case manager is key to the integration of care across settings in the most seamless and cost-effective manner. Case managers in the primary mental health arena implement treatment interventions that focus on case identification and treatment protocols for known mental health problems. Examples of case identification might include tobacco use, depression screening, and drug and alcohol testing. Furthermore, the identification of physical health problems by mental health case managers provides another important arena for integration between primary care providers and mental health case managers (Satinsky, 1996).

The most visible of the APN roles is that of the NP. Because of their economic appeal as well as their biomedical knowledge base, NPs are sought by employers in a wide range of settings. In addition, policymakers and the public are familiar with the NP role, making it more attractive and marketable. Further, because several studies indicated that between 60 percent and 90 percent of all primary care visits are stress-related (Benson, 1996) and cannot be detected and treated effectively with the treatments the medical profession relies on, psychiatric APNs would offer an important perspective, given their tradition of client advocacy and holistic practice (Moller and Haber, 1996). Clearly, behavior patterns have been shown to have a great impact on disease. Together with changing clients' behavior patterns such as drinking, smoking, or other substance abuse, it is essential to establish new patterns of behavior that cope with stress and anxiety, thereby reducing the rate of relapse. Psychiatric APNs are uniquely qualified for this role.

Autonomy: The Key to the Nursing Role

The marketplace still does not distinguish effectively among the various mental health practitioner roles in nursing. Discussions of the NP workforce have addressed the numbers needed in primary care to balance the supply and demand of physicians. Analyses have tended to overlook the roles that NPs play in mental health care (Harper and Johnson, 1998). A master's-prepared psychiatric nurse is able to function in the roles of both case manager and primary mental health provider. The skill sets for each role are indeed similar: health assessment, management and knowledge of complex delivery systems, therapy/counseling expertise, and prescriptive authority. Market-driven changes, however, will present renewed opportunities for a variety of roles for nursing that include case managers who coordinate care and aggressively manage clients along care path; nurses as leaders of multidisciplinary teams who develop plans for comprehensive care that focuses more on the behavioral aspects of care; and APNs as physician substitutes (Coile, 1995). There is no question that the future of nursing will be shaped by market forces in ways never before considered even as remote possibilities.

A main source of difference of the health care marketplace is the degree of **autonomy** the APN seeks and/or desires. In addition, much of the role blurring among psychiatric APNs as case managers, CNSs, or primary care providers has to do with the age-old political resistance to nursing's professional autonomy. Objections to autonomy have been tied to quality-of-care issues, even though there is extraordinary evidence documenting that master's-prepared nurses provide care that is *as good as physicians' care and superior in some respects* (Harper and Johnson, 1998).

Since the inception of managed care, there is renewed interest in the use of APNs as vital components of innovative delivery models. In a recent survey of managed care companies in New York and Connecticut that investigated the extent to which NPs are utilized in their client services, it is remarkable that 44 percent of the 28 companies surveyed listed NPs as primary care providers. Nonetheless, because of the high visibility of Columbia-Presbyterian Hospital's practice of all-APN primary care practice, the New York Medical Society has launched an intensive campaign to undermine public confidence in NPs (Harper and Johnson, 1998).

It is clear that the trend is toward greater autonomy for all APNs. In 34 states and the District of Columbia, legislation provides for some degree of prescriptive authority for APNs; 45 states have granted prescriptive authority for NPs, certified nurse-midwives (CNMs), and nurse anesthetists (Kaas and Markley, 1998). Also, 32 states permit prescriptive authority for NPs with a collaborating physician, whereas in 8 states and the District of Columbia, substitutive authority is granted, which requires neither collaboration nor supervision by a physician. it is also clear that increased autonomy for NPs has increased access to primary care for many individuals and families (Kaas and Markley, 1998).

Nursing's political struggle to achieve greater autonomy has recently made great advances. The Balanced Budget Act of 1997 further expanded direct Medicare reimbursement for NPs and CNSs to include all nonhospital sites, and it removed any requirement for physician involvement. In addition, nursing's progress in this direction seems assured by a confluence of interests that includes health care organizations, insurers, legislators, physicians, and nurses themselves (Sheffler, 1996).

Well over a decade ago, Claire Fagin (then Dean of the University of Pennsylvania School of Nursing) predicted, in the midst of ubiquitous concerns over cost and access, that Marcus Welby, in the near future, would be a nurse. Now, as managed care uses fewer physicians, that scenario is on the horizon. There is a renewed interest on the part of policymakers as well as managed care companies to examine nurses' potential as autonomous primary care providers who will provide care that is more accessible, high quality, and less expensive.

In fact, APNs are being used with increasing frequency in primary care settings (Harper and Johnson, 1998). Knowledge, expertise, and clinical judgment characterize their practices rather than title in managed care settings, however. Thus, it is important to distinguish how nurses are prepared for these roles because credentialing can be key in distinguishing quality. Increasingly, APNs are becoming certified in their specialty areas. Although many employment settings do not require certification, the specialty organizations in nursing as well as the American Nurses Association have been successful in communicating the importance of achieving a standard measure of excellence in specialty practice. Because of this trend, MCOs may succeed in sorting out the long and protracted controversy over appropriate levels of credentialing in the nursing profession, a controversy that has been a barrier to the profession's ability to serve the American public more fully (PEW, 1995b). Increasingly, MCOs are requiring nurses to be prepared at the graduate level and certified in their specialty areas. Similarly, most state legislation requires a master's degree, national certification, pharmacology education, current registered nurse status, and a collaborative agreement with a physician to qualify for prescriptive privileges (Kaas and Markley, 1998).

Supporting Data for the Advanced Practice Role

Ample studies support the idea that NPs can provide high-quality, cost-effective care (Sheffler, 1996). Costs per episode of care were found to be at least 20 percent less when NPs rather than physicians provided care in a landmark Office of Technology Assessment study. Additionally, the care provided by the APN was of equal competence and resulted in greater client satisfaction.

Sheffler (1996) reported that 38 studies of NPs and 15 studies of CNMs demonstrated the following:

- NPs provided more health promotion activities such as client education and exercise programs than physicians.
- NPs ordered more laboratory tests than physicians, and the costs of the tests were 8 percent lower than those ordered by physicians.
- NPs scored higher on quality-of-care measures than physicians (these measures examine diagnostic accuracy and completeness of the care process).
- The average cost for an NP visit was 3 percent less than the cost of one to a physician.

Evidence documenting the effectiveness of NPs as primary care providers (PCPs) has existed for over two decades. Most of the debate over the potential for widespread utilization of NPs as PCPs tends to be political in nature, reflecting the resistance of the medical community (Safriet, 1992). But even as managed care evolves with deliberate speed, the problems of cost, quality, and access will drive the need for a fundamental restructuring of existing health care delivery systems and the effective use of health care personnel in new ways (PEW, 1995b). The shift is already evidenced in the increasing use of psychiatric NPs as primary therapists.

In a recent study of physician staffing levels, which extrapolated HMO staffing levels to the entire physician workforce, it was observed that HMOs appear to use more NPs than the overall U.S. health care system (Sheffler, 1996). Another study by Marder, Gaumer, and Minkovitz (1991), using a GMENAC-type model that incorporates clinical experts' judgments about appropriate client utilization patterns (rather than actual utilization rates), estimated that NPs could assume responsibility for 630 million visits, or slightly more than one-third of the 2.1 billion annual U.S. primary care visits.

In this intensely competitive and price-sensitive environment, the system would clearly benefit from the use of other professionals who would be trained more quickly and less expensively than physicians and who would provide health care of similar or better quality at lower costs (PEW, 1995b). Many have suggested that APNs are particularly well suited to serve as PCPs in managed care. For psychiatric NPs who also provide basic health care and adult health NPs skilled in treating uncomplicated mental health and addictive problems, opportunities are increasing throughout the United States. This role is a more economic option not only because of lower salary expenses but because of nursing's prevention and wellness orientation and the comprehensiveness of nursing's approach.

Limits of the Medical Model: The Case of Mental Health and Substance Abuse

There is renewed interest in the use of NPs as primary providers of care in the new firmament of managed care for economic reasons. Expenditures for mental health and substance abuse reached nearly $80 billion in 1996 (Harper and Johnson, 1998). That increase represents a doubling of expenditures over a 10-year period. It is also important to emphasize that the nursing model of practice and the aims of managed care are congruent, representing a host of new opportunities in the managed care arena. Nursing practice differs substantially from medicine in prevention and wellness orientation and its focus on the well-being of the total person. As diagnosis and cure, the chief aims of medical science, are challenged by (1) the prevalence of chronic illness (which by definition cannot be cured), (2) public unease with the primacy of the medical model, and (3) economic incentives for prevention and wellness, the appeal of NPs as PCPs is strengthened.

Because there is a growing recognition of the need for more integrated approaches to care that include a new framework for conceptualizing the determinants of health, nursing models present many exciting possibilities. How a problem is framed will determine which kinds of evidence are given weight and which are disregarded. At present, perfectly valid data, which consist of important observations bearing directions and important questions, drop out of scientific consideration when the medical model provides no set of categories in which to place them.

This observation is particularly striking in the case of mental health. Although mental symptoms as well as substance abuse and alcohol disorders are prevalent in clients visiting their PCPs, many mental health problems are mostly found at the edges of the medical model and reflect its limitations. Consider the following:

- Mental illnesses are more common than cancer, diabetes, or heart disease.
- More than 5 million Americans suffer an acute episode of mental illness each year.
- Depression has been on the rise since 1960. According to one study, 718 million Americans will be diagnosed with depression at a cost of $50 billion a year (Rochefort and Goering, 1998).
- Heavy alcohol consumption has continued to be high since the late 1960s, with a current prevalence of 18 percent of the general population (National Institutes of Alcohol Abuse and Alcoholism, 1998).
- Alcohol and substance abuse are key factors in the development of biomedical problems such as heart disease and cancer.

- Psychiatric conditions such as schizophrenia and manic depression fill 21 percent of all hospital beds, more than any single physical illness such as cancer or heart disease (Blount, 1998).
- Substance-related problems are evident in 35 percent to 50 percent of clients hospitalized under another diagnosis (Blount, 1998).

Many of these problems have their roots in psychosocial origins that are not in concert with the approach of the medical model. The vast majority of health care dollars spent in the United States is for people with chronic conditions. A recent study found that 59 percent of direct and indirect costs of all illnesses could be attributed to chronic conditions (Freudenheim, 1996). If managed care has done a poor job in responding to chronic illness, its track record in the area of mental health has been abysmal. The services essential to caring for the mentally ill, including counseling and therapy, rehabilitation, medication, and supportive care, are much more than the medical model has offered, especially under managed care.

The psychological component is a powerful one in the care of substance abuse and addictions. Addiction functions in a person's life to remove intolerable realities through a series of obsessive-compulsive experiences. Gradually, the addiction becomes a priority in the person's life, becoming more important than anything or anyone else and creating destructive consequences, which the addict denies or ignores.

The treatment of individuals with addictive disorders requires a comprehensive approach that involves an intense biospsychosocial treatment, including a spiritual component. Assessment and treatment interventions must be based on a biopsychosocial approach that integrates an informed assessment of physical health, mental health, and psychosocial factors. When such an approach is implemented early by providers of primary care such as APNs, morbidity of the conditions is greatly decreased.

APNs must be able to recognize symptoms of depression, mental illness, and substance abuse. Failure to identify and treat the underlying issues can result in increased costs and higher rates of medical utilization. Far too many primary care practitioners do not even ask about drinking patterns and do not question clients about use of other substances. A seminal study, the *Commonwealth Fund Survey of Women's Health* (1993), found that two-thirds of women with checkups in the past year were not asked about current drinking patterns. In spite of extensive research linking stress to illness and the interplay of emotions and spirituality, most medical practitioners assume that physical causes can explain all diseases and that pharmacological treatments are the only ones that count (de Gruy, 1996).

Nursing's Challenges and Opportunities

Advanced Practice Nursing Models of Care

Advanced practice nursing is based on a conceptual model that is comprehensive and that addresses the psychological, social, and spiritual aspects of well-being as equal to or greater than the medical perspective. Nursing models of care are prevention-oriented, emphasizing nursing theory psychology and sociology of health. In fact, nursing leaders in mental health have been prominent in advancing new models of health in the last two decades. In addition, research programs have grown out of clinical practice and frustration with the disease model of health and illness. Nursing research is aimed at an understanding and integration of the biopsychosocial aspects of well-being and the identification of outcomes of intervention that include these aspects.

Nursing education rarely limits its focus to care derived from the medical diagnosis, and the science of nursing has developed in relation to prevention and wellness. Newer holistic theorists such as Barbara Dossey are attempting to build an empirical base for the holistic phenomena involved in achieving positive health status. Dossey and Gazzetta consider the client as a biopsychosocial, spiritual entity (Dossey, Keegan, Gazzetta, and Kolkmeier, 1995). They do not dismiss the traditional elements of the medical model; rather, their theoretical perspectives supplement and enhance the understanding of the individual in health and illness.

Despite the remarkable conceptual work of APNs outside the medical model, in order to have a far-reaching impact on current systems of managed care, further work must clarify and integrate the conceptual bases of advanced practice nursing with health care as it is currently provided. The different APN models—the CNS, NP, and CNM—have evolved in the context of the health care delivery system, but the conceptual bases of these roles must be clarified and understood by purchasers and consumers. These roles are essentially variations based on the same unifying clinical principles and core competencies. **Consumer education** must be provided so that clients have information upon which to base choices among the various practitioners.

Medical leaders have finally begun to elaborate on the need for a stronger emphasis on the social and psychological aspects of illness, and to emphasize behaviors that can be healthful (Tarlov, 1992). Medical science has enhanced the prevention of some diseases, and it can cure others and alleviate symptoms or slow the progress of many more; however, it is now increasingly understood that health is dependent on a range of factors that lies outside the traditional practice of medicine. Leaders in medicine such as Herbert Benson, Andrew Weil, Norman Shealy, and Dean Ornish speak vociferously about the vital components of stress, dietary factors, and spirituality on health and well-being. Alternative therapies are increasingly accepted by the public. It is projected that, by the year 2000, $40 billion will be spent out-of-pocket on alternative therapies.

It is critical that the nursing profession devise strategies to explain to the public the common elements of advanced practice nursing in biomedical, psychological, and spiritual realms. Nursing has had a pioneering and prominent influence in shaping the biopsychosocial model, yet to date nursing's voice is eclipsed by those of other professionals and lay people. Managed care programs employ nurses successfully as case managers in disease management, and they understand why nursing skills are critical to the health of their populations. Yet, when it comes to the more powerful gatekeeper PCP role, resistance continues. This happens even though nursing models of care offer more in contrast to medicine in the customer-driven world of managed care. As health economist Eli Ginzberg (1998) recently commented, because of the urgent need for more attention to the chronically ill, clients will invariably require more care from nurses, as well as treatment in ambulatory settings, in clinics, and in homes.

Striking differences have been found in the diagnostic and therapeutic styles of NPs as compared with physicians. An important study conducted by researchers at Kaiser Permanente found that NPs delivered almost twice the amount of preventive services and three times the amount of prenatal care as did physicians. In a 1991 study (Safriet, 1992), twice as many physicians opted to write a prescription, whereas only 20 percent of the NPs chose to do so. NPs more often recommended either a change in diet or counseling to help the client deal with stress; for example, appropriate interventions when a client complains of gastritis include assessment and advice about limiting high intakes of aspirin, caffeine, alcohol, and tobacco.

The fact that more nurses than physicians elicit the basic historical information necessary to make an intelligent treatment plan for clients has inescapable implications for both the quality of care and its costs. It is essential to recognize that managing the health of enrolled populations will require, in the final analysis, a new approach based on the determinants of health. Managed care calls for a new, truly comprehensive approach for which there is currently no knowledge premise or framework that exists in medicine for such practice.

Aside from the tentative response of the medical community toward nurses performing as PCPs, a major obstacle in nursing's progress has been what the PEW report (1995a) referred to as the "Labyrinthine professional definitions, educational pathways and practice patterns." The infrastructure of the nursing profession is confusing from the outside and creates friction from the inside, circumstances that have the effect of stalling responses to the challenges of the emerging system. This is unfortunate for NPs and tragic for the consumer because in many ways nurses are the best-prepared professionals to respond to a system in constant flux (PEW, 1995a).

Nursing's Current Discussions with Managed Care Organizations

In spite of the confusion surrounding education and credentialing in nursing, some MCOs are moving toward listing nurses as PCPs in their directories. In these instances, organizations seem convinced that NPs, with their own panels of clients, provide the advantages of lower costs and decreased utilization of expensive tests and medical procedures.

In New York State, many members of the New York University and Columbia University's nursing faculties are listed with several MCOs as PCPS and mental health providers. The credentialing criteria proposed to ensure quality are the master's degree with certification in a specific practice area. The New York State Coalition of Nurse Practitioners concurs with these criteria and is establishing a network of NP practices throughout the state. CNMs have long practiced in hospital-related and independently maintained service centers, such as the Maternity Center Association.

In California and other regions of the United States, the situation has been different. Progress has been thwarted as NPs find that no managed care system will contract with or list an NP as a PCP. A multicoalition action group made up of several nursing organizations is meeting to devise a strategy to address the problem. Nurses have fought for new practice authority in the reimbursement arena, and this episode could well be precedent-setting for nursing's future role in managed care.

REINVENTION OF NURSING

The PEW Health Professions Commission (1995b) recommended that all health professions revise their strategic plans to accommodate the enormous impact of the market-driven changes in health care; nursing is no exception. First, the learning opportunities available to students and practitioners should incorporate an economic and political understanding of the new system dynamics. Schools remain open and creative in the face of the opportunities offered by market-driven change. Second, schools and the profession must develop new relationships and partnerships with these market-driven institutions. Those partnerships, which will be equally vital to education, service, and research, will form a better understanding and provide the foundation for deeper collaboration. In many ways, graduate nursing education has been very progressive in developing curricula that combine biopsychosocial, multicultural, life span, and gender-centric frameworks. Although curricula for mental health and substance abuse include disease management, they must expand beyond the biomedical framework to include primary prevention and health promotion, to create links among specialties that fragment the individual, and to facilitate health across the life span to diverse populations. In large measure, graduate programs in advanced practice nursing are already structured to accomplish this objective. A further approach is to freely integrate appropriate levels of mental health and substance abuse prevention, detection, and treatment into advanced practice education in all specialties.

THE FUTURE

If managed care is to embrace nurses in the roles of autonomous care providers, several challenges lie ahead. In 1994, the PEW Health Professions Commission recommended expanding the use of NPs and called for a doubling of the NP workforce by 2005 (PEW, 1995a). In its recent primary care report, the Institute of Medicine explicitly recognized NPs as an integral part of the primary care team (Sheffler, 1996). In addition, the recent passage of direct Medicare reimbursement for NPs reflects nursing's capabilities as well as its political strength.

To a large extent, nursing schools have responded vigorously to society's increased demand for PCPs. The number of academic institutions with NP tracks increased from 101 in 1990 to 202 in 1995. In effect, the number of clinical tracks doubled in the three-year period. Furthermore, the largest growth occurred in specialty tracks.

The trends in spending and use of mental health and substance abuse services portend an increased demand for APNs to use their mental health and substance abuse skills in a wide variety of roles. Mental health and substance abuse expenditures grew from $39.5 billion in 1986 to $79.3 billion in 1996, an average annual rate increase of 7.2 percent. In comparison, the Consumer Price Index grew by 3.5 percent annually over this period. Broad-based skills across nursing specialties can increase early detection and lower expenditures on long-term conditions requiring rehabilitation and tertiary care.

Preparing nurses to function as the primary providers of care requires major attitudinal changes. Creative risk-accepting leadership from the nursing schools and the profession will be required to assume such roles in a large-scale way. Before the onset of managed care, nursing researchers pointed to the need to redesign nursing education, especially to empower nursing students through encouraging more analysis, critical thinking, and risk taking (Allen and Jewel, 1996). Yet, it has been pointed out that a major problem in creating change in nursing education is the system in which it is embedded. "The oppression of clients and nurses in a hierarchical health care system and faculty within bureaucratic, traditional universities create the need for change to occur both internally and externally" (PEW, 1995). Hospitals and many other health care institutions often operate in regimens and hierarchical ways that encourage obedience and dependence in nurses. These institutions are the laboratories for students and the workplace for faculty. Change must occur at this level as well as in employing institutions.

Nurses must continue to become more knowledgeable about the economic and political levels of change. In so doing, we can become drivers of change rather than responders. Many pressing questions loom in the future of substance abuse treatment that nurses should be involved in shaping and answering; these include the delineation of boundaries between primary care and specialty care and the fiscal and quality implications of these decisions. Also, studies of carve-outs and carve-ins are needed to determine the benefits and risks of integrating mental health, substance abuse, and medical care.

For nurses, radical transformation in health care delivery can be effectively used to promote consumer choice, which may be nursing's greatest challenge. There is no question that once consumers have been exposed to the notion of having a nurse as their primary provider of care and educated about the merits of the situation, they are very satisfied customers.

The fact remains, however, that clients of all ages identify a family physician as their usual source of care. To many providers, managed care seems like a crisis that will last forever; to many Americans, quality of care hangs in a precarious state. Americans are very dissatisfied with the quality of care they are receiving (Hart, 1998). Most importantly, many policymakers believe the current insurance system in our country threatens access to health services for thousands of Americans. Although efforts have been initiated by Congress and policymakers to address consumer concerns about managed care, the jury is still out. During this time, there are many opportunities and a great need for nursing's voice in addressing the challenges to come.

REFERENCES

Allen, D., and Jewel, B. (1996). Restructuring nursing education. *Nursing Outlook 40*, 44–45.

Benson, H. (1996). *Timeless Healing*. New York: Firestone Press.

Blount, A. (ed.). (1998). *Integrated Primary Care*. New York: W.W. Norton and Company.

Coile, R.C., Jr. (1995). Integration, capitation and managed care: Transformation of nursing for the 21st century health care. *Advanced Practice Nursing Quarterly 1*(2), 77–82.

Commonwealth Fund Survey of Women's Health. (1993). New York: Louis Harris and Associates.

de Gruy III, F. (1996). Mental health in the primary care setting. In M.S. Donaldson, S. Molla, K. Yordy, K.N. Lohr, and N.A. Vanselow (eds.), *Primary Care: America's Health in a New Era*. Washington, DC: National Academy Press.

Dossey, B.M., Keegan, L., Gazzetta, C.E., and Kolkmeier, L.G. (1995). *Holistic Nursing: A Handbook for Practice* (2nd ed.). Gathersburg, MD: Aspen Publishers.

Freudenheim, E. (1996). *Chronic Care in America: A 21st Century Challenge*. Princeton, NJ: Robert Wood Johnson Foundation.

Friedman, R., Meyers, P., Sobel, D., Caudill, M., and Benson, H. (1995). Behavioral medicine, clinical health psychology and cost offset. *Health Psychology 6*, 283–298.

Ginzberg, E. (1998). The changing health care environment. *Journal of the American Medical Association 279*(7), 110.

Goode, E. Your mind may ease what's ailing you. *New York Times,* April 18, 1999, Ideas and Trends.

Harper, D., and Johnson, J. (Winter 1998). The new generation of nurse practitioners: Is more enough? *Health Affairs,* 158–164.

Hart, G. (August 1998). American health survey. *The Wall Street Journal,* Special Section.

Kaas, M.J., and Markley, J.M. (1998). A national perspective on prescriptive authority for advanced practice psychiatric nurses. *Journal of the American Psychiatric Nurses Association 4*(6), 190–198.

Kuttner, R. (February 25, 1999). The American health care system. *The New England Journal of Medicine 340*(8), 664–668.

Lamm, R.D. (May/June 1996). The ethics of excess. *Public Health Reports,* 218–224.

Marder, W.D., Gaumer, G.L., and Minkovitz, C.S. (1991). GMENAC Revisited: Updated Projections for Selected Specialties. Cambridge, MA: ABT Associates. Unpublished paper.

McDaniel, S.H., Campbell, T.L., and Seaburn, D.B. (1995). Principles for collaboration between health and mental health providers in primary care. *Family Systems Medicine 13,* 283–298.

McEwen, S.S., and Stellar, E. (September 1993). Stress and the individual. *Archives of Internal Medicine 19,* 2093–2101.

Moller, M., and Haber, J. (1996). Advanced practice psychiatric nursing: The need for a blended role. *Online Journal of Issues in Nursing* (http://www.nursingworld.org/ana/ojin/tpc1-7.htm).

National Institute on Alcohol Abuse and Alcoholism. (1998). *Drinking in the United States.* Bethesda, MD: U.S. Department of Health and Human Services.

New York Times. (December 26, 1998). Insurance plans skirt requirement on mental health coverage, pp. A1, A20.

Pert, C.B. (1998). *Molecules of Emotion.* New York: Scribner.

PEW Health Professions Commission (1995a). *Health Professions Education and Managed Care: Challenges and Necessary Responses.* San Francisco: University of California, San Francisco Center for the Health Professions.

PEW Health Professions Commission (1995b). *Critical Challenges: Revitalizing the Health Professions for the Twenty-First Century.* (1995). San Francisco: University of California, San Francisco Center for the Health Professions.

Rochefort, D.A., and Goering, P. (September/October 1998). More a link than a division: How Canada has learned from U.S. mental health policy. *Health Affairs 17*(5), 110–164.

Safriet, B.J. (1992). Health care dollars and regulatory sense: The role of advanced practice nursing. *Yale Journal of Regulation 9,* 419–485.

Satinsky, M.A. (1996). Advanced practice nurse in a managed care environment. *Advanced Practice Nursing,* 126–144.

Schuster, M.A., McGlynn, A., and Brook, R.H. (1998). How good is the quality of health care in the United States? *The Milbank Quarterly 76*(4), 517–563.

Sheffler, R.M. (1996). Life in the kaleidoscope: The impact of managed care on the U.S. health care work force and a new model for the delivery of primary care. In M.S. Donaldson, S. Molla, K.D. Yordy, K.N. Lohr, N.A. Vanselow (eds.), *Primary Care: America's Health in a New Era.* Washington, DC: National Academy Press.

Simon, G., Ormel, J., von Korff, M., and Barlow, W. (1995). Health care costs associated with depression and anxiety disorders in primary care. *American Journal of Psychiatry 152,* 352–357.

Spiegel, D. (1999). Healing Words. *JAMA 28*(14), 1328–1329.

Tarlov, A. (November 1992). The coming influence of a social sciences perspective on medical education. *Academic Medicine, 67*(11).

3

Drug Policy in America: Ethical Implications for Practice

Robert Granfield, PhD
Kevin Ryan, PhD

LEARNER OUTCOMES

On completion of this chapter, the learner will be able to:

1. Gain a critical understanding of the social history of American drug legislation, particularly as it relates to the health professions.
2. Understand how the medical profession lost control of controlled substances.
3. Develop insight into the political nature of drug laws and their related ambiguity.
4. Gain knowledge of the scheduling of controlled substances.
5. Critically analyze the ethical dilemmas associated with the medical use of controlled substances.
6. Reflect on the future direction of American drug policy as it relates to practice by health professionals.

KEY TERMS

Drug Enforcement Administration (DEA)   medical marijuana
Harrison Narcotic Act   Uniform Controlled Substances Act

Federal control over narcotics began in 1914 with the passage of the **Harrison Narcotic Act.** Despite calls for, and passage of, state legislation seeking to control the distribution of narcotic drugs in the years prior to the Harrison Narcotic Act, the health care professions had been in a position to determine when, how much, and to whom such drugs were delivered. This was viewed by most as medical territory and was jealously guarded against state interference. Numerous factors, however, led to the entry of the federal government into the drug control field. Among these were a popular belief that the number of narcotic addicts was increasing exponentially, the emergence within the health care professions themselves of voices calling for government action (undoubtedly related to status concerns in the rapidly professionalizing fields of medicine and pharmacy), and the embarrassment that occurred when the United States took the lead in international efforts to control narcotic distribution and was criticized for failing to do so at home. The Harrison Narcotic Act was itself a compromise between government and health care interests, and it was understood by many at the time as a law permitting the distribution of narcotics, albeit with registration and taxation, rather than a prohibition model.

This chapter examines the medical profession's loss of control over prescribing controlled substances. It explores recent developments within drug legislation, beginning with the Controlled Substances Act of 1970, and examines the implications for health care practitioners. The failures of criminalization efforts are discussed; medical literature on the therapeutic benefits of controlled substances is reviewed. A discussion of the ethical dilemmas that health care workers face in recommending that clients use illegal substances for their therapeutic potential concludes the chapter.

Criminalization and the Loss of Medical Autonomy

From the perspective of the health professions, the Harrison Narcotic Act is particularly interesting. It divided drugs into four distinct classes: Class A contained drugs that were highly addictive; Class B contained drugs that were considered to possess little addiction potential; and Classes X and M contained exempt narcotics, or patent medicine containing narcotics. In its original form, the act was a tax measure written to license and tax those who imported and dispensed opium and cocaine products. The act was a public health and revenue-generating law. It required purchasers of narcotics to use standardized order forms and to file copies of those purchase orders with the local Internal Revenue office. In addition, the act required all those dealing with narcotics, including manufacturers, importers, distributors, wholesalers, and physicians, to be registered with the federal government. Musto (1987) points out that, by 1916, approximately 221,000 people were registered, of whom 124,000 were physicians. Thus, the act originally left much of the power of distribution in the hands of professionals.

Granting control of narcotic distribution to the medical profession extended its professional jurisdiction into matters of drug abuse and addiction (Abbott, 1988). Physician control of narcotics distribution symbolized early efforts toward the medicalization of these problems. Not unlike the transformation of definitions of alcohol problems from immoral behaviors to illnesses (Conrad and Schneider, 1980), the original Harrison Narcotic Act extended physicians' monopoly over the distribution of narcotics. Under the act, physicians possessed autonomy for the prescription of narcotics as well as the medical reasons for such prescriptions. However, although the act permitted physicians to prescribe narcotics in treatment, it was silent about whether doctors could prescribe narcotics to addicts. Lindesmith has pointed out that the medical profession at the time reacted to the Harrison Narcotic Act with a certain amount of hostility and was divided over the issue of prescribing narcotics to addicts (1965, p. 147):

> Numerous editorials and comments criticizing the manner in which the Harrison Act impinged on doctors appeared throughout the country at this time. In a number of instances clinics were sponsored and supported by local medical bodies, which also resisted government orders closing them down. All of this demonstrates beyond any reasonable doubt that the government's program of closing all avenues of legal access to drugs to addicts did not have the undivided support of medical authorities at the time, and that the latter were in fact engaged in bitter controversy on the question.

At first, physicians who prescribed narcotics to addicts went unchallenged. In *United States v. Jin Fuey Moy* (1916), the U.S. Supreme Court ruled that the Harrison Narcotic Act was a revenue measure and could not be used to prosecute a physician for prescribing maintenance doses of opiates to a patient. Further, the Court held that the regulation of the practice of medicine was a power reserved to the states. However, this interpretation was challenged by law enforcement authorities three years later, first in *United States v. Doremus* (1919), which held that federal control over the dispensing of opiates was constitutional. More striking, however, was the Court's decision in *Webb v. United States* (1919). There the Supreme Court upheld a lower court conviction of Tennessee physician W. S. Webb for conspiracy to violate the Harrison Narcotic Act. Webb's violation stemmed from his practice of prescribing narcotics to narcotic-addicted individuals. Justice Day, delivering the majority opinion, wrote that prescribing narcotics to known addicts for the purpose of maintaining an addiction was not appropriate medical practice:

> If a practicing and registered physician issues an order for morphine to an habitual user thereof, the order not being issued by him in the course of professional treatment in the attempted cure of the habit, but being issued for the purpose of providing the user with morphine sufficient enough to keep him comfortable by maintaining his customary use, is such an order a physician's prescription under exception? [T]o call such an order for the use of morphine a physician's prescription would be so plain a perversion of the meaning that no discussion of the subject is required (*Webb v. United States*, 1919).

From the beginning, federal law enforcement authorities, anxious to extend the sphere of their professional influence, had interpreted the Harrison Narcotic Act as a prohibition law and had engaged in a vigorous campaign of arresting not merely addicts but also physicians and pharmacists who prescribed and dispensed narcotics to addicts. The result of *Webb* was that law enforcement was legitimized, and the treatment of narcotics users passed out of the hands of health care professionals into the hands of law enforcers where it has remained ever since.

The decision in *Webb* stimulated a brief movement for government-sponsored clinics to dispense opiates (Musto, 1987). These were especially common in large cities. In New York, for example, the city clinic in 1920 had 7,500 clients; other sites treated between 2,500 and

3,000 clients. These clinics, however, appear to be the last gasp of the medical establishment in attempting to medicalize the treatment of narcotics use. In 1921, most of the clinics were closed by order of Levi Nutt, head of the Narcotic Division of the Prohibition Unit within the Bureau of Internal Revenue. Nutt contended that the Harrison Narcotic Act prohibited the sale and consumption of opiates and other drugs, no matter what the circumstances, and criminal charges should be brought against physicians who prescribed to addicts as well as against black market suppliers. The AMA fought against the usurpation of physicians' rights to prescribe narcotics when medically appropriate. In 1921, the AMA's council on Health and Public Instruction asserted:

> In the opinion of your committee, the only proper and scientific method of treating drug addiction is under such conditions of control of both the addict and the drug, that any administration of habit-forming narcotic drugs must be by or under the direct personal authority of the physician, with no chance of any distribution of the drug of addiction to others, or opportunity for the same person to procure any of the drug from any source other than the physician directly responsible for the addict's treatment (AMA, 1963).

In the years that followed the *Webb* decision, physicians were increasingly arrested and prosecuted for their unwillingness to discontinue prescribing narcotics to treat addicts as clients as opposed to criminals. Two decades after the *Webb* decision, it has been estimated that 25,000 physicians were arraigned on narcotics-selling charges, and 3,000 served prison sentences (Goode, 1989). The principal effect of the Supreme Court's decision and subsequent law enforcement's assault on the medical profession was effectively to remove health care professionals from at least one major form of addiction treatment. Narcotics use and addiction were now clearly the province of law enforcement officials, not health care professionals. The practice of harassing and prosecuting physicians had become so firmly entrenched that even when the Supreme Court reversed *Webb* in *Linder v. United States* (1925), the arrest of doctors and pharmacists continued unabated (Rouse and Johnson, 1990). As Goode points out, the arrest of physicians at this time resulted in "driving most physicians out of the practice of treating addicts. . . . The few who continued to do so, whether for idealistic or mercenary reasons . . . were charged with 'trafficking' in narcotics" (1989, p. 219). Thus, the movement to medicalize the drug use problem came to a halt.

The United States was an exception to the general pattern of worldwide narcotics policy, wherein a public health approach predominated in the 1920s and 1930s. For example, in England, Parliament established the Rolleston Committee (composed of nine medical professionals) whose 1926 report became the basis of British policy until the 1970s. The report explicitly provided for the distribution of narcotics and other drugs to addicts who either were seeking to withdraw gradually or were unable to withdraw because of the severity of withdrawal symptoms. The difference between England and the United States seemed primarily to be the existence in the former of a united medical community that stood firm on the view that addiction is a disease requiring treatment rather than a vice demanding punishment, as viewed by the latter. In addition, Britain did not have a prohibition movement or a police organization with the authority and the inclination to interfere with the physician–client relationship (Rouse and Johnson, 1990).

A Brief History of Drug Control Since 1970

Despite the expansion of treatment facilities devoted to alcohol and drug treatment (Weisner and Room, 1978), the 1970s saw increased criminalization of drugs and drug users. Motivated in large part by increases in crime as well as shifts in political ideology toward conservatism, the decade witnessed a significant expansion of law enforcement efforts in this area. On October 27, 1970, the Harrison Narcotic Act was effectively removed from the books with the passage of the **Uniform Controlled Substances Act.** Although there were provisions in this act to increase research into the prevention and treatment of drug abuse, it was principally a law enforcement measure. This new act established a uniform federal code requiring persons involved in the manufacture, distribution, and dispensing of scheduled drugs to obtain a registration from their state.

Perhaps the most important drug policy of the 1970s, the Uniform Controlled Substances Act had wide-ranging effects in both law enforcement and the health care profession. The act increased the number of prosecutable drug offenses. For instance, it made possession of drugs with the intent to distribute a criminal act. It also legalized no-knock entry policies, giving the police increased law enforcement license. Following the legal issue of a search warrant, an authorized agent could now forcibly and without warning enter private premises if he or she felt that evidence might otherwise be disposed of, or if the warrant permitted such action. In addition, the act led to the 1973 creation of the **Drug Enforcement Administration (DEA),** extending to law enforcement agents increased powers at home and abroad (Nadelmann, 1993). Although the areas of prevention and treatment benefited from the drug legislation of the 1970s, the greatest emphasis was placed on law enforcement, thus continuing a trend that had been established 50 years earlier.

The decade of the 1980s saw continued preference for criminalization over medicalization. Public Law 97-86, enacted in 1981, resulted in substantial revisions in the long-standing Posse Comitatus statute (Wisotsky, 1990). Prior to this law, all military involvement in civil law enforcement was prohibited unless authorized by the Constitution or by a specific act of Congress. Under the new law, the use of military personnel in civilian enforcement activities, particularly in the area of drug trafficking, became permissible. This Department of Defense Authorization Act, as it became known, resulted in the dramatic expansion of military surveillance in foreign countries, increased military expenditures for sophisticated tracking technology, and the escalation of military incursions into foreign countries such as Panama for the purpose of destroying drug laboratories and arresting drug traffickers. In 1984, the Comprehensive Forfeiture Act was passed, extending the boundaries of seizure and forfeiture of profits derived from drug distribution. Similar to the previous decade, the 1980s placed far greater emphasis on law enforcement than on public health.

The movement toward increased criminalization has greatly affected drug users as well as health care professionals. The consequences of defining drug use as a criminal problem as opposed to a medical problem have been well documented. As drug policy scholars have pointed out, constituting drug use as a criminal problem has led to increased incarceration (approximately 30 percent of the more than 1 million prisoners are felony drug offenders), increased crime, and increased violence on the streets (Brecher, 1972; Currie, 1993; Nadelmann, 1989; Ryan, 1994; Wisotsky, 1990). There have also been numerous medical consequences, including users' increased health problems resulting from toxic reactions to impure substances, exposure to toxic agents (such as paraquat sprayed on marijuana), and, perhaps most problematic for the health care industry, contraction of infectious diseases such as acquired immunodeficiency syndrome (AIDS) and hepatitis. The medical consequences that result from violence that frequently erupts during illegal drug transactions add to these costs. Health care professionals are all too aware of the fact that handguns have become increasingly common in the illegal drug trade. As a highly profitable and unregulated enterprise, the illegal drug industry frequently turns to violence to resolve trade disputes (Goldstein et al., 1997). Such widespread violence places great burdens on health care professionals and inflates the costs of an already expensive health care system.

Current Drug Laws and Health Care Professionals

Although the costs of a criminalization policy are well known, another consequence receives little attention: The decision to adopt a punitive rather than a public health policy has limited health care professionals' ability to have a voice in drug policy matters, which has led to conceptual ambiguity in the law. The power to reclassify controlled substances, for instance, rests in the hands of law enforcement authorities, ultimately the administrator at the DEA, rather than public health officials. Neither the current nor previous DEA administrators have had medical backgrounds, most having been in either legal or law enforcement professions. In regard to controlled substances, law enforcement officials have greater control over the body politic than do health care professionals. This control often undermines a health care worker's efforts to treat drug abusers, as has been the case with crack-using pregnant women who fail to seek prenatal medical services for fear of being arrested (Norton-Hawk, 1994). Indeed, the construction of drug problems within a criminal justice framework has significant real-world implications for health care professionals.

According to the Uniform Controlled Substances Act, passed in 1970, Schedule I drugs (those most strictly regulated, being all but totally unavailable legally, even for research purposes) must meet three criteria. Substances must have (1) a high potential for abuse, (2) no accepted medical use in treatment in the United States, and (3) lack of safety for use under medical supervision. In the original act, there were more than 80 substances designated as Schedule I drugs, including such substances as acetylmethadol, alphameprodine, benzethidine, heroin, ibogaine, marijuana, mescaline, morpheridine, normethadone, peyote, psilocybin, and tetrahydrocannabinol. Many more drugs have been added to Schedule I since the passage of the act. Schedule II substances are drugs with great abuse potential but limited medical use. Drugs in this category include cocaine, fentanyl, and methadone. Schedule III substances are those that are designated as having less abuse potential and accepted medical usage. Drugs in this category include amphetamines, certain barbiturates, lysergic acid diethylmide (LSD), and phencyclidine. Schedule IV drugs include those substances for which the abuse potential is low, such as barbital, phenobarbital, and methylphenobarbital.

Schedule V drugs are those substances that contain limited quantities of narcotic agents and that have been deemed as having minimum abuse potential.

DEA spokespersons have stated that the term "currently accepted medical use" is defined by the existence of an approved New Drug Application or an exemption from such approval granted by the Food and Drug Administration (FDA). Both of these options are in the hands of the FDA. Procedures used to classify drugs, however, have not received unanimous support from the medical profession. For instance, in the legal response during the methylenedioxymethamphetamine (MDMA) hearings, the DEA concluded, "The DEA would be derelict in allowing a substance [that] has not been found by the FDA to be safe and effective for use to have an accepted medical use for treatment in the United States, merely because a handful of physicians are of the opinion that it may have therapeutic usefulness." However, it is exactly this criterion—the view of physicians, even a minority, that a substance has therapeutic utility—that is held sufficient by both the medical community and the courts. An extensive review of court opinions was brought together by Administrative Judge Young during the public hearings held concerning the scheduling of MDMA (ecstasy), and extensive analysis of the term "currently accepted medical use" was made. Judge Young concluded that the medical community should define medical practice, even when it is conducted by a small handful within that community. Despite the fact that MDMA was considered medically useful by some physicians, particularly psychiatrists, and despite Judge Young's recommendations, DEA administrators pursued the government's own political agenda, classifying MDMA in Schedule I and asserting it had no current medical value and great abuse potential.

A broader examination of events surrounding MDMA reveals the political nature of the scheduling process. MDMA received extensive law enforcement attention in 1985 as the result of the widespread media coverage of ecstasy. The media reports implied a dramatic increase in the use of the drug; within a very short period of time, the drug drew the attention of the DEA, which viewed ecstasy as a dangerous and abused designer drug with no therapeutic value. Various psychiatrists opposed drug enforcement officials as well as others who saw ecstasy as a valuable therapeutic adjunct with minimal harm under carefully monitored use. The drug was subjected to the emergency scheduling provisions of the Uniform Controlled Substances Act, which permits the DEA to schedule substances on a temporary basis pending further consideration prior to permanent scheduling. In 1985, MDMA was placed in Schedule I on a temporary basis. In response to the challenges made by the therapeutic proponents, three federal administrative law hearings were held in 1985. Beck and Rosenbaum (1994) point out that what emerged from these hearings was the relative dearth of information about the drug, including a lack of research concerning its benefits and/or harms. In general, both sides were limited to offering anecdotal evidence and extrapolations from preliminary animal studies. Those with the most experience with the drug, a small number of therapists on both the East and West Coasts, began using MDMA as a therapeutic adjunct in 1976. They found it was effective in facilitating communication, acceptance, and fear reduction, but they were reluctant to publish any preliminary findings, worrying that doing so would trigger a law enforcement response that would block further research.

In the hearings, the government attempted to prove that MDMA fit all three criteria for placement in Schedule I: a high abuse potential, no currently accepted medical use, and lack of safety under medical supervision. Researchers and therapists contended that Schedule I placement would destroy any hope of evaluating MDMA's therapeutic potential, as had occurred with the criminalization of other substances in the late 1960s. Several psychiatrists testified on behalf of MDMA's therapeutic potential, claiming that the drug was safe and a valuable therapeutic tool in the treatment of a wide range of problems.

DEA attorneys criticized the anecdotal nature of the therapists' evidence and contended that the preliminary studies of the drug's effects were inadequately controlled, making them scientifically unsound. Despite this, however, the DEA administrative law judge, in his findings and recommendations, generally concurred with the proponents of MDMA. Citing currently accepted medical use and safety and noting minimal evidence of significant abuse or problems, the judge recommended placement in Schedule III. This would have permitted extensive research into the effects of the drug, including its potential for abuse, and would have allowed continued therapeutic use. The DEA, however, rejected the judge's recommendation and sought to place MDMA permanently into Schedule I on November 13, 1986 (Beck and Rosenbaum, 1994). Several legal challenges ensued, even though the DEA was faulted for its actions on various technical grounds, the DEA administrator once again ordered the permanent placement of MDMA into Schedule I as of March 23, 1988 (Beck and Rosenbaum, 1994).

The story has been much the same for marijuana. Although there is no consensus in the American Medical Association (AMA) or other health care professionals' associations, such as the American Nurses' Association, American Public Health Association, or National Association of Social Workers, on the medicinal benefits of this substance, there is enough consensus among health care professionals to warrant reclassification. The medical literature on the utility of marijuana in the treatment of various ailments is quite extensive (Grinspoon and Bakalar, 1995). There is substantial evidence that **medical marijuana** is useful in treating glaucoma as well as alleviating discomfort associated with chemotherapy. In fact, until the latter part of the 1980s, several hospitals were legally prescribing marijuana.

Marijuana has been found to be beneficial in relieving clients suffering from a host of medical problems. In one study, for instance, of 56 clients who received no relief from antiemetic drugs, 78 percent became symptom-free when they smoked marijuana (Vinciguerra et al., 1988). Among clients, anecdotes describe the benefits of marijuana (Grinspoon and Bakalar, 1995). Many doctors and nurses, knowing the potential of marijuana to relieve some clients' nausea and vomiting associated with chemotherapy, have treaded dangerously close to the boundaries of ethical practice by recommending its use. Health care professionals may be in violation of ethical principles if they encourage clients to engage in illegal activity. Thus, the desire to help individuals often evokes dilemmas for health care professionals. For instance, principle 3 of the AMA's *Principles of Medical Ethics*, which maintains that "A physician respect the law," suggests that a conflict might exist between providing sound client care and following the code of professional ethics. Such unethical practice appears to be widespread. In one study of oncologists, 44 percent indicated that they had recommended the illegal use of marijuana to at least one client. Many of these physicians did so because they believed that smoked marijuana was more effective than other antiemetic drugs, including Marinol or oral synthetic THC (Doblin and Kleiman, 1991).

In addition to its utility in relieving side effects from chemotherapy, marijuana has been found beneficial for glaucoma. Since 1971, it has been relatively well established that marijuana reduces intraocular pressure (Hepler and Frank, 1971). In many instances, the inevitable end result of glaucoma is blindness. Frequently, clients who hear about the medical benefits of marijuana are forced to violate the law. As one glaucoma sufferer explained,

"I accept that an illegal, medically prohibited weed may help me not go blind." Many others, including those who suffer from epilepsy, multiple sclerosis, AIDS, chronic pain, and migraines, report similar sentiments about the relief gained from marijuana (Grinspoon, 1993). Moreover, reports of the medicinal qualities of marijuana have been known for centuries. The substance has been used much longer for its medicinal qualities than for its mind-altering effects (Abel, 1980).

Since 1976, several clients throughout the country had been involved in the so-called compassionate IND (investigative new drug) program that gave some individuals access to legal marijuana. Law enforcement agents harassed many who participated in this program. The practice of providing legal marijuana to persons suffering from medical problems was terminated in 1992 by the Bush administration. As Trebach and Zeese have noted, "Only 13 disease sufferers had survived the arduous process of securing a government supply of marijuana at the time of the closing" (1992, p. 218). By 1994, there were only 8 survivors from the original group who continued to receive legal prescriptions for marijuana.

The recognition of the medical benefits of marijuana has led to efforts by groups such as the National Organization for the Reform of Marijuana Laws, the Drug Policy Foundation, and the Physicians Association for AIDS Care to petition for the rescheduling of marijuana. Public hearings commenced in the summer of 1986 and extended through the next two years. As was the case with MDMA, Administrative Judge Young again reviewed the evidence on "currently accepted medical use" and again found that approval by a significant minority of physicians was sufficient to meet that standard. Young additionally concluded, "There is no lack of accepted safety for use of it under medical supervision and that it may lawfully be transferred from Schedule I to Schedule II" (Drug Enforcement Agency, 1988). This recommendation was rejected, however, by the DEA administrator, and marijuana remains in Schedule I.

Since then, other associations such as the National Association of People with AIDS and the California Medical Association have expressed support for the rescheduling of marijuana to allow its use in medical circumstances (Trebach and Zeese, 1992). In California as well as in Arizona and Maine, laws have recently been enacted allowing the use of marijuana for medical purposes. Among the supporters are the National Nurses Society on Addictions and the California Nurses' Association. California Governor Wilson, as well as the federal government, opposed this legislation despite its broad-based support among the medical communities. In addition to support from these medical communities, the Federation of American Scientists recently petitioned DHHS Secretary Donna Shalala to expedite research on the medical use of marijuana. Reacting to public attention over the medical marijuana movement, the DEA has claimed that no one major medical association has recommended marijuana for treatment purposes (Sauer, 1995) and continues to assert vociferously the dangers of marijuana use.

A number of other state medical associations have endorsed rescheduling controlled substances for medical use. For instance, nurses in the state of Colorado are presently considering such an endorsement. The 1995 Colorado Nurses' Association (CNA) House of Delegates proposed that the CNA recognize the therapeutic use of cannabis, and that it support efforts to end federal policies that prohibit or unnecessarily restrict marijuana's legal availability for legitimate health care uses. Delegates considered the following:

Marijuana is a Schedule I drug, which prohibits it from being prescribed for or used by patients. Criteria for a Schedule I designation are: the drug has no therapeutic value; the drug is not safe for medical use; and the drug has a high abuse potential. There is overwhelming evidence that marijuana does NOT meet these criteria. As a medicine, marijuana has been found to be effective in such areas as the treatment of glaucoma, by reducing intraocular pressure; the reduction of nausea and vomiting caused by chemotherapy; in stimulation of appetite for AIDS patients; and for controlling spasticity in spinal cord injury patients. Marijuana has been found to be remarkably non-toxic. It is considered virtually impossible to overdose with the drug in its natural state. The estimated lethal dose is 20,000 to 40,000 times a normal dose. Thirty-five states have recognized marijuana's therapeutic potential and have passed legislation supporting its value. However, the Drug Enforcement Administration has failed to remove marijuana from the Schedule I category. Marijuana must be placed in a less restrictive Schedule and made available to patients who may benefit from its use.

At the present moment, history is repeating itself. The government has continued to usurp the authority of the medical and nursing professions to decide what constitutes accepted medical use. The decision to control physician practices with regard to marijuana, as well as the government's unwillingness to reclassify the substance or even to hold open hearings with independent medical professionals, highlights the ideological issues of lawmakers. These politicians and law enforcement agents prefer to maintain a criminal policy regarding substances despite medical evidence supporting medicalization of these drugs. Such efforts to control medical practice are not unlike the days during the *Webb* era when doctors were prosecuted by law enforcement agents for engaging in practices that they deemed medically justifiable.

While the government delays action, people afflicted with life-limiting ailments are moving forward. Unfortunately, many who desire to purchase marijuana for medical purposes are forced to buy in an illegal and often inflated market. Robert Randell, a leading advocate of medical marijuana and a glaucoma sufferer, has said, "Leaving sick and dying people to the tender mercies of self-described drug dealers is not an appropriate response" (Sauer, 1995). In dozens of cities around the country, cannabis clubs have formed in order to provide the sick with affordable access to marijuana. These "buyers' clubs," sometimes referred to as the "green cross," break the law to provide marijuana to the sick. In San Francisco, for example, one buyers' club has attracted more than 2,000 persons, 70 percent of whom suffer from AIDS (Batz, 1994; Wilkie, 1995). Another club, Cannabis Hemp AIDS Medical Project (CHAMP), opened in Pittsburgh (Batz, 1994). Like the health care collectives of the past, sufferers throughout the country are pursuing alternative treatment options, which in this case are being restricted by law enforcement.

The reluctance of the government to reschedule marijuana stems from claims about the substance's high abuse potential (linked to addiction and withdrawal) and the belief that marijuana use leads to use of drugs of higher addictive potential. However, even the terminology "high abuse potential" has never been clearly defined within the Controlled Substances Act. The classification of Schedule I and II drugs requires that there be a high abuse potential. For a drug to be placed in Schedule III, the potential must be lower than in I and II. A Schedule IV drug must be low relative to that of III; a Schedule V must be low relative to IV. Such a standard, based on relative magnitude of abuse potential, in the absence of clear medical evidence amounts to no standard at all. What does accepted safety actually mean? What are the procedures taken to prove the lack of safety? These questions are rarely addressed in the law: The final decision rests with high-level law enforcement officials, not health care professionals.

Another standard can be seen in the justification of the Schedule I placement for alpha-methylfentanyl, a synthetic heroin substitute that quickly became a true health hazard. The reports of several deaths from China White (a street name for alpha-methylfentanyl) were taken to imply a high abuse potential, although the deaths could have just as easily been attributed to a lack of safety associated with its use or to sleazy practices of street dealers. Yet, in answer to a question, "Why was alpha-methylfentanyl singled out from its many derivatives that might have a high abuse potential?" (see 46 FR 46799), government officials stated that although the other derivatives "may have pharmacological properties [that] are commensurate with a potential for abuse, they have not been specifically studied to determine whether they have an abuse potential nor is there evidence that the other derivatives are being abused" (46 FR 46799).

Another example of ambiguity is found in the proposed invocation of the emergency scheduling law to MDMA in 1985 (50 FR 23118), which applies to both the abuse and the hazard factor. Here, the reported neurotoxicity of methylenedioxyamphetamine (MDA) was a major argument supporting the scheduling of MDMA, a different compound. The FDA considers any use of an unapproved drug an example of drug abuse. Yet, a recent survey published by the American Medical Association includes no such approval clause.

Medicalization and Ethical Decisions

This brief review suggests that many health care professionals prefer a medicalized approach to psychoactive drug use over the current policy of criminalization. According to Levine, a medicalized approach would be a policy that could allow substances to "be obtained on the prescription of a physician; when thus acquired, their possession or use would no longer be considered a criminal offense" (1993, p. 319). In Levine's view, such a policy would reduce the public health costs to individuals as well as society. Indeed, medicalized views of drug use have been gaining popularity in Europe. According to one study, a majority of British doctors favor a change of law to allow marijuana to be prescribed. A poll of almost 70 percent of the 290 members of the British Medical Association indicated that they believed marijuana should be made available for therapeutic purposes (*The Gazette-Montreal,* 1994). One Italian physician (Del Gatto, 1988) argues that the following therapeutic effects could result from the medicalization of narcotics: (1) a decrease in the number of drug-related deaths; (2) a reduction in the rate of illness; and (3) an improvement in the drug addict's everyday life, due to decreased criminal and deviant behavior. Such a medicalized policy has the distinct advantage of accomplishing these effects while simultaneously maintaining a mechanism for social control, such as increasing access to treatment services. Although many health care professionals would probably not endorse legalization or medicalization for recreational use, based on the data reported above, many would and do support medicalization for therapeutic purposes. Some may support it for pathological use "within the context of a fully developed physician-client relationship in which the client recognized his dependency as undesirable and wanted to cooperate with the physician in a mutual effort either to end the dependency or, at the very least, to mitigate its destructive effects" (Levine, 1993, p. 334).

Until the time that a medicalized drug policy officially replaces the present criminalized approach, the ethical dilemmas faced by health care workers with regard to the use of controlled substances for medicinal purposes are great. Although many medical organizations have endorsed the medical use of marijuana, it remains a Schedule I controlled substance that is subject to strict enforcement. Currently, the ethical principles advanced in medical, nursing, and social work professions provide little guidance in this matter. Unfortunately, ethical standards within many professions are vague and ambiguous, often lacking direction in actual situations. Lawyers, for instance, frequently complain that the ethical principles of the profession are not sufficient to guide professional conduct on a daily basis. In fact, many of the ethical dilemmas experienced by lawyers are not even addressed in the code of professional conduct (Granfield and Koenig, 1994).

In regard to medicine and nursing, ethical codes may conflict with one another in the case of marijuana. Nurses, for instance, are expected to maintain competence in nursing and exercise informed judgment, yet they also are expected to safeguard individuals and the public when safety is affected by the illegal practice of any person. Does recommending marijuana use for medical purposes in light of the government's unwillingness to reschedule marijuana due to its belief it is a dangerous substance constitute a breach of the ethical code for nurses? What obligations do nurses and physicians have to a client when they recommend that he or she violate a federal law? There are numerous cases in which clients have received prison sentences for using marijuana to relieve their pain and suffering because of the court's reluctance to accept a medical necessity defense (Goldin, 1995; Kramer, 1995). During the 1980s, Daniel Murphy, an arachnoiditis sufferer, began using marijuana to alleviate pain and spasticity. In 1994, Murphy was arrested and sentenced to five years in prison for possessing marijuana. In the court case, there was no indication where he had learned about the therapeutic effects of marijuana; however, he had obtained information that directed his self-medication. Because the courts have not consistently recognized medical necessity in controlled substances cases, what are the ethical obligations of nurses and physicians to their clients to whom they recommend the use of such substances?

There are numerous other instances in which physicians, acting on behalf of their clients' interests, risk ethical and legal sanctions. Physicians who write prescriptions for narcotics and/or needles in order to maintain an addiction are in violation of ethical as well as criminal codes. Such laws exist in part to protect the public from the practices of unscrupulous physicians who sell prescriptions for monetary gain or satisfaction of prurient appetites. However, it is also just as conceivable that physicians could write prescriptions for syringes to safeguard addicts against AIDS. In such a scenario, a physician is acting in the interest of public health, yet places the client as well as himself or herself at grave risk of criminal prosecution. Despite the success of needle exchange programs, many AIDS activists, including health care professionals, have been arrested for illegally distributing needles. Physicians who write prescriptions for needles to addicts are subject to similar criminal sanctions as well as license revocation. Similarly, if a nurse participates in a needle-bleaching program to reduce the spread of AIDS, he or she risks criminal liability as sanction for unprofessional conduct. Such ethical dilemmas derive from a criminal justice policy that fails to exempt health care professionals from criminal sanctions for prescribing controlled substances.

Ethical dilemmas also confront medical social workers. Social workers should not make medical recommendations; they nonetheless experience ethical dilemmas about medical use of controlled substances. It is quite possible that a social worker could enter into a professional relationship with an adult who is using marijuana daily for medical purposes and who is the parent of young children. Does this social worker violate ethical responsibility if he or she fails to report this to the proper authorities? According to the Child's Bill of Rights in Colorado, a child has a right to live in an atmosphere that is free of abuse of controlled substances, and the Colorado Children's Code instructs social workers to report abuse and neglect that threaten the health or welfare of a child. How far does a social worker's ethical authority extend? Does it include acceptance of a parent's practice of allowing a child with incurable cancer to smoke marijuana to alleviate the discomfort from chemotherapy and to experience improved quality of life for his or her remaining years? Does this constitute child abuse or simply the sound decision of a parent whose autonomy and self-determination the social worker should protect? What are the legal ramifications for a social worker who fails to inform the authorities in such cases? Policies that criminalize substances that possess therapeutic qualities give birth to such ethical dilemmas.

Conclusion

The history of American drug policy is one of conflict among the three ideologies of social control, law enforcement, and public health. Although the use of law enforcement to control alcohol consumption was partially relinquished with the repeal of national prohibition, law enforcement has maintained a prohibitionist policy on other drugs. The criminal justice system, through the DEA, retains primary control over drugs other than tobacco and alcohol.

The shift in alcohol policy from criminalization to medicalization was influenced by a number of factors including the delegitimization of the law and increasing lawlessness, the financial and labor control needs of the rich and powerful, and the demands by the medical profession to treat excessive alcohol consumption as a disease (Conrad and Schneider, 1980; Kobler, 1973; Levine, 1985). The respectability and power of the antiprohibitionist groups (including health care professionals), as well as the failures of prohibition, ultimately led to an uncoupling of alcohol from control by law enforcement.

The history of alcohol policy offers some insight into potential directions for current drug policy. Although it is doubtful, given the present political climate, that radical changes in drug policy will occur, it is clear that the legitimacy of drug policy reformers is changing. There are presently a number of individual advocates of decriminalization, including Nobel Prize winner Milton Friedman, George Schultz, William F. Buckley, noted biologist Stephen Jay Gould, and Baltimore Mayor Kurt Schmoke. More importantly, perhaps, a number of organizations have endorsed drug policy reform measures that reduce law enforcement's hegemonic control over drugs. Among these organizations are the Drug Policy Foundation in Washington, D.C., the Lindesmith Center, and the Princeton Working Group on the Future of Drug Policy, as well as an assortment of law enforcement agencies. As Levine and Reinarman maintain, "Although all this does not yet constitute a grass-roots movement for fundamental change in our drug laws, nevertheless the list of credible critics of drug prohibition who advocate some form of drug regulation regime (instead of prohibition) has grown surprisingly long and their arguments have gained a certain momentum" (1993, pp. 186–187).

Important advocates of drug policy reform are members of the health care professions, particularly medicine and nursing. Throughout the country, health care professionals are challenging current drug policy. These professionals are calling for the medical use of illicit drugs, particularly marijuana. For the most part, the experience and expertise of health care providers have not been incorporated into the official assessment of drug policy. Throughout contemporary drug policy's history, the medical utility of drugs has been determined by law enforcement officials and politicians. In the past several years, members of the health care professions have been reasserting their claim over drugs and mobilizing for change. For the moment, the efforts of these groups and associations to loosen law enforcement's grip on drugs have been unsuccessful; however, while unsuccessful, these efforts have gained increasing media attention, thereby forcing the government to consider their challenge.

The future of drug policy is uncertain, but it is clear that more moderate reforms stand a greater chance of success than more radical ones (Levine, 1993). Subsequently, a policy that turns the control of drugs over to health care professionals is likely to receive more support than the present approaches to legalization. With this in mind, health care professionals need to initiate discourse on what a medicalized drug policy would contain in their professional associations, the workplace, journals, and schools. Central questions to be explored are whether medical and nursing practice should be limited by law enforcement, what should be limited, and whether health care professionals rather than law enforcement make the best determinations. If health care professionals articulate clear statements about their roles in drug policy, this will assist them to regain jurisdiction over certain drugs that was lost more than 75 years ago.

Case Study

Ron is a 41-year-old computer technician who was diagnosed with multiple sclerosis eight years ago. When Ron's mobility is optimal, he uses crutches; days with more impaired mobility require that he switch to his wheelchair. His colostomy bag is positioned high on his abdomen and the smell often ruins his appetite. At night, he lies in bed and tries to sleep, but his body twitches as his muscles fight the disease. Although Ron has tried various drugs, including marijuana derivatives such as Marinol for pain relief, he is unable to find any comfort. In the course of his most recent medical checkup, Ron inquires whether there are any other medications that might be available to relieve his symptoms because his work and personal life have become extremely limited. As a nurse, you are aware of the recent federal guidelines that ban health care practitioners from recommending marijuana use, but you also wish to help Ron relieve his suffering.

1. What factors influence a decision to recommend or not recommend the use of marijuana for medicinal purposes?
2. Should a nurse bring this particular problem to the attention of the client's physician?
3. What are the pros and cons associated with having a client such as Ron use marijuana?
4. What are the ethical issues involved in this case?
5. If you choose to recommend marijuana use, what precautions might you take to protect the client, your organization, and yourself from potential prosecution?

CRITICAL THINKING QUESTIONS

1. Several states have passed or are considering new laws allowing the medical profession to prescribe controlled substances such as marijuana and heroin. What advantages and disadvantages are associated with such a law?

2. In some states, the state nursing associations have endorsed changes in the scheduling of controlled substances. How does such legislative activity on the part of nurses influence policy directions?

3. What positions have been taken by state nursing associations on the medical use of marijuana?

4. Should health professionals influence greater control over prescription rights to controlled substances not presently available? If so, what strategies should the health professions take to regain control?

5. What curricular changes in medical and nursing education would expand knowledge about controlled substances?

6. Identify the ethical dilemmas that surround limitations on the availability of substances that have medical benefits.

7. Do the health professions have an obligation to contest and challenge punitive measures implicit in American drug policy? If so, how and in what ways?

8. What would be the medical implications of a legalized drug policy, such as the one that applies to alcohol use and tobacco?

9. In what ways might a punitive approach to drug use be antithetical to the principles of health care?

10. Several states have sought to prosecute women who use drugs during pregnancy despite unclear evidence that controlled substances have detrimental effects on a fetus. Should medical communities endorse policies that prosecute women for alcohol and drug use during pregnancy?

REFERENCES

Abbott, A. (1988). *The System of Profession.* Chicago: Chicago University Press.

Abel, E. (1980). *Marihuana: The First Twelve Hundred Years.* New York: Plenum Press.

American Medical Association. (1963). *Narcotics Addiction: Official Actions of the AMA.*

Batz, B. (1994). "AIDS weapon: Pot." *The Chicago Tribune,* December 5, p. 7.

Beck, J., and Rosenbaum, M. (1994). *Pursuit of Ecstasy: The MDMA Experience.* Albany, NY: State University of New York Press.

Brecher, E. (1972). *Licit and Illicit Drugs.* Boston: Little Brown.

Conrad, P., and Schneider, J. (1980). *Deviance and Medicalization: From Badness to Sickness.* St. Louis, MO: Mosby.

Currie, J. (1993). *Reckoning: Drugs, the Cities and the American Future.* New York: Hill and Wang.

Del Gatto, L. (1988). The chains of prohibition and the freedom of the physician. In *The Cost of Prohibition on Drugs.* Rome, Italy: CORA.

Doblin, R., and Kleiman, M.A.R. (1991). Marihuana as anti-emetic medicine: A survey of oncologists' attitudes and experiences. *Journal of Clinical Oncology 9,* 1275–1280.

Drug Enforcement Agency. (1988). In the Matter of Marijuana Rescheduling Petition, Docket 86-22, Opinion, Recommended Ruling, Findings of Fact, Conclusions of Law, and Decision of the Administrative Law Judge, September 6. Washington, DC: Author.

The Gazette-Montreal. (1994). MDs want to prescribe cannibus. January 31, B-1.

Goldin, D. (1995). Marijuana cure: Rx for arrest. *New York Times,* September 10, Section 13, p. 8.

Goldstein, P., Brownstein, H., Ryan, P., and Belluci, P. (1997). Crack and homicide in New York City: A case study in the epidemiology of violence. In C. Reinarman and H. Levine (eds.), *Crack in America: Demon Drugs and Social Justice.* Berkeley: University of California Press.

Goode, E. (1989). *Drugs in American Society.* New York: McGraw-Hill.

Granfield, R., and Koenig, T. (1994). Does ethical training matter?: Between ethics in the books and ethics in action. Paper presented at the Law and Society Association Meeting, Phoenix, AZ, June 2.

Grinspoon, L., and Bakalar, J. (1995). *Marijuana: The Forbidden Medicine.* New Haven, CT: Yale University Press.

Hepler, R.S., and Frank, I.M. (1971). Marihuana smoking and intraocular pressure. *JAMA 217,* 1392.

Kobler, J. (1973). *Ardent Spirits: The Rise and Fall of Prohibition.* New York: G. P. Putnam.

Kramer, B. (1995). Marijuana prescription lands man behind bars. *The Providence Journal,* August 12, 1A.

Levine, H. (1985). The birth of American alcohol control: Prohibition, the power elite, and the problem of lawlessness. *Contemporary Drug Problems 12,* 63–115.

Levine, R. (1993). Medicalization of psychoactive substance use and the doctor–patient relationship. In R. Bayers and G. Oppenheimer (eds.), *Confronting Drug Policy: Illicit Drugs in a Free Society.* New York: Cambridge University Press.

Levine, H., and Reinarman, C. (1993). From prohibition to regulation: Lessons from alcohol policy for drug policy. In R. Bayers and G. Oppenheimer (eds.), *Confronting Drug Policy: Illicit Drugs in a Free Society.* New York: Cambridge University Press.

Lindesmith, A.R. (1965). *The Addict and the Law.* Bloomington: Indiana University Press.

Musto, D. (1987). *The American Disease: Origins of Narcotic Control.* New York: Oxford University Press.

Nadelmann, E. (1989). Drug prohibition in the U.S.: Costs, consequences, and alternatives. *Science 245,* 939–947.

Nadelmann, E. (1993). *Cops Across Borders: The Internationalization of U.S. Criminal Law Enforcement.* University Park: Pennsylvania State University Press.

Norton-Hawk, M. (1994). Unintended consequences: The prosecution of maternal substance abuse. In P. Venturelli (ed.), *Drug Use in America: Social, Cultural, and Political Perspectives.* Boston: Jones Bartlett.

Rouse, J.J., and Johnson, B. (1990). Hidden paradigms of morality in debates about drugs: Historical and policy shifts in British and American drug policies. In J. Inciardi (ed.), *The Drug Legalization Debate.* Newbury Park, CA: Sage.

Ryan, K. (1994). How we lost the war: Explorations of U.S. drug policy and its consequences. *Criminal Justice Review 19,* 79–99.

Sauer, M. (1995). Herbal medicine club serves up potent pot to ease the deathly ill. *San Diego Union-Tribune,* May 11, E-1.

Trebach, A., and Zeese, K. (1992). Medical marijuana fight heats up. In A. Trebach and K. Zeese (eds.), *Strategies for Change: New Direction in Drug Policy.* Washington, DC: Drug Policy Foundation Press.

Vinciguerra, V., Moore, T., and Brennan, E. (1988). Inhalation marijuana as an anti-emetic for cancer chemotherapy. *New York State Journal of Medicine 88,* 525–527.

Weisner, C., and Room, R. (1978). Financing and ideology in alcohol treatment. *Social Problems 32,* 157–184.

Wilkie, D. (1995). Medical marijuana: Political pot boils. *San Diego Union-Tribune,* June 16, A-1.

Wisotsky, S. (1990). *Beyond the War on Drugs: Overcoming a Failed Public Policy.* Buffalo, NY: Prometheus Books.

Cases Cited

Linder v. United States, 268 U.S. 5 (1925).

United States v. Doremus, 249 U.S. 86 (1919).

United States v. Jin Fuey Moy, 241 U.S. 402 (1916).

Webb v. United States, 249 U.S. 96 (1919).

4

Policy and Educational Developments in Nursing

Laina M. Gerace, RN, PhD
Marie Talashek, RN, EdD, CS, FAAN

LEARNER OUTCOMES

On completion of this chapter, the learner will be able to:

1. Report the evolution of government policies on substance abuse, with implications for nursing practice.
2. Discuss the treatment implications of federal policy in relation to substance abuse and dependence.
3. Describe principles for nursing organization involvement with impaired professional practice.
4. Analyze opportunities that nursing organizations have created to influence policy development in the area of substance abuse.
5. Describe major activities undertaken by nursing organizations in relation to education and policy on substance abuse and dependence.

KEY TERMS

Americans with Disabilities Act (ADA)	impaired nursing practice	polypharmacy
breathalyzer	mandatory reporting	position statement
cooperative nondisciplinary alternative program	peer assistance network	

Historical Background

Nurses have always cared for individuals with drug and/or alcohol problems; however, nursing diagnoses and interventions have only recently supported standards for practice with these populations. Early documentation shows that Florence Nightingale noticed that soldiers drank excessively on the front during the Crimean War and that they dissipated their pay checks on alcohol because recreation was limited and postal service to send money home was erratic. Based on this observation, she oversaw the organization of recreation halls and obtained supplies for healthy recreation. Whether she linked drunkenness to mental health or simply observed that unstructured time could lead to drinking, she took steps to limit the growth of alcohol-related problems.

Nurses specializing in the treatment of alcohol and other drug problems first began meeting in a formal way under the auspices of the National Council on Alcoholism (NCA), which earlier had sponsored a similar group for physicians. The National Nurses Society on Alcoholism was officially convened as a component of the National Council on Alcoholism and supported in 1975 by the American Nurses' Association (ANA). The initial goals of this specialty organization were to (1) advocate for programs that would improve the care and treatment of alcohol-abusing clients and families and (2) become involved with public policy and issues of social concern about alcohol use and alcoholism.

Membership was limited to registered professional nurses interested in the clinical practice of addictions care. The organization's name was formally changed to the National Nurses Society on Addictions (NNSA) in 1983 and now comprises more than 20 regional chapters. The group became independent from the NCA in 1981 and since has worked closely with the ANA in the development of two important monographs: *The Care of Clients with Addictions: Dimensions of Nursing Practice* (1987) and *Standards of Addictions Nursing Practice with Selected Diagnoses and Criteria* (1988). The organization's newsletter merged with a journal in 1996 to create the *Journal of Addictions Nursing,* for nurses treating drug and alcohol problems. Other organizations for nurses interested in the field include the Drug and Alcohol Nurses Association (DANA), founded in 1979, the National Consortium of Chemical Dependency Nurses (NCCDN), and the California Association of Nurses in Substance Abuse (CANSA). DANA and CANSA have now merged with NNSA, expanding membership and decreasing the number of specialty organizations. These organizations form a loose coalition to explore topics and issues of interest to the field.

The role of nursing in caring for clients with drug and alcohol problems was a theme within the overall fabric of nursing until the mid-1970s. With the establishment of specialty organizations that focus on nursing care of addicted clients came assurance that committed monies would be available to their professionals and the public.

Policy Perspectives

Health care providers find the extent of the destructive effects of alcohol, tobacco, and other substance misuse or abuse evident in their client populations to be potentially overwhelming. The problems of drug use appear to be embedded in social behavior; consequently, social attempts to regulate or control the supply and distribution of illicit substances have had little effect on the availability of various mind-altering substances. Because people seek to alter consciousness, the notion of a drug-free world is a myth. The use of alcohol, drugs, and tobacco is a central element within the social structure, and efforts to rid the world of these substances may be unrealistic. A more realistic social goal appears to be managing accessibility of psychotropic substances in the environment to reduce the harmful consequences of their use. Relevant questions posed about these issues are: How do we develop the social capacity to regulate demand for and use of potentially damaging substances? How do we prevent misuse? How do we deal with those individuals who abuse and become dependent on substances?

Supply Reduction and Demand Reduction

In the broadest sense, there have been two approaches to societal regulation of substance use and abuse: supply reduction and demand reduction. Supply reduction refers to control or interruption of the manufacture, distribution, and sale of substances. Supply reduction falls under the realm of law enforcement, security maintenance, and international agreements. The so-called War on Drugs costs the United States an estimated $75 billion per year of public money and is the reason for the incarceration of nearly 50 percent of the more than 1 million Americans who are imprisoned. Yet these efforts have had virtually no effect on drug sales and profits or the prevalence and incidence of dependence.

Demand reduction relates to decreasing people's need and desire for substances through health care, community awareness, prevention and education, and the influence of social values. Efforts directed at reducing demand include primary prevention, early detection and treatment, and recovery and relapse prevention. Demand reduction is implemented at various national, state, and local levels. Mechanisms include policies, programs, and educational and health care prevention efforts. These activities hold more promise of influencing individuals, families, and groups in making responsible decisions about alcohol, drug, and tobacco use.

Governmental Regulatory Policies

Federal policies include laws that control the supply and limit consumer demand for drugs. These policies are essentially punitive in nature and relate to acquisition, possession, and use of illegal substances, as well as dealing for profit. Although many of these laws seem reasonable and appear to reflect public values (such as drunk-driving laws), some of these laws are viewed by public health professionals as counterproductive. One example of this is state laws that enforce prosecution of addicted pregnant women for child abuse. Laws relating to substance use that are generally endorsed by health providers include those that protect the welfare and promote the rehabilitation of substance-abusing clients. Two of these are discussed here.

FEDERAL DRUG AND ALCOHOL ABUSE ACT (42 U.S. CODE OF FEDERAL REGULATIONS, SECTIONS 290EE-3 AND 290DD-3)

This federal law protects confidentiality of identification, information, and records for clients receiving treatment for substance abuse. The protection extends to clients receiving consultation and referral for substance abuse problems. There are at least six specific circumstances that delineate situations in which confidentiality does not need to be maintained:

1. Prior written release of information provided by the client
2. Internal reporting within a treatment unit
3. Suspected child abuse
4. Court orders
5. Departure of a mentally ill (dually diagnosed) client against medical advice
6. Cases of medical emergency

To be in compliance with the law, all treatment programs need policies and procedures that address client confidentiality. By law, these must be disseminated to health care providers and clients. Visitors and telephone contacts are properly screened, and information should not be given to anyone, including legal authorities (e.g., police, probation officers, and attorneys) without the client's permission.

Legal protections help clients seeking treatment because privacy is ensured. In the case of breach of privacy, lawsuits or malpractice and disciplinary action by the licensure board *can be applied*. The advanced practice nurse (APN) has a key role in explaining privacy protection to clients under the provider's care and in ensuring that others adhere to these standards. Employee assistance programs must similarly limit information given to employers.

AMERICANS WITH DISABILITIES ACT OF 1990 (ADA) (PUBLIC LAW 101-336)

Persons with mental or physical disabilities have traditionally received very little protection from inequitable situations in the workplace. The **Americans with Disabilities Act (ADA)** prohibits discrimination by employers, regardless of whether there is receipt of federal funds, on the grounds of a handicapping condition. Individuals who qualify as having disabilities must be able to perform essential functions of their jobs. Specific accommodations needed by handicapped individuals must be provided by employers as long as they do not impose undue hardship on the organization or company. *Current illegal use of drugs or alcohol* is not included within the scope of the ADA, but once an employee is diagnosed with a substance-related illness and is actively participating in or has completed a drug rehabilitation program and is no longer engaged in illegal use of drugs or alcohol, that employee is protected by the ADA. An employer may ban the use of alcohol and illegal drugs in the workplace and require that employees not be under the influence of drugs or alcohol in the work environment. In fact, federal policies require a drug-free workplace for the granting of funds for a range of educational, research, treatment, and support services.

APNs should advise clients that legal protection is not afforded in the workplace if they continue to abuse alcohol or drugs on the job. On the other hand, the ADA ruling protects clients in treatment and recovery from unfair discrimination due to a diagnosis of addiction.

Professional Organization Policies

The nursing profession needs to continue to define its role within the larger context of demand reduction and to set priorities as efforts are directed toward clearly articulated goals. APNs should provide leadership in this area. The problem of substance abuse has rarely received adequate attention from any group of health professionals, including nurses. *A prominent reason includes denial of the scope of the problem, which in turn supports a reluctance to develop clear policies and education about the extent of the substance use and abuse problem.* The definition of a clear professional role is compromised by widely held negative attitudes, such as viewing substance-related problems as moral failings or being pessimistic about the effectiveness of treatment and recovery. Such attitudes are based on a lack of knowledge and clinical experience.

Nursing has made strides in this area by developing policies, standards, and curriculum materials dealing with both impairment within the profession and primary, secondary, and tertiary prevention with clients despite these obstacles. The major policy efforts for nursing are concentrated in professional impairment, standards of care and position statements, and curriculum and educational developments.

Professional Impairment

Professional impairment refers to professional practice that is negatively affected by substance abuse, cognitive deficiencies, and/or psychological/emotional problems. Although the problem of impairment is not unique to any professional or occupational group, it becomes a critical safety issue for individuals who work in professions in which provision of direct service to others is a priority. **Impaired nursing practice** often comes to the attention of nursing administrators or APNs with substance abuse expertise. It is important to understand the issues central to impaired nursing practice and to develop competence in the identification, treatment, and monitoring of professionals with addiction problems.

SCOPE OF THE PROBLEM

The prevalence rates for addiction in society provide some basic estimates of the scope of this problem in nursing. It is estimated that about 6 percent to 8 percent of nurses are substance-dependent (Haack and Hughes, 1989; Hughes and Smith, 1994). The work of Trinkoff and associates (1991) provides better insight into the extent of the problem. In an annual survey on the regulatory management of addicted/dependent nurses, it was found that, in 43 out of 52 states reporting, over 1,000 nurses had substantiated complaints against them related to substance dependence or abuse. Over 900 of these complaints resulted in disciplinary action against their licenses (Trinkoff, Eaton, and Anthony, 1991). These statistics emphasize the importance of policy development for professional impairment within nursing.

POLICY DEVELOPMENT

During the 1980s, the ANA and the addictions specialty organizations worked in concert on the issue of impaired professional practice. The prevalence of substance abuse and psychological dysfunction among nurses was highlighted in 1982. At that time, the ANA was the key organization that responded to requests for assistance by state associations that sought to assist nurses with licensure problems related to substance abuse and mental health. A landmark resolution was passed in 1982 declaring that the profession needed to address the misuse of alcohol and other drugs, as well as emotional and psychological dysfunction, in its own members (Table 4-1). This resolution called for ongoing collection and dissemination

TABLE 4-1 1982 ANA Resolution.

American Nurses' Association

Resolution #5

Sponsored by the Division on Psychiatric and Mental Health Nursing Practice

Adopted June 29, 1982, by ANA House of Delegates

Action on Alcohol and Drug Misuse and Psychological Dysfunctions Among Nurses

WHEREAS, There are people in the United States among whom are registered nurses whose functioning is impaired because of misuse of alcohol and other drugs or because of emotional and psychological dysfunction; and

WHEREAS, The membership of the American Nurses' Association recognizes its professional responsibility to colleagues and to those they serve; and

WHEREAS, Misuse of alcohol and other drugs and emotional and psychological dysfunction can impair the individual's ability to meet the requirements of the Code for Nurses; and

WHEREAS, Timely and effective intervention can contribute to the restoration to health of the nurse, the maintenance of standards for nursing practice, [the] adherence to the Code for Nurses, and the safety of the public; therefore, be it

Resolved, That ANA, in collaboration with other health care organizations and interested groups, develop guidelines for establishing programs of assistance and intervention for those nurses whose functioning is impaired because of misuse of alcohol and other drugs or because of emotional and psychological dysfunction; and be it

Resolved, That ANA encourage nursing administrators and other employers of nurses to offer appropriate treatment antecedent to disciplinary action in the same manner as with other health problems and to maintain options for continuing or subsequent employment; and be it

Resolved, That ANA establish mechanisms for continuing collection and dissemination of information that includes statistical data, status of program implementation, significant educational and research activities, and legal and ethical issues as related to the impaired nurse.

Source: Reproduced, with permission, from the American Nurses' Association. (1983). *Summary of Proceedings.* Washington, DC: ANA, p. 242.

of information, including educational and research activities related to impaired practice. Policy guidelines were published in a monograph. In response to the leadership of the ANA, the addictions and other specialty organizations developed policy statements to advocate for treatment rather than termination of nurses with such problems. NNSA and DANA established committees to address the issues, and many state nurses' associations developed peer assistance and outreach programs.

PROFESSIONAL ISSUES

Neither education and membership in a profession nor clinical knowledge about the potential harmful effects of alcohol and other drugs protects an individual from becoming a drug abuser or addict. Nurses and other health professionals have the same vulnerabilities and possess the same risk factors as others in relation to the development of addiction. The stress and responsibilities of nurses in particular roles may place them at increased risk, although the implications of research findings about this factor are unclear. The availability of prescription narcotics and other analgesics appear to be a workplace factor of importance. At the very least, nurses are no more immune to these problems than others (U.S. Department of Health and Human Services, 1982).

Nursing as a profession assumes responsibility for self-regulation both through the development of professional standards and a code of ethics and through membership in professional organizations. Because strong protective networks exist among nursing colleagues, behaviors such as problem drinking or drug use are sometimes tolerated even when performance is affected and professional standards are threatened. It is often the case that health care professionals enter treatment at advanced stages of addiction with their licenses intact and while continuing to practice. Few practitioners who perform while impaired receive feedback from professional colleagues about excessive drinking or drug use (Hughes and Smith, 1994). Failure to identify impaired practice and exert peer pressure suggests an ongoing need for APNs to educate members of the profession about impairment within its own ranks. It also suggests that organizational policy is not interpreted at levels that influence the thinking of frontline practitioners.

COOPERATIVE NONDISCIPLINARY ALTERNATIVE PROGRAMS

Prior to the concerted professional action in the form of the 1982 resolution, nurses identified as addicted or abusing alcohol or drugs were reported to the state boards of nursing and were disciplined by censure, suspension, or revocation of their professional license. Because few nondisciplinary alternatives were available, substance-dependent nurses often progressed in their illness because colleagues, sensitive to the punitive outcomes, were reluctant to report them. When they were reported, it led to disciplinary action similar to that taken for incompetence or fraudulent behavior. This approach did not acknowledge the illness or those nurses' need for treatment.

Given the scope and frequency of this problem, the Committee on Chemical Dependency Issues of the National Council of State Boards of Nursing (NCSBN) developed model guidelines for a nondisciplinary alternative (also known as diversion) program for chemically impaired nurses (NCSBN, 1997). These guidelines seek to protect public safety by providing a plan that helps the chemically impaired nurse enter treatment voluntarily. A **cooperative nondisciplinary alternative program** offers a confidential voluntary alternative to license discipline for nurses whose practice is impaired by alcohol, drug abuse, or psychiatric illness. It is important to note that not all states have formal cooperative nondisciplinary alternative programs. Through organizational work and legislative action, APNs can promote development of such programs at the state level.

The model guidelines recommend the development and passage of state legislation that defines the intent to rehabilitate and supports the return to practice for nurses whose function is impaired by use of alcohol or other drugs. It is further recommended that a diversion evaluation committee be established within the state. The functions of a diversion committee include evaluation of nurses who request participation in the program and review of treatment programs as well as program monitoring. Systems for monitoring nurses with impairment problems, from entry into treatment through recovery and reentry to practice, are also described. Table 4-2 describes the objectives of the cooperative nondisciplinary alternative model. Samples of documents, such as a monitoring contract, counselor report, and policies on body fluid testing and monitoring, are included in the guidelines.

TABLE 4-2 Objectives of a Cooperative Nondisciplinary Alternative Program for Chemically Impaired Nurses.

The objectives of the program are as follows:

1. To ensure public health and safety through a program that provides close monitoring of nurses who are impaired due to chemical dependency.

2. To decrease the time between the nurse's acknowledgment of a problem with chemical dependency and the time she/he enters a recovery program. Early entry into a recovery program will allow the nurse to practice in a manner that will not endanger public health and safety and will redirect the nurse's energies to the provision of patient care much sooner.

3. To provide a program for affected nurses to be rehabilitated in a therapeutic, nonpunitive, and confidential process.

4. To provide a voluntary alternative to the traditional disciplinary process.

5. To reach nurses who may be affected by chemical dependency but who are not being reached through the current disciplinary system.

6. To provide a program that can refer nurses to services that are within their economic means.

Source: Reprinted by permission of the National Council of State Boards of Nursing. (1994). *Model Guidelines: A Nondisciplinary Alternative Program for Chemically Impaired Nurses* (pp. 4–5). Chicago: NCSBN.

PEER ASSISTANCE NETWORKS

Peer assistance networks, which usually are organized and function within the state nursing organizations, are the organizational structures through which reporting and requests for assistance in relation to problems of abuse and/or addiction are often initiated. Peer assistance programs are maintained through volunteer activity and collaborating organizations. State nurses' associations often provide staff support. Table 4-3 lists the goals that underlie peer assistance networks. Peer assistance networks are also effective resources in the development of policies related to reentry of the nurse to the workforce following treatment. In conjunction with health services or employee assistance programs, peer assistance groups can develop guidelines to support the nurse as well as protect patient safety.

Recovering nurses can be vital contributors to peer assistance networks. In order to participate as a peer advocate or sponsor, recovering nurses are requested to be drug and alcohol free for at least two years. Recovering nurses have unique assets that are invaluable in helping impaired nurses. They can readily identify common signs that may suggest addiction in another health professional. Through empathetic approaches, they are often able to constructively deal with denial and other defenses and effectively confront troubled colleagues. Advanced practice psychiatric nurses and certified addictions nurses and counselors are also active in peer assistance work. They serve as consultants and educators and may provide direct service through referral, assessment, and treatment.

ASSESSMENT OF STATE-LEVEL IMPLEMENTATION

Although nursing has made headway in dealing with professional impairment, more work remains. Cooperative nondisciplinary policy development needs to be launched in some

TABLE 4-3 Peer Assistance Network Goals.

1. Assist registered nurses experiencing job performance and personal problems related to chemical use, mental illness, or other disabilities by providing preliminary information, counseling, and referral to self-help and treatment resources.

2. Motivate registered nurses to assess personal alcohol and drug use and enter appropriate treatment programs as necessary.

3. Educate families, employers, and individuals about the signs, symptoms, and consequences of impaired professional practice.

4. Educate individuals and groups about policies, procedures, and/or cooperative alternative nondisciplinary programs available to nurses experiencing drug, alcohol, and/or psychiatric problems.

5. Promote nonpunitive rehabilitative approaches and supportive professional networks to assist nurses experiencing substance abuse and psychiatric problems.

states and strengthened in others. Resources should be provided with outcomes that provide information on success as well as problems.

A survey of policies from state nursing associations revealed that state-level implementation of the ANA policy guidelines for the impaired nurse is inconsistent (Gerace and Talashek, 1992). When all state-level policies were reviewed, only a handful of policies were judged as comprehensive; quite a few states have inadequate guidelines for professional impairment. Some policies were found to have punitive wording (e.g., if a nurse is "found guilty of substance abuse"). On the other hand, the best policies give evidence that organizations use resources such as epidemiological data about professional impairment, signs and symptoms of impairment, and documentation of impairment. These policies include case examples, return-to-work guidelines, and referral sources. Many states still do not have sophisticated policies and implementation plans.

Mandatory reporting poses important challenges. **Mandatory reporting** is in effect in about 25 states, where nurses are legally required to report any colleague who uses alcohol or drugs at work or who is addicted. APNs need to be aware of mandatory reporting requirements within the states in which they practice and should obtain information on ways to assist colleagues in difficulty and still be legally compliant.

RECOGNITION AND REPORTING OF PROFESSIONAL IMPAIRMENT

Impaired nursing practice is a common problem. In one study of 195 chief nurse executives, 80 percent reported having made one or more disciplinary decisions about a chemically dependent nurse, the majority of whom reported experiences with 1 to 5 nurses (Hughes, 1995). The profession has been responsible about educating its members on recognizing and reporting chemical dependence through publications and workshops. Typically, these educational efforts include how to identify job performance problems that may result from signs and symptoms of substance abuse. Signs that an employee is experiencing problems fall into three general areas: (1) decline in job performance and decreased professionalism, (2) changes in personality and emotional expression, and (3) drug diversion behavior (Hughes and Smith, 1994). Table 4-4 describes some of the common signs and symptoms.

TABLE 4-4 Indicators of Behavioral Changes Linked to Chemical Dependency.

Job Performance

- Excessive use of sick time, especially following days off. (This is most common in alcohol dependency.)
- Absence without notice or last-minute requests for time off.
- Long breaks or lunch hours.
- Frequent or unexplained disappearances from the unit.
- "Job shrinkage" (i.e., the nurse increasingly does the minimum work necessary for the job).
- Increasing difficulty meeting schedules or deadlines.
- Sloppy or illogical charting.
- Excessive number of mistakes—frequent medication errors or misjudgments in patient care.
- Smell of alcohol on breath.
- Excessive use of breath mints, chewing gum, or mouthwash.
- Elaborate implausible excuses for behavior.

Behavior

- Emotional lability (or instability) (e.g., the nurse becomes unusually quiet or irritable or has frequent mood swings).
- Inappropriate verbal or emotional responses such as snapping at colleagues, uncontrolled anger, or crying.
- Diminished alertness (perhaps appearing dazed or preoccupied), confusion, or frequent memory lapses.
- Increasing isolation from coworkers (e.g., the nurse eats alone, avoids informal staff get-togethers, or requests transfer to the night shift).

Diversion

- Consistent volunteering as the medications nurse or frequent signing out of more controlled drugs than coworkers.
- Frequent reports of medication spills or other waste.
- Failure to obtain cosignatures.
- Reports reflecting excessive use of PRN medications.
- Discrepancies in end-of-shift medication counts.
- Evidence of tampering of vials or other drug containers.
- Creation of opportunities to be alone to open the narcotics box or cabinet or disappearance into the bathroom after opening it.
- Increase in patients' complaints of unrelieved pain.
- Defensiveness when questioned about medication errors.
- Consistent early arrival at and late departure from work.
- Volunteering to work with patients who receive regular or large amounts of pain medication.

Source: Adapted, with permission, from Hughes, T.L., and Smith, L.I. (1994). Is your colleague chemically dependent? *American Journal of Nursing 94*(9), 31–35.

Standards of Care and Position Statements

Nursing has also developed standards of client care and position statements that have contributed to alcohol and other drug prevention and intervention. These documents attest to the nursing profession's concern with appropriate care for clients with substance abuse problems.

STANDARDS OF CARE CERTIFICATION

Two key addictions specialty nursing organizations, NNSA and DANA, collaborated with the ANA to develop standards of practice for the care of addicted clients. Outcomes of collaboration between the two organizations (DANA is now incorporated into NNSA) include the two-volume publication *Nursing Care Planning for the Addicted Client* (1989, 1990) and *The Core Curriculum for Addictions Nursing* (1990). These educational resources are used to help nurses prepare for addictions certification and are aids for curriculum integration and continuing education.

The NNSA has developed a certification exam. This examination is based on a broad perspective on addictions and contains approximately 200 multiple-choice items on biological, psychosocial, cognitive, and spiritual problems resulting from concurrent diagnoses; depressant, stimulant, and hallucinogenic substances; and process addictions (e.g., eating disorders, gambling, sexual addiction, and codependence). To qualify for the certification examination, a candidate must document a minimum of two years' experience in addictions nursing as a staff nurse, administrator, teacher, consultant, counselor, or researcher. In addition, the candidate must hold an unrestricted RN license in the United States, its possessions, or Canada and have at least three years' experience practicing as a registered nurse (Addictions Nursing Certification Board, 1996). One of the problems associated with one exam for nurses with a range of educational backgrounds is its validity only as a broad general knowledge measure. At the same time, the examination does not evaluate a level of specialty expertise that parallels the master's degree–level certification of other nursing specialties.

POSITION STATEMENTS

Position statements are not considered policies in the strictest sense, but they do provide proactive guidance in specific areas and thus are important; they can serve as a first step for legislation or policy development. In recent years, the American Nurses' Association has drawn on the work of task forces made up of experts with clinical knowledge and research backgrounds in formulating a policy that is the basis of legislative efforts. The ANA and other specialty nursing organizations have developed position statements related to aspects of substance abuse. The goals of these statements are to provide referents for practice standards, views on current issues of concern to the field, and rationales for organizational political action. Six of these position statements are summarized here.

Opposition to Prosecution of Pregnant Women for Drug Abuse (1991)

One area of great concern is the treatment of pregnant women identified as misusing alcohol and other drugs. The serious, debilitating effects of substances on mother, fetus, and infant are well documented. However, an increasing number of women are being arrested and prosecuted solely because they used drugs while they were pregnant. They often receive more severe sentences than those imposed on men and nonpregnant women. A current trend is for states to consider laws to make drug use a felony subject to punishment by imprisonment. These punitive approaches discourage drug-abusing women from seeking early prenatal care, thereby decreasing opportunities to deal effectively with perinatal substance abuse. ANA's position statements supporting (1) opposition to criminal prosecution of women for use of drugs while pregnant and (2) support of treatment services for alcohol- and drug-dependent women of childbearing age preceded the above policy statement, which was formulated in response to punitive state legislation.

Both the ANA (1991a) and the Association of Women's Health, Obstetric, and Neonatal Nurses (AWHONN) (1991) have developed position statements in support of nonpunitive treatment of pregnant women. Both organizations are committed to prevention and treatment as primary solutions to perinatal substance abuse and addiction. Both support an increase in research to test innovative programs tailored to the needs of women of childbearing age.

Abuse of Prescription Medications (1991)

The nursing profession is concerned about overprescription and misuse of certain categories of prescribed medications, such as antianxiety medications (e.g., the benzodiazepine class), especially for women, adolescents, and the elderly. In a position statement, the ANA (1991b) supported the comprehensive assessment and referral to nonpharmacologic treatments of women and others seeking relief from anxiety and depression, rather than the overreliance on prescription medications with high potential for abuse and addiction. Elderly persons experience tolerance and intoxication at lower does of medication, yet as a group, they are recipients of two-thirds of all drugs prescribed in the population and frequently overuse prescription and over-the-counter (OTC) medications. The ANA opposes fraudulent or incompetent prescribing by health care providers and misuse of prescribed medications by nurses themselves.

Polypharmacy and the Older Adult (1990)

Polypharmacy is defined as the concurrent use of several prescription and/or OTC medications. The elderly use more medications than younger people and often require several medications, thus increasing the potential for adverse reactions, drug interactions, and administration errors. Indeed, thousands of deaths are attributed to adverse medication reactions and interactions in the elderly population annually. The health risks associated with polypharmacy and the escalating costs of medications require that the elderly have necessary and effective medication treatment at reasonable cost with decreased risk and maximum benefit (ANA, 1990).

ANA's 1990 position statement on polypharmacy and the older adult recommends heightening awareness of health professionals regarding principles of prescribing for older adults and deterring unnecessary administration of multiple medications. The appropriateness of prescription medications needs to be evaluated periodically. To minimize adverse effects, the ANA recommends that older adults receive the fewest number of necessary medications. In the older adult, alcohol consumption should consistently be assessed for its interaction with prescribed drugs. A medication profile should be initiated on admission of older adults to any health care setting, and the ANA supports nurses in actions to communicate, document, and refuse to give medications that, by nursing judgment, may adversely affect their older clients.

Promotion of Comfort and Relief of Pain in the Dying Patient (1995)

Nurses concerned with addiction often worry about administering pain medications, especially to clients with chronic pain problems associated with illnesses such as sickle cell anemia and cancer or to terminally ill clients. Nurses are often concerned with the development of tolerance to pain medications in clients and its implications for potential addiction, and they may withhold needed medication out of ignorance about the nature of addiction and drugs. Although the ANA has not addressed administration of pain medications in clients with chronic pain, a position statement on pain and comfort measures in dying clients was approved (ANA, 1995). This statement addresses concerns about intractable pain that can occur in dying clients and the distress experienced by their families during the dying process.

Overwhelming pain can cause sleeplessness, loss of morale, fatigue, irritability, restlessness, withdrawal, and other serious problems for dying patients. The ANA holds that assessment and management of pain should be based on a thorough understanding of the individual client's personality, culture and ethnicity, coping style, and emotional, physical, and spiritual needs, as well as an understanding of the pathophysiology of the disease state. The ANA (1995) states that because tolerance to narcotics can develop in clients, both adults and children may require very high doses to maintain adequate pain control. The depressant side effects of pain medications should not be an overriding consideration in their use for dying clients as long as such use is consistent with a client's wishes. The statement is as follows: "The increasing titration of medication to achieve adequate symptom control, even at the expense of maintaining life or hastening death secondarily, is ethically justified. Nurses should not hesitate to use full and effective doses of pain medication for the proper management of pain in the dying patient" (ANA, 1995, p. 2). Guidelines on pain management of clients with chronic pain problems and of clients who are addicted or in recovery remain to be incorporated into medical and nursing care. Drug-seeking clients present a complex array of challenges to pain management.

Prevention of Tobacco Use in Youth (1997)

Although tobacco use among adults has recently declined, an increase in teenage smoking and the initiation of tobacco use at earlier ages are major barriers to the reduction of tobacco-related morbidity and mortality. Indeed, smoking in adolescence, especially by females, is increasing. All APNs need to be aware of the trends and factors contributing to this increase in tobacco addiction. Recent data from the Centers for Disease Control (CDC) support that an increased number of youth are smoking; the Surgeon General describes smoking among the young as a "pediatric epidemic" (ANA, 1997). Organized nursing, including specialty nursing organizations and the ANA, favors prevention and control of tobacco use in youth and all populations as well as policy development and other initiatives in support of federal and state legislation for educational programming.

Drug Testing for Health Care Workers (1994)

A 1994 ANA position paper on drug testing for health care workers was formulated following a presidential mandate that all federal agencies become drug-free. This mandate led to the development of numerous private contracts with federal agencies for workplace surveys related to drug testing as well as methods and techniques for use in public and private industry. The ANA opposes random drug testing of health care workers in the absence of evidence of misuse of drugs. Analysis of body fluids using urine, **breathalyzers,** or blood tests are supported when there is reasonable suspicion and objective evidence that job performance is or has been impaired by substance abuse. Examples include impaired mental status, injury to employees or clients, or verbal altercations of a violent nature. The use of random urine screening is considered an invasion of legal rights and personal dignity of the professional. This policy does not discourage agreements for random screening of those health care workers whose licenses were voluntarily surrendered while in treatment or nurses in recovery when random urine testing is a provision of the return-to-work contract.

Curriculum and Educational Developments

During the 1980s, concern has been expressed over the lack of education and clinical training among all health professionals about substance use and addiction and standards of client care in this area (Gerace, Sullivan, Murphy, and Cotter, 1992; Murphy, 1989). Lobbying and consultation with agencies of the National Institutes of Health have resulted in a number of federal programs to promote education and training for health care professionals, including nurses.

NATIONAL EFFORTS TO IMPROVE NURSING EDUCATION

Three federal institutes—the Office of Substance Abuse Prevention, the National Institute of Drug Abuse, and the National Institute of Alcohol and Alcoholism—funded the development of three model curricula for educating undergraduate and graduate nursing students about substance abuse in 1987. The Ohio State University School of Nursing (Burns, Thompson, and Chaconne, 1989), the Division of Nursing of New York University (Naegle, 1991), and the University of Connecticut (Church, Fisk, and Neafsey, 1990) produced the models, composed of multiple learning modules appropriate for integration into standing nursing curricula or continuing education. In addition, a Center for Substance Abuse Prevention (CSAP) curriculum on Prevention of Alcohol, Tobacco, and Other Drug Problems was established. These curricula provide extensive resources for basic, graduate, and continuing education for nursing.

Another federal initiative of importance was the Faculty Development Programs in Alcohol, Tobacco, and Other Drug Problems. Initiated in the early 1980s, these programs provided funds to approximately 30 schools of medicine, nursing, social work, and psychology to support the education of faculty and the development of addictions care as a subspecialty. Academic faculty whose primary clinical specialties were in other areas (such as obstetrics, medical-surgical nursing, and pediatrics) were supported in substance abuse educational programs, teaching, and research. This initiative was directed at raising the level of knowledge about alcohol, tobacco, and other drugs (ATOD) among all faculty members, preparing researchers, and increasing institutional initiatives for research and publication in the field (Gerace, Sullivan, Murphy, and Cotter, 1992). The foregoing efforts have contributed to the rather limited knowledge base available to practicing health professionals, although there is much to be done before standard practices in the care of clients and families with addiction problems are consistently implemented. The most recent initiative in this area is a funded Human Resources Service Agency (HRSA) cooperative interdisciplinary program with the Association of Medical Educators and Researchers in Substance Abuse (AMERSA). This program will train health professionals from multiple disciplines with ATOD education.

CONTINUING EDUCATION

Attention has also been directed to increasing the knowledge of nurses already in practice. In fact, nurse educators have recommended that position statements guide the development of educational curricula or continuing education in substance abuse and that educational offerings in this area be required to include content on cultural competence. Cultural competence is seen as increasingly important; lack of cultural knowledge and awareness can create obstacles to effective assessment of and intervention for clients with substance abuse problems.

Early recognition of signs and symptoms of substance misuse was emphasized by Brown and Talashek (1992). For example, a number of signs and symptoms have been noted as generalizable across a variety of chemical addictions (see Table 4-4). In addition, patterns of increasing use, craving, tolerance, withdrawal symptoms, and reinstatement following a period of abstinence also characterize addictive behaviors. Because nurses work in a variety of acute and primary care settings and are often the frontline professional, they potentially play important roles in early detection and intervention.

Several evaluation studies based on these efforts to prepare nurses for clinical practice in this area have been published. Talashek, Gerace, Miller, and Lindsey (1995) found that family nurse practitioner (NP) graduate students significantly improved their skills in identification of substance-abusing clients after an educational intervention. When asked to assess a standardized client with a hidden substance abuse problem, these students performed better than NPs with several years of experience. Gerace, Hughes, and Spunt (1995) found in clinical studies that educational efforts extended over three years improved knowledge and confidence in nurses practicing in acute and primary care settings. These efforts point to the importance of incorporating knowledge and skills training as part of basic and ongoing education for professional nurses.

Conclusion

It is important for a profession to develop and articulate goals and priorities related to decreasing people's demand and desire for using psychoactive substances. Clearly, nursing has taken steps to define its role in the larger arena known as demand reduction of alcohol and other drugs. The contributions of nursing in the areas of professional impairment, prevention and intervention, and education of its professionals are admirable; however, there is a need for more initiatives at the actual implementation level. In order to accomplish this goal, resources are needed in terms of budget, expertise, and planning. The profession should continue to promote and facilitate research and fund community, educational, and clinical projects. Such projects, if carefully crafted and peer reviewed, are needed to actualize the effects of nursing at the bedside, in the primary care setting, and in the community.

Case Study

While working in a midsize community hospital located in a small Midwestern city, Nurse S.J. was observed diverting narcotics, that is, actually taking drugs from hospital supplies or from a patient designated to receive them for her own use. She was immediately discharged from her job by the nursing director and hospital administrator. Ms. S.J. soon learned that the entire staff of physicians, nurses, and others heard the details of this event and that information about it was being circulated in the community. Ms. S.J. entered substance abuse treatment and is currently in aftercare and engaged in recovery. Through an attorney, Ms. S.J. is now appealing to be reinstated in her job and is suing the hospital for back pay and damages to her reputation. Her claim states that she was a competent nurse with excellent periodic evaluations and that her practice was impaired due to the serious chronic illness of addiction. She claims her civil rights were violated through the release of confidential information and slander. The lawsuit led to the discharge of the nursing supervisor and resulted in serious morale problems in the other nursing staff. The supervisor also reported that she was treated unfairly by the hospital administration. Her position is that she could have called the police and had Ms. S.J. arrested for diverting narcotics; instead, she protected Ms. S.J. and her license by discharging her from her job.

1. Analyze the steps leading to the lawsuit. What other decisional options would have provided better outcomes in this situation? How could appropriate steps be delineated if the supervisor had access to state or national nursing association policy statements?
2. List examples of policies and procedures that hospitals need to develop in order to deal fairly with professionals whose practice is impaired by drugs or alcohol. What legal information undergirds the development of appropriate policies?
3. Identify policy provisions or legal tenets that help to answer questions regarding the potential violation of the nurse's rights.
4. What provisions serve as references in deciding if the supervisor's rights were violated?
5. What nursing organizational resources, should they exist, could be accessed in addressing issues for concern for the nurse and for the supervisor?
6. Discuss state and federal legislation that provide guidelines for making ethical and legal decisions in such cases.

CRITICAL THINKING QUESTIONS

1. What steps taken by the American Nurses' Association to address impaired practice might be applied to substance abuse education?
2. Identify some ways in which nursing organizations can assist with the evaluation of diversion legislation.

3. Discuss the implications for treatment and care delivery that derive from certification of nurses in this specialty.
4. Which approaches to clinical education might prove most meaningful to advanced practice nurses in general practice areas?
5. Analyze some strategies by which nursing colleagues can support the nurse reentering the workforce.

REFERENCES

Addictions Nursing Certification Board. (1996). *Examination Information Booklet.* Raleigh, NC: Author.

American Nurses' Association. (1990). *Position Statement on Polypharmacy and the Older Adult.* Washington, DC: Author.

American Nurses' Association (1991a). *Opposition to Criminal Prosecution of Women for Use of Drugs While Pregnant.* Washington, DC: Author.

American Nurses' Association. (1991b). *Position Statement on Abuse of Prescription Drugs.* Washington, DC: Author.

American Nurses' Association. (1994). *Position Statement: Drug Testing for Health Care Workers.* Washington, DC: Author.

American Nurses' Association. (1995). *Position Statement on Promotion of Comfort and Relief of Pain in Dying Patients.* Washington, DC: Author.

American Nurses' Association. (1997). *Position Statement on Prevention of Tobacco Use in Youth.* Washington, DC: Author.

American Nurses' Association and National Nurses Society on Addictions. (1987). *The Care of Clients with Addictions: Dimensions of Nursing Practice.* Kansas City: American Nurses' Association.

American Nurses' Association and National Nurses Society on Addictions. (1988). *Standards of Addictions Nursing Practice with Selected Diagnoses and Criteria.* Kansas City: American Nurses' Association.

Association of Women's Health, Obstetric, and Neonatal Nurses. (1991). *Opposition to Criminal Prosecution of Women for Use of Drugs While Pregnant.* Washington, DC: Author.

Brown, R.L., and Talashek, M.L. (1992). *Developing Clinical and Teaching Skills on Screening, Assessment, and Brief Intervention for Alcohol and Drug Problems: Teaching Module.* Washington, DC: Association for Medical Education and Research in Substance Abuse.

Burns, E.M., Thompson, A., and Chaconne, J. (1989). *An Addictions Curriculum for Nurses and Other Helping Professionals.* New York: Springer.

Church, O.M., Fisk, N.B., and Neafsey, P.J. (1990). *Curriculum for Nursing Education in Alcohol and Drug Abuse. Project NEADA.* Storrs: University of Connecticut, School of Nursing.

Gerace, L.M., and Talashek, M. (1992). Substance abuse policies in U.S. nursing organizations. *Proceedings of the 36th International Congress on Alcohol and Drug Dependence.* Glasgow, Scotland: Author.

Gerace, L.M., Hughes, R.L., and Spunt, J. (1995). Improving nurses' responses toward substance-misusing patients: A clinical evaluation project. *Archives of Psychiatric Nursing 9*(5), 286–294.

Gerace, L.M., Sullivan, E., Murphy, S.A., and Cotter, F. (1992). Faculty development and curriculum change in substance abuse. *Nurse Educator 17*(1), 24–29.

Haack, M., and Hughes T.L. (1989). *Addiction in the Nursing Profession: Approaches to Intervention and Recovery.* New York: Springer.

Hughes, T.L. (1995). Chief nurse executives' responses to chemically dependent nurses. *Nursing Management 26*(3), 37–40.

Hughes, T.L., and Smith, L.I. (1994). Is your colleague chemically dependent? *American Journal of Nursing 94*(9), 31–35.

Jack, L. (ed.). (1989). *Nursing Care Planning with the Addicted Client. Volume I.* Skokie, IL: National Nurses Society on Addictions.

Jack, L. (ed.). (1990a). *Nursing Care Planning with the Addicted Client. Volume II.* Skokie, IL: National Nurses Society on Addictions.

Jack, L. (ed.). (1990b). *The Core Curriculum for Addictions Nursing.* Skokie, IL: National Nurses Society on Addictions.

Murphy, S. (1989). The urgency of substance abuse education in schools of nursing. *Journal of Nursing Education 28*, 247–251.

Naegle, M.A. (1991). *Substance Abuse Education in Nursing* (Vol. 1). New York: National League for Nursing Press.

National Council of State Boards of Nursing. (1994). *Report of the Committee on Chemical Dependency Issues.* Chicago: Author.

National Council of State Boards of Nursing. (1997). *Chemical Dependency Handbook for Boards of Nursing.* Chicago: Author.

Talashek, M.L., Gerace, L.M., Miller, A.G., and Lindsey, M. (1995). Family nurse practitioner clinical competencies in alcohol and substance abuse. *Journal of the American Academy of Nurse Practitioners 7*(2), 57–63.

Trinkoff, A., Eaton, W., and Anthony, J. (1991). The prevalence of substance abuse among registered nurses. *Nursing Research 40*(3), 172–175.

U.S. Department of Health and Human Services. (1982). *Target Alcohol Abuse in the Hard-to-Reach Workforce.* Rockville, MD: National Institute on Alcohol Abuse and Alcoholism.

5

Developing Culturally Informed Strategies for Substance-Related Interventions

Carolyn D'Avanzo, RN, MSN, DNSc
Patricia Dunn, EdD, LCSW, ACSW
Jane Murdock, RN, EdD
Madeline Naegle, RN, CS, PhD, FAAN

LEARNER OUTCOMES

On completion of this chapter, the learner will be able to:

1. Compare and contrast the models used to describe the processes of acculturation and assimilation of immigrant populations.
2. Identify the factors that affect the acculturation and assimilation of immigrant populations.
3. Discuss methodological research problems that limit the validity of available data on substance use among minority populations.
4. Discuss the patterns of acculturation of European American, African American, Hispanic American, and Asian American immigrant populations and their relation to alcohol, tobacco, and other drug use.
5. Discuss the patterns of alcohol use within major European American, African American, Hispanic American, and Asian American immigrant populations.
6. Summarize the characteristics of the various population subcultures that are most successful in preventing alcohol abuse.
7. Discuss the implications for providing culturally sensitive care.
8. Describe principles for the development of culturally relevant advanced practice nursing interventions.

KEY TERMS

acculturation	assimilation	race
African Americans	Hispanics/Latinos	stages of change
Asian Pacific Islanders	historical context	

The composition of American society is changing. By the year 2000, more than one-quarter of the U.S. population will consist of ethnic minorities; by 2080, minorities will account for 51.1 percent of the total population. The predominant racial minorities in the United States—African, Hispanic, Asian, Pacific Islander, Native, and Eskimo Americans—differ widely in history and experiences of society, politics, and economics (Hickey, 1996). As these groups grow in number, these differences emerge as issues that, if not acknowledged, have the potential to compromise the effective delivery of human services. It is estimated that, by 2080, Hispanics will account for 23.4 percent, blacks 14.7 percent, and Asians and others 12 percent of the entire population. Nursing and other professional groups are recognizing the importance of preparing practitioners to deliver care that acknowledges the diversity of beliefs, attitudes, traditions, and lifestyles of different racial and ethnic groups, the practice of various religions, and the variations in lifestyles linked to sexual orientation and gender. Diversity is defined as differences rooted in health status, age, gender, experience, or other aspects of sociocultural or socioeconomic positions (Kavanaugh and Kennedy, 1992). Diversity is manifested in language, physiology, and physical characteristics; vulnerabilities to illness; and a range of behavioral patterns associated with health and illness. The diverse nature of populations for whom nurses care precludes the notion that any standard approach to assessment and treatment will be effective with members of all groups. It is important that efforts be made to care for clients in ways that match clients' perceptions of the health problem and its treatment. Recognizing differences as well as developing approaches to care that take differences into consideration is often referred to as culturally sensitive or culturally competent care. An American Academy of Nursing expert panel in 1997 defined culturally competent care as that which is sensitive to issues related to culture, race, gender, and sexual orientation (AAN, 1997). The Academy's report was subsequent to guidelines for the implementation of curricula on cultural competence published by the American Nurses' Association in 1986 and the position that all nurses should be educated in the provision of culturally competent care through theoretical and experiential learning experiences.

Organizational positions on the importance of skills in cultural competence are supported by data indicating that poor-quality client care results from the lack of knowledge and sensitivity. Money is wasted; clients are often misdiagnosed, do not receive adequate pain relief, and are alienated from the health care delivery system when providers overlook the many individual variations that are associated with racial backgrounds, religious beliefs, and cultural practices (Andrews, 1992). Theoretical frameworks within which to understand cultural differences have been proposed by Leininger (1996), Spector (1996), and Campinha-Bacote and associates (1996). All these frameworks identify effective and culturally meaningful nursing care as the desired outcome, although each varies in its components and the importance of components to learning the process. Leininger's Sunrise Model considers the influence of technological, religious and philosophical, kinship and social, political and legal, economic, and educational factors, as well as cultural values and lifeways, as important to understanding what well-being is for a particular person, family, group, or community (Leininger, 1991). Spector details an interactional model that includes social organization, time, space, communication, environmental control, and biological variations and framing, interacting with religion, ethnicity, and culture to influence health traditions of a unique cultural being (Spector, 1996). These models identify the many factors that influence the decision to use substances, which substances are used, and the patterns of use, abuse, and dependence on drugs.

These many determinants require that a comprehensive assessment related to cultural background be part of prevention, assessment, and treatment of substance-related problems. Members of all major ethnic groups report problems with illicit drugs, alcohol, and cigarette use (see Figure 5-1). These are considered in the application of a culturally competent model of care espoused by Campinha-Bacote. This nursing model identifies four components or processes of cultural competence (Campinha-Bacote, Yahle, and Langenkamp, 1996):

1. *Cultural awareness*—the deliberate cognitive process in which the nurse is appreciative of and sensitive to the values, beliefs, lifeways, practices, and problem-solving strategies of a client's culture
2. *Cultural knowledge*—the process in which the nurse seeks out and obtains a sound educational foundation concerning the worldviews of different cultures and the resources available that are congruent with the clients' ethno-religious and cultural heritage
3. *Cultural skill*—the process of learning how to conduct a cultural assessment
4. *Cultural encounter*—the process that allows the nurse to directly engage in cross-cultural interactions with clients from culturally diverse backgrounds

Cross-cultural care refers to global, interdisciplinary, and generic approaches to individuals, families, or groups considered by self or others as different in race, cultural heritage, or sexual orientation. Nurses throughout the world deliver care to many cultural groups in a variety of settings. Educating them to care competently for people of different backgrounds is a major educational mandate for the twenty-first century.

General Considerations for Assessment

Cultural, racial, and religious traditions are linked to variations in patterns of substance use among cultural groups throughout the world. Research findings on these patterns are largely descriptive. Zane and Huh-Kim point out that too often addictive behavior research focuses on a descriptive level of use patterns in various ethnic groups. Ethnic differences refer to variations in those personal-social characteristics (e.g., social class) that an individual tends to have simply by being a member of a certain ethnic group. Cultural differences imply differences in attitudes, values, and perceptual constructs as a result of different cultural experiences (Zane and Huh-Kim, 1994).

Within nursing the cultural approach has received considerable emphasis in recent years. The culturological assessment, as described by Leininger (1978), is a systematic appraisal or examination of individuals, groups, and communities as to their cultural beliefs, values, and practices to determine explicit needs and intervention practices within the cultural context

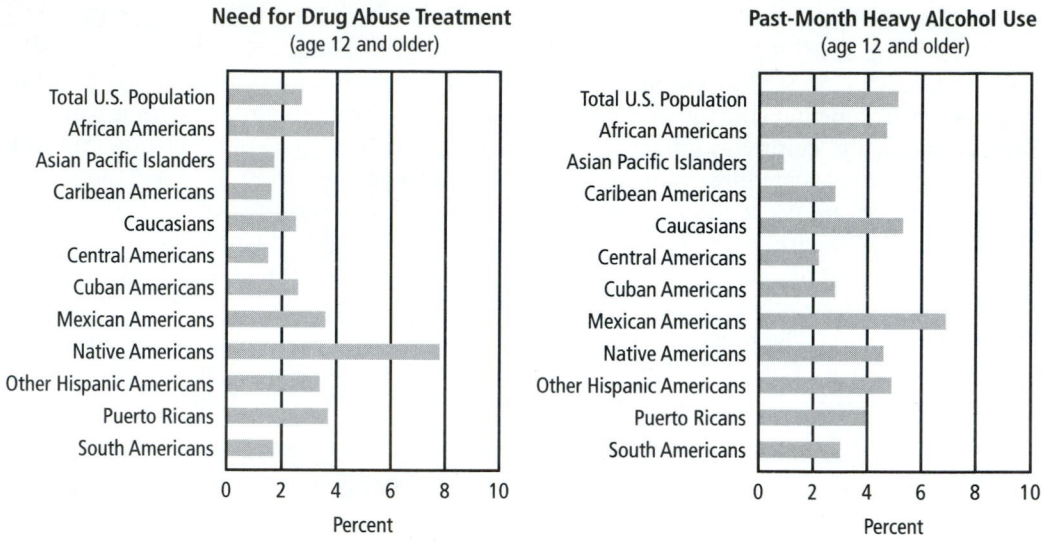

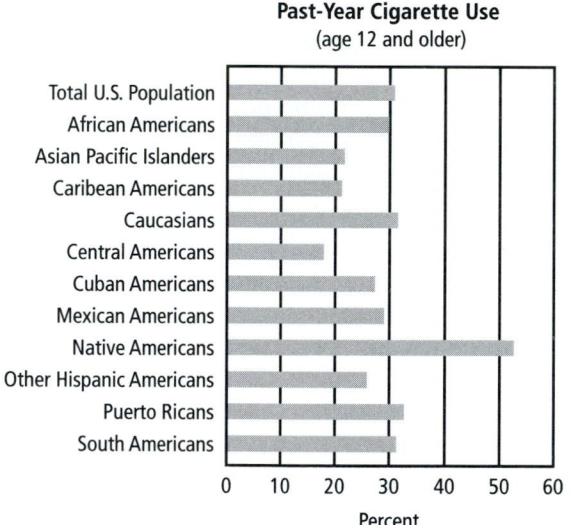

FIGURE 5-1 Racial/Ethnic Subgroups' Substance Use

Source: Substance Abuse and Mental Health Services Administration. *SAMHSA Fact Sheet.* July 6, 1998.

(Leininger, 1996). She suggests that the guiding principles for an accurate culturological assessment are that the nurse (1) maintain a broad, objective, and open attitude about individuals and their cultures; and (2) avoid seeing individuals as all alike (Leininger, 1978). A cultural assessment of every client is needed and should not be limited to individuals of ethnic or racial groups different from that of the provider. Educating providers to abide by such recommendations is difficult because each person enters a health profession with culture-bound definitions of health and disease. These beliefs are often not congruent with, or may even be antithetical to, clients' beliefs and traditions about prevention and treatment of illness. Providers must develop awareness of their own perspectives and biases and acquire education about a range of cultural practices. Numerous factors shape client assessment and include factors such as the circumstances surrounding a newcomer's status as immigrant or refugee, length of residence in this country, and concerns about immigration status and/or one's illegal status. For cultural groups recently emigrated included in studies on substance use, the degree of acculturation or assimilation has been an important factor in trends to use various drugs as well as the amounts of drugs used and social circumstances in which drugs are used. As members of newly emigrated groups have begun to acquire the traditions and practices of the dominant culture, substance use has increased consistently.

Assessment must necessarily include traditions and the practice of drug use, but also all cultural factors that relate to stigma, health problem disclosure and identification, treatment, and legal and social sanctions. The client's beliefs about health practices may include the use of treatments and practices that differ from Western traditions, such as folk medicine, specific foods or diets imbued with healing potential, and the role of the family in care.

Many members of minority groups are not fluent in English, and language poses barriers to both assessment and treatment. Many non-Western languages, in particular, do not possess cultural equivalents of numerous Western psychological constructs. A culturological and health assessment may not be possible without the assistance of an interpreter; even then, the interpreter may lack the facility to understand any distortion of the translations (Marcos, 1979). Sue and Sue (1987) note that the inclusion of an interpreter expands the assessment process to a triadic situation, thereby increasing the risk for miscommunication and inaccurate diagnoses. Every practitioner should be knowledgeable about translation resources at the clinic or institution where assessments are performed. Use of an interpreter who is not a family member is optimal, as family members may omit or modify sensitive issues such as shameful behavior or issues related to sexuality that they perceive as shameful or damaging to the family. When a translator is not available, supplementing family translations by using nonverbal communication in the form of drawings or educational material presented in the native language is recommended.

Culturally Competent Nursing Care

Given the amount of intragroup variation in all populations represented in the United States, it is important to assess the degree to which the client's subgroup cultural values and beliefs may enhance or deter his or her ability to seek out and participate in an effective treatment plan, as well as how family, friends, and coworkers may be able to offer support in the treatment process.

Depending on generational assignment and the degree of assimilation and acculturation, an individual may be influenced to a greater or lesser extent by his or her subcultural values and beliefs. One way to determine this is to screen for what Spector (1996) calls heritage consistency—how closely a particular person's lifestyle reflects that of his or her cultural group. The closer an individual matches his or her ethnic group's views and lifestyle, the greater will be the group's influence on the person's beliefs and practices.

Spector (1996) has identified the following 12 factors that, when present, indicate higher levels of heritage consistency:

1. Childhood development occurred in the person's country of origin or in an immigrant neighborhood of like ethnic group in the United States.
2. Extended family members encourage participation in traditional religious or cultural activities.
3. The individual engages in frequent visits to his or her country of origin or to the old neighborhood in the United States.
4. Family homes are within the ethnic community.
5. The individual participates in ethnic cultural events, such as religious festivals or national holidays, sometimes with singing, dancing, and costumes.
6. The individual was raised in an extended family setting.
7. The individual maintains regular contact with the extended family.
8. The individual's name has not been Americanized.
9. The individual was educated in a parochial (nonpublic) school with a religious or ethnic philosophy similar to the family's background.
10. The individual engages in social activities primarily with others of the same ethnic background.
11. The individual has knowledge of the culture and language of origin.
12. The individual possesses elements of personal pride about his or her heritage.

General principles for assessment include recognition that the individual seeks treatment for a specific complaint and that symptoms, whether singly or in a constellation, have personal and cultural significance for the individual. A suggested model to assist the practitioner in understanding the value clients place on symptoms and/or treatments is proposed by Kleinman (1978). Kleinman's model to explain symptoms has the eight following questions (1978, p. 256):

1. What do you call your problem? What name does it have?
2. What do you think has caused your problem?
3. Why do you think it started when it did?
4. What does your sickness do to you? How does it work?
5. How severe is it? Will it have a long or short course?
6. What do you fear most about your sickness?
7. What are the chief problems your sickness has caused you?
8. What kind of treatment do you think you should receive? What are the most important results you hope to receive from the treatment?

Models of Acculturation and Assimilation

Acculturation and assimilation are helpful concepts in understanding how immigrants adapt to a new society. **Acculturation** is the process whereby newcomers assume American cultural attributes, such as English language, manners, and values. **Assimilation** is the process of newcomers' incorporation into social networks (e.g., work, residence, leisure, and families) of the host society (Gordon, 1964). Many immigrants experience only limited acculturation and practically no assimilation during their lifetimes. Factors that affect these processes are ethnicity, class, gender, and the character of settlement.

The most important factor is the willingness of the dominant ethnic group to accept foreigners. Because the dominant group wields political and social power, it decides who to include and who to exclude. Religion, language, and nationality impede the integration of immigrants into the mainstream. Social class also strongly affects interactions among various ethnic groups. A high degree of residential, occupational, and leisure segregation severely limits acculturation across class and ethnic lines. Gender is a factor; variations exist among groups as to the degree to which women, for example, are restricted to traditional roles or have the freedom to pursue opportunities. The density and location of immigrant settlements influence the rate and character of incorporation into the mainstream culture. Concentrated urban settlements and isolated rural settlements, by limiting contacts between immigrants and others, tend to inhibit the processes of assimilation and acculturation (Vecoli, 1995).

A key variable in these processes is the determination of immigrants themselves to give up their cultures and become simply Americans. Many cling to their traditions and beliefs, maintaining a sense of peoplehood (Gordon, 1964). Relatives and friends often regroup in a new environment to provide mutual assistance and to maintain their customary ways. They establish churches, societies, newspapers, and other institutions, all of which sustain their cultural identities. They take from American culture that which they need and keep from their traditional culture what they value (Vecoli, 1995).

A number of models have been used to describe the processes of assimilation and acculturation as they play out in American society. Prior to the twentieth century, *caste systems* based on race and industrialization dictated, in the case of the former, who would be free and who would not and, in the case of the latter, who would have power, wealth, and status and who would be laborers. A model of *Anglo-conformity* or *Americanization* was a major influence, particularly in the American public school system where conformity to mainstream American middle class values and behaviors has been a key characteristic. Another model/metaphor, the *melting pot,* conceives of a society in which foreign elements are "melted" into the mix, blending with and changing the mainstream into a new American race. The model of *cultural pluralism* provides an alternative to the melting pot view. In this model, while sharing a common American citizenship allegiance to democratic values, ethnic groups maintain and foster their cultures. The metaphors employed for the cultural pluralism view have included a symphony orchestra, a flower garden, a mosaic, and a stew or salad (Abramson, 1979; Glazer and Moynihan, 1963; Gleason, 1979; Kallen, 1924, 1956; Novak, 1972; Vecoli, 1995).

The various explanatory models continue to influence the discussion of multiculturalism in this country. Multiculturalism can be defined as "the most common way in which the ideology or philosophy of cultural pluralism is put into practice" (Cordiero, Reagan, and Martinez, 1994). Although the cultural pluralism model has received the most support, no model captures fully the dynamism and complexity of the processes involved. Leading scholars assert that a more refined explanatory model is needed, one that affirms both the existence of an American identity and the existence of ethnic subgroups, with neither one precluding or dominating the other (Gleason, 1979; Mann, 1992; Vecoli, 1995).

The following chapter sections provide information and history, and they highlight principles basic to understanding variations of alcohol and other drug use in four general categories of persons: European Americans, African Americans, Hispanic Americans, and Asian Americans. Some important considerations in reviewing the material include the understanding that major ethnic or racial categories are composed of numerous subgroups. The subgroups are made up of populations whose members share regional origins, ethnic backgrounds, basic language, and religious traditions. All vary from one another and cannot any longer be considered to consist of persons descended from one particular group. Asians, for example, are groups composed of numerous ethnic strains and hundreds of religions. Latinos, or persons of Hispanic origin, may share a basic language, but traditions, health practices, and cultural beliefs range widely.

European Americans

The white majority population in America is made up of the descendants of European immigrants who made the United States their home and who, through assimilation and acculturation, have taken on an American identity. However, although they may share a common American identity, they continue to be influenced by the cultures of their countries of origin. Certain aspects of their heritage endure through migration and are resistant to the effects of education, whether they are first, second, or third generation in this country, or how self-conscious they may be of their ethnic identity. Ethnically linked traits, religion, alcohol consumption, and political behavior, for example, have been shown to have remarkable durability despite pressures to assimilate (Greeley, McCready, and Theisen, 1980).

Studies of ethnic variation within the white European American population went out of style in the 1940s and 1950s, as they went against the prevailing melting pot ideology. In addition, any emphasis on ethnic differentiation was uncomfortably reminiscent of the Nazi racist ideology and its genocidal consequences (Room, 1985). Alcohol studies were the exception. Beginning with Robert Bales's study (1944) of Irish and Jewish drinking habits, there is a rich body of literature focusing on the different patterns of drinking among English, Irish, Italian, Jewish, and Polish Americans. The sections that follow focus on these five population subgroups, emphasizing their patterns of migration and acculturation and their patterns of alcohol use. Because no similar body of literature links drug abuse to ethnic heritage in the European American population, the focus in these sections will be exclusively on alcohol use.

English Americans

MIGRATION AND ACCULTURATION

The English were the first non-native Americans to settle in the United States, seeking the religious freedom, economic opportunities, and cheap land in the New World. By the time of the American Revolution, English institutions and English-trained officials, clergymen, merchants, landlords, and professionals dominated the government and social structures. Subsequent waves of immigration increased the English American population, until it peaked in the latter part of the nineteenth century. Throughout, churches were central to ethnic identity with the Episcopal, Methodist, and Baptist churches being most influential.

English immigrants had little difficulty assimilating American life and suffered little discrimination. Faced with few language barriers and a familiar legal and political system, they had little inclination to establish ethnic organizations, newspapers, or political organizations. In comparison with other new immigrants, they were more willing to separate from the community of their fellow immigrants, more willing to intermarry, and more enthusiastic in embracing the culture. For the most part, they were absorbed into mainstream American life within a generation, becoming identified with the white Anglo-Saxon Protestant majority that exerted so much influence and power in the early history of the country (Hanft, 1995).

PATTERNS OF ALCOHOL USE

In the colonial period (1620–1775), alcohol was widely and heavily consumed. Toddlers drank alcohol with their parents; regular use was seen as healthful for everyone. Taverns were integral to community life, and there was widespread agreement over proper drinking behavior. Social control was strong, and drunkenness was not tolerated. The Revolutionary War was followed by social upheaval, a relaxation of antidrunkenness laws, and an increase in drinking problems (Hanson, 1995).

Protestant churches exerted a strong influence on drinking patterns. The Methodist creed on alcohol, first put forth by John Wesley in 1739, was the most stringent. It labeled alcohol consumption and drunkenness as sinful behavior and not to be allowed. This creed also influenced other prominent Protestant religious groups, such as the Baptists, Presbyterians, and Congregationalists, to strongly oppose alcohol use and to view drunkenness as sinful. Both the Episcopal and Lutheran churches did not oppose moderate drinking. From the midnineteenth century on, abstinence and a religious-oriented lifestyle became touchstones of middle-class respectability and the status symbol separating the Protestant middle class from the lower working class, most of whom at that time were Catholic Irish and German immigrants (Ames, 1985).

Irish Americans

MIGRATION AND ACCULTURATION

Some Irish immigration occurred during the seventeenth and eighteenth centuries, but it was the Irish potato famine of 1845–1851 that brought the greatest wave of Irish migration to the United States. About 4 million Irish immigrants came to this country in the latter half of the nineteenth century, settling primarily in the large cities of the Northeast (Rapple, 1995).

Major changes in the Irish family structure precipitated this mass migration. Prior to the famine, Irish children married at an early age and acquired a small segment of the family landholding to provide for their subsistence. A single landholding could then be subdivided many times, depending on the size of the family. This soon became an escalating economic problem, one that the potato famine exacerbated dramatically. Within 20 years, a shift in the patterns of land use took place. The economic need to consolidate the landholdings led to a new system of inheritance, and the practice of passing the land from father to eldest son at the time of his marriage was instituted. The father, the mother, and the son, as well as his wife and children, shared the household; other siblings had to find subsistence away from the landholding. Many immigrated; others sought work in Irish cities (Stivers, 1976, 1985).

This created major changes within the Irish family. Because parents wished to retain title to the landholding as long as possible and marriage was dependent on the acquisition of land, sons married late, if at all. Most marriages were designed to attract a bride with an appropriate dowry and were arranged rather than spontaneous. Hence, the average age at marriage increased, the marriage rate decreased, the percentage that remained permanently unmarried increased, and (driven by the prevailing sexual norms of Irish Puritanism in which chastity is highly valued) the percentage that chose celibacy increased. This led to the phenomenon of the bachelor group in the Irish culture, which provided a context for all nonwork and nonfamily activities, characterized by a constantly shifting set of friendships and associations. It removed much of the stigma attached to being single. Both emotional and recreational needs were provided for within the bachelor group.

Family interaction patterns were affected. The primary relationship between father and son was distant and austere, as was the relationship between husband and wife. The husband's primary obligation to his wife was to provide economically for a household in which she was in charge of domestic life, child rearing, and religious practice. There was often little warmth or communication in the relationship, and most married men sought and were welcomed into the membership of the bachelor group. Upon immigration, Irish American families retained these characteristics. Life was harsh for most immigrants; many lived in substandard housing or in shantytowns and were frequently discriminated against on the basis of their Irish origin and their Catholicism. Parochial schools, charitable societies, workers' organizations, and social clubs aided them in their entry into mainstream society. However, negative stereotypes characterizing the Irish as pugnacious, drunken semisavages were common and endured for most of the nineteenth century. Some important advantages, however, were that they arrived in great numbers, most spoke English, and their culture was similar in many ways to the dominant culture. This allowed them to blend in far more easily than some other ethnic groups. The influx of even poorer southern and eastern European immigrants helped the Irish attain greater acceptance (Rapple, 1995).

PATTERNS OF ALCOHOL USE

In the late eighteenth and early nineteenth centuries, drinking behavior and attitudes were similar in England, Scotland, Ireland, and much of Northern Europe. Drinking rituals pervaded occupations, professions, and virtually every rite of passage from birth to death. In other countries, drinking practices and attitudes toward drinking were changed dramatically by the temperance movement. In Ireland, however, after the Prohibition era ended, old drinking patterns reemerged. Previous convivial uses of alcohol returned and were expanded to include emergent bachelor groups. Taking a drink in the company of bachelor group members in the local pub newly marked the rite of passage from boyhood to manhood. Attaining male identity was thus intimately bound to an ethic of hard drinking. Although hard drinking was approved of, drunkenness was not condoned, and the Church defined intemperance as a mortal sin. The man who could hold his own after a full night's drinking achieved high status in the bachelor group.

Irish Americans demonstrated similar drinking patterns. Together with the Church, the saloon became a focal point of community life, particularly political life. The Irish political machine drew its power from the network of street gangs and social clubs that had their origin in the drinking world of the saloons. In the Irish American neighborhood, a priest's power covered mainly religious and family concerns; the political boss had power in politics and business.

Hard drinking was part of the group identity of the ward boss and of Irish American men in general. Ultimately, drink acquired spiritual value, and hard drinking became symbolic of Irish identity rather than just male identity. The implication for Irish Americans was that the more one drank, the more Irish one became (Stivers, 1976, 1985).

Italian Americans

MIGRATION AND ACCULTURATION

From 1876 to 1924, over 4.5 million Italian immigrants came to the United States, clustering heavily in the cities of the Northeast and Midwest. The overwhelming majority (over 75 percent) were from southern Italy, a socially backward and economically depressed area. They were artisans, small landowners, sharecroppers, or farm laborers with little education, from the peasant population of a virtually feudal society. They brought strong family-centered values and an intense identity with the local community, so much a part of their peasant culture.

Around 90 percent of them congregated in urban areas where they followed kin and village-based chain migration networks to form Little Italys. They limited their association primarily to kin and fellow villagers, and the discrimination they experienced at the hands of the majority culture intensified their isolation. They were overwhelmingly Roman Catholic. Their faith was a personal folk religion of feast days and peasant traditions that often had little to do with formal dogma or rituals. As such, their practices differed greatly from those encountered in America's Irish-dominated Catholic Church. This led to demands for separate parishes, intensifying their isolation still further. Within these communities, they created a network of Italian language institutions, newspapers, theaters, churches, and mutual aid societies, which helped to fuel this emerging Italian American ethnic culture. The cultural patterns of Little Italys were constantly evolving, expressing a dynamic interplay between Old World celebrations or rituals and new inventions forged in the New World. Columbus Day celebrations and festivals honoring patron saints became the focal point of culturally based celebrations (Pozzetta, 1995).

The traditional Italian family was father-headed but mother-centered. In public, the father was the uncontested authority figure; wives were expected to defer to their husbands. At home, however, females exercised considerable authority as wives and mothers and played central roles in sustaining familial networks. Male children occupied a favored position of superiority over females, and strong family mores governed female behavior. Above all, protection of female chastity was critical to maintaining family honor. World War I, World War II, and the Cold War all hastened the pace of Italian American integration into mainstream American society. With each successive generation, marriage outside the ethnic community has increased, and movement away from the old urban settlement areas and the Italian language institutions founded by the immigrants has continued.

A resurgent Italian ethnicity emerged in the 1960s and 1970s, and Italian Americans retain distinguishing characteristics. They display a pronounced family loyalty, still relying heavily on personal and kin networks in residential choices, visiting patterns, and general social interaction (Pozzetta, 1995).

Patterns of Alcohol Use

Since Greek and Roman times, the Mediterranean area has been a major region for the production and consumption of wine; wine continues to be the principal beverage. Wine is symbolically related to the blood of Christ in the celebration of the mass. This linking of blood and wine has led to an elaborate health belief system closely associating wine with food, nourishment, good digestion, strength for hard work, good blood, the making of new blood, and general well-being and good health (Simboli, 1985). Wine is consumed daily (in moderation), usually around mealtimes by the whole family, including young children. Drunkenness is frowned upon and is relatively uncommon.

First-generation Italian Americans reflected these beliefs in their lives in the New World. They often made their own homemade wine for family consumption with meals. Wine was consumed in moderation for its social and presumed nutritional value rather than for its psychological effects. Children continued to be introduced to drinking wine at an early age at home. Some drinking went on in cantinas, but meal-based usage predominated.

Several studies over a span of the last 40 years have evaluated changes in these traditional drinking patterns with successive generations of Italian Americans (Blane, 1977; Greeley and McCready, 1975; Jessor, Young, Young, and Tesi, 1970; Lolli, Serianni, Golder, and Luzzatto-Fegiz, 1958; Simboli, 1985). All have documented that Italian American drinking is related to generational membership. From the first generation through the succeeding ones, there has been a decline in traditional patterns of wine drinking and an increase in the consumption of other types of alcoholic beverages outside of mealtimes. Despite this, traditional values continue to provide some protection from alcoholism and its more serious consequences. The rate of occurrence of alcoholism remains lower in the Italian American population than in other ethnic groups (Simboli, 1985).

Polish Americans

Pattern of Migration and Acculturation

Although Polish immigrants participated in the early colonization of the United States, their numbers were relatively small. Since then, three distinct waves of immigration have occurred. The first and smallest wave, from 1800 to 1860, was precipitated by the partitioning of Poland and brought intellectuals and lesser nobility to New York and Chicago. The second most significant wave took place between 1860 and World War I. These immigrants in search of a better economic life tended to be from rural areas. They clustered in industrial cities and towns of the Midwest and mid-Atlantic states where they became steelworkers, meatpackers, miners, and (later) autoworkers. The third wave lasted from the end of World War I through the end of the Cold War; again it comprised dissidents and political refugees. The influx of such large numbers, over 2.5 million between the midnineteenth century and World War I, created friction with the white Anglo-Saxon Protestant mainstream society. The fact that Polish immigrants were strongly Catholic intensified the discrimination they experienced. As a result, Polish Americans formed tight links with each other, relying on ethnic cohesiveness not only for moral support but for financial support as well. Polish fraternal, national, and religious organizations helped to maintain a Polish identity and also helped to obtain insurance and home loans.

Despite increasing assimilation and acculturation to mainstream American society, Polish Americans maintain a strong ethnic identity. The Polish family structure remains distinctly nuclear and patriarchal; until recently, Polish Americans tended to marry within their community. Now this is changing, and a strong ethnic identity is maintained less through shared traditions or folk culture than through national pride. However, the Poles still maintain traditions in those ceremonies for which the community holds great value, such as weddings, christenings, and funerals (Jones, 1995).

PATTERNS OF ALCOHOL USE

Traditional attitudes toward alcohol use in peasant Poland treated it as a necessary part of socializing and a symbol of hospitality. Alcohol was a well-integrated feature of peasant life and was used for a variety of purposes including sealing contracts, marking life events, and celebrating. Children were socialized to drinking at a young age (8–10 years), and drinking occurred after, rather than during, meals. The drink of choice was distilled spirits, typically vodka or whiskey. Drinking was primarily a male activity, and alcohol was associated with virility and manhood; both heavy drinking and drunkenness were tolerated. Sanctions only occurred when drinking resulted in the neglect of the individual's moral duties toward family and church.

Weddings and ethnic festivals for first-generation Polish Americans were accompanied by heavy drinking, but much of the drinking was done after work in ethnic saloons and Polish American social clubs. Saloons and social clubs offered a wide range of services and recreation including access to foreign newspapers and writing materials, communication with relatives and friends in the home country, a labor exchange, and credit, as well as pool, billiards, and card games; they were designed primarily as sanctuaries for males. They differed from the village taverns in Poland, which were the focus of community and family gatherings.

Drinking patterns of first- and some second-generation men included standing rounds and frequent drinking of toasts. The practice of standing rounds was not only a way of establishing a reputation among one's peers; it also served to build status within the ethnic community. It was common for groups of 6 to 10 men to come in after work, each buying the others a round of boilermakers (a glass of beer with a shot on the side) until each man had consumed as many as 10 shots of whiskey and 10 glasses of beer. Few engage in this practice today, but the drinking of toasts has persisted (Freund, 1985). After Prohibition, Polish social clubs served as a partial substitute for saloons.

Jewish Americans

MIGRATION AND ACCULTURATION

Jewish migration to the United States occurred as early as 1654, but the number of immigrants was relatively small. The largest migrations occurred in three waves between 1826 and 1941. The first wave, accounting for up to 150,000 people, included German Jewish immigrants from Central Europe who were escaping social unrest in their homelands. The second and largest wave, between 1881 and 1924, accounted for over 4.5 million people and included young, working-class Jews from Eastern Europe. The third wave, of 150,000 people, included middle-class, middle-aged professionals and businesspeople escaping from Nazi Germany. The early immigrants and those in subsequent waves experienced little discrimination, with the former group settling in large cities on the eastern seaboard and the latter contributing to westward expansion. They were eager to assimilate into American society and did so with little difficulty. Beginning in 1881, with the large-scale immigration of Eastern European Jews, anti-Semitism became a problem. These immigrants tended to be poor, and they settled in tight-knit communities where they retained the traditions and customs from the Old World. They consciously avoided assimilation into American culture and continued to speak Yiddish. As a result, they were stereotyped as clannish, greedy, vulgar, and physically inferior. This discrimination reached a peak in the 1930s and did not decrease significantly until the end of World War II when the atrocities of the Nazi Holocaust became widely known.

Immigrant Jews have passed on Jewish traditions in the home, in religious schools, and through observation of the Sabbath, a day of rest, contemplation, and family and community togetherness. Courtships, marriages, births, weddings, and funerals are accompanied by important rituals and traditions shared by all Jews despite their countries of origin, level of orthodoxy, or level of acculturation to mainstream American society. For the most part, these traditions have remained to the present day and play a large part in maintaining a Jewish identity (Kamp, 1995; Snyder, 1958).

Patterns of Alcohol Use

In the traditional Orthodox Jewish culture, alcoholic beverages, particularly wine, have a symbolic role in religious celebrations associated with rites of passage, weekly Sabbath observances, and annual holy days and festivals. The first rite of passage—and the first drinking occasion in the life of a Jewish boy—is his circumcision. During the ceremonial operation, a benediction is pronounced over a cup of wine; the child is given a name and also given a few drops of the wine. Other rites (e.g., Bar Mitzvah, marriage, and funerals) also incorporate wine in either a celebratory or a symbolic role. Similarly, during the annual cycle of holy days and festivals, wine is an important part of the celebrations. Unlike other cultures in which festivals are seen as times for pleasure seeking and convivial drinking, however, in the Jewish culture true rejoicing and festivity are integral with worship and contingent on conformity with religious customs and fulfillment of ritual obligations (Snyder, 1958). The Sabbath celebration has the greatest impact on establishing the cultural definition of drinking for the individual in the Jewish culture. The Sabbath, being a weekly occurrence, has an inescapable, recurrent impact on the Jewish child brought up in a religious home. The Sabbath begins and ends with a ritualistic benediction of a cup of wine and the consumption of the wine in ritualistic, symbolic ways.

In the Jewish culture, Jews do not drink with the aim of getting drunk or feeling good. Drinking is not sought for its psychological effects. Rather, Jews develop a ritual attitude toward drinking in which drinking for the effect of alcohol is alien to them (Bales, 1944). As a result, although few Jews abstain from alcohol, the rate of alcoholism among Jews is lower than in any other cultural group (Greeley, McCready, and Theisen, 1980).

Several additional factors influence this low incidence of alcoholism. First, the Jewish family maintains a permissive drinking culture in which drinking is permitted, but excessive drinking is not. Second, the Jewish tradition of drinking with food may provide some protection from the more serious consequences of alcohol consumption. Finally, moderation in Jewish drinking may be a defense against retaliation from the majority Gentile world. Discrimination against Jews has been common throughout history; maintaining sobriety may have closed one additional avenue for potential persecution (Snyder, 1958).

Although there is some evidence to suggest that assimilation into the mainstream culture increases the risk of alcoholism among Jewish Americans, the rate of alcoholism remains relatively low. The influence of traditional cultural values remains strong, and the influence of outside pressure is moderated. Even when associating with the Gentile world, Jews have developed a repertoire of avoidance strategies (e.g., nursing drinks over long periods or switching to similar-appearing nonalcoholic drinks after the first drink) in instances where they are pressured to drink more than they wish to drink (Glassner and Berg, 1985).

Other Subcultures

Although the literature describing European American subcultures is limited to those already reviewed, the international literature provides information about drinking practices in other European countries (e.g., there is a rich body of literature describing French drinking practices). Although to a certain extent, the French mimic the Italian practice of drinking wine with meals, the French have traditionally experienced higher rates of drinking problems than the Italians. In both countries, wine is consumed copiously by the entire population, and children are initiated early into the drinking customs. There the similarity stops. The Italians are relatively free of problems associated with drinking, but the French experience a high incidence of drunkenness and alcoholism (Sadoun, Lolli, and Silverman, 1965). The rates of death from alcoholism and cirrhosis of the liver in France have been among the highest in the world. This may be related to the differences in attitudes. In Italy, drunkenness is socially unacceptable; in France, intoxication is viewed as a sign of manhood, and there is a wide tolerance for copious drinking. French American drinking practices are more difficult to document. French migration to the United States has been sporadic and characterized by the migration of individuals rather than groups. Immigrants were accepted by, and assimilated rapidly into, the mainstream culture (Hillstrom, 1995).

Similarly, the drinking patterns of Swedish Americans and those from other Scandinavian countries have not been well documented. The same is true of German Americans. However, some generalizations can be drawn from the international literature. Drinking in the Scandinavian countries, as in Poland, is characterized by the separation of drinking from dietary functions, a preference for distilled spirits, the deliberate use of alcohol to produce intoxication, and the concentration of heavy drinking in a relatively small portion of the male population (Babor, 1992).

In Germany, permissive attitudes toward drinking and drunkenness have prevailed throughout German history and persist today. Since the 1800s, clear-cut patterns have emerged. There are preferences for wine in the wine-growing regions, for spirits in East Germany, and for beer in Bavaria; however, beer is the first choice of frequent and regular drinkers. The German pub is the place where men gather, and "to hold one's drink" is a highly valued virtue of manhood (Voght, 1995).

Summary

Hanson (1995) has provided an insightful summary of the characteristics of those cultures that are most successful in preventing alcohol abuse. The members of these cultures tend to:

1. View alcohol as a natural, normal part of life about which they have no ambivalence.
2. Teach their young by example how to drink in moderation.
3. Encourage drinking among family and friends rather than in same-gender settings.
4. Discourage heavy episodic drinking.
5. Sanction negatively and promptly any unacceptable drinking behaviors.
6. Respect the decision of those who choose not to drink and not pressure them to drink.
7. Be free of the belief that alcohol can solve problems, signify adulthood, grant power, or confirm manhood.

Using these characteristics as screening criteria, it can be inferred that of the five sub-cultural groups reviewed here, Jewish Americans, followed closely by Italian Americans, would experience the fewest problems with drinking, and that Irish Americans, English Americans, and Polish Americans would experience the greatest number of problems. This problem-based ranking has been substantiated in a number of studies (Cahalan, Cisin, and Crossley, 1969; Greeley, McCready, and Theisen, 1980; Vaillant, 1995).

African Americans

Those persons who identify themselves as non-Hispanic African Americans in the United States comprise approximately 12 percent of the total U.S. population (U.S. Bureau of Census, 1997). These **African Americans** are a varied people comprising populations whose ancestors came as slaves from various African regions and tribes. On arrival, they were different in their spoken languages, their religions, and their values. Other more recent arrivals came from Haiti, other Caribbean Islands, South America, and the African continent. Attempts to understand current alcohol, tobacco, and other drug use and misuse among African Americans must include an understanding of the collective and historical experiences of African Americans. This knowledge provides the context for prevention and treatment approaches to be examined and designed. In this chapter, the use of the terms blacks and African Americans reflects the social context of various eras.

Historical Context

An **historical context** is the best perspective from which to understand current use of alcohol, tobacco, and other drugs by African Americans. The use of alcohol began in Africa, was involved in the enslavement of Africans, and relates to drinking and other drug use patterns among African Americans in the United States.

PRECOLONIAL AFRICA

Africa has always been culturally complex and diverse; in spite of this, there has also existed a certain cultural unity reflected in worldviews and normative assumptions held by Africans (Asante, 1987; Maquet, 1972). The use of fermented beverages has a long tradition among non-Islamic Africans (Christmon, 1995; Herd, 1985b; Umunna, 1967). Wine and beer were made from grain, nuts, vegetables, or fruits and had low alcohol content. Consumption of fermented beverages was an integral part of religious, social, healing, and agrarian rituals of the time. Stimulants made from kola nuts and vegetables were also used in rituals and as healing medicines (McNeese and DiNetto, 1994). Intoxication and related disruptive behaviors were neither accepted nor tolerated (Christmon, 1995; Herd, 1985a). Community norms indicated who could drink, how much, and under which circumstances. Hence, although alcohol and other drug use were an integral part of non-Islamic African culture, it was not a social problem (Grey, 1996).

ALCOHOL'S ROLE IN ENSLAVEMENT

Alcohol played a significant and devastating role in the U.S. slavery system. Rum distilled from West Indies molasses was shipped to West Africa and traded for slaves who were subsequently sold in South Carolina, other southern states, or the West Indies. For 20 gallons of rum, a slave trader could purchase a muscular young man. This profitable exchange eventually led to the encouragement of the use and abuse of liquor on the West African coast. This interaction of events came to be known as the slavery triangle.

ALCOHOL AND OTHER DRUG USE DURING SLAVERY

There are ambiguous and conflicting accounts in the literature about the use of alcohol during slavery. Frederick Douglass (1892) described the use of alcohol during holidays, particularly the days between Christmas and New Year's, times when alcohol was provided to slaves by their owners. Slaves were encouraged to drink until they were drunk to prevent them from planning insurrections. Wright and colleagues (1990) described alcohol as being an integral part of slaves' lives, with weekend drinking being regarded as a reward for hard work. However, the revolt of Nat Turner in 1830 resulted in the passage of laws that levied stricter controls on drinking and prohibited blacks from owning stills.

Under the conditions of slavery, alcohol was alternately forbidden and supplied in generous amounts; excessive drinking, however, was not a problem (Herd, 1985a). Drinking by overseers and owners themselves did create problems for their charges (von Wormer, 1995).

Not all blacks were slaves. Some were born free, and others bought their freedom. Free blacks lived mainly in urban areas. Class differences emerged based on skin color (light versus dark), roles on plantations (house slave versus field slaves), religion (Catholic versus African-Methodist or African-Baptist), ethnicity (Latin Negroes of Creole descent versus American Negroes), or socioeconomic (elite free blacks versus poor blacks). These socioeconomic differences produced class differences as well as different attitudes and behaviors toward alcohol use. Active members of the Methodist and Baptist churches were likely to be abstainers, disapproving of drinking alcohol, whereas elite free blacks were likely to use alcohol as a symbol of wealth (Grey, 1996).

There is a paucity of information on the use of other drugs among slaves. Tobacco during this period was commonly molded into plugs and chewed or held in the lower lip. It was also ground into powder and sniffed or held in the lower lip. Little was written detailing the extent and pattern of its use among blacks.

The Civil War

During the Civil War, laws restricting the use of alcohol by blacks were unenforceable, but following the Civil War, in southern states blacks were again prohibited from owning firearms and using alcoholic beverages (Brown and Touley, 1989). According to Koren (1899), profuse drinking and public drunkenness were not uncommon in the ranks of some former slaves; most blacks, however, practiced moderation. In fact, blacks as a collective exhibited comparatively low rates of alcohol use, drunkenness, and drinking-related problems. Because chronic drunkenness was so rare among African Americans, they were thought to be physiologically immune from prolonged inebriety (Koren, 1899).

Opium was widely used for therapeutic and recreational purposes among the general population in the United States in the 1800s. Morphine, the active ingredient in opium, was isolated in 1803. But it was not until 1856, with the invention of the hypodermic syringe, that morphine became a widely accepted therapeutic drug. Although use of the syringe was introduced too late for the American Civil War, pills and powder were distributed to soldiers, leading to widespread dependence among returning veterans. The extent to which morphine addiction was prevalent among black veterans is not clear.

The Reconstruction and Migration Periods

The political gains granted after the Civil War were lost following Reconstruction. The Supreme Court disbanded the Civil Rights Act, and the doctrine of separate but equal was created. By 1910, most blacks in the South had been disenfranchised (Franklin, 1974). Their political, economic, and social maltreatment caused the initiation of a mass migration from the South into the industrial cities of the North. Their numbers in cities such as Washington, Baltimore, New York, and Philadelphia increased radically (Franklin, 1974). Most of these migrants were forced into ghettos because of discrimination, unmarketable skills, and economic instability (Brown and Touley, 1989). Families and relationships were often disrupted. Further, the elite blacks already established in the North were not receptive to the throngs of poor, uneducated blacks from the rural South. Even the black church, a source of comfort and tangible support, was overwhelmed with the influx of these migrants. Drinking became a means of the migrants' coping with an environment devoid of support (Herd, 1985c).

African Americans aligned themselves with the temperance movement of the 1800s because of its antislavery emphasis and its compatibility with their own cultural patterns of abstinence and moderation. When the temperance movement shifted its political base from the northern abolitionists to poor rural southern whites who supported white supremacy and protection of white women, African Americans detached themselves from the antiliquor movement and went North to avoid violence (Brown and Touley, 1989). Alcohol became a major factor during the Depression for the working poor, as manifested by their involvement in bootlegging, speakeasies, and rent parties (Herd, 1985c). Individual entrepreneurship in the form of nightclubs and liquor stores influenced the development of an African American entertainment culture. Among those who migrated to the North, there was an upsurge of alcohol-related illness and death compared to those blacks who remained in the South. The urbanized African American born in the early 1900s contributed to the high alcohol statistics of the 1950s to 1970s (Brown and Touley, 1989; Daniels, 1980; Herd, 1985b).

Cigarettes began to be massed-produced in the late 1880s and grew in popularity after World War I. By 1918, cigarette consumption had surpassed all other forms of tobacco consumption, and the epidemic of smoking had begun. Cigarette sales in the United States increased from 45 billion in 1920 to 80 billion in 1925 and to 180 billion by 1940 (Levinthal, 1996). Heavy smoking contributed to increased morbidity and mortality rates among African Americans migrating from rural to urban areas.

At the beginning of the 1900s, marijuana use also became a noticeable phenomenon. Although cannabis or hemp was imported to the New World by the Spaniards in the 1500s and cultivated for its use as a commercial source for making ropes, twine, ship sails, and containers of all kinds, it was not until the 1920s that the smoking of cigarettes made from the cannabis leaf was introduced by Mexican immigrants who came north seeking work. Some attribute the use of marijuana as a recreational drug to a response to Prohibition that made good liquor hard to obtain. The working class turned to growing marijuana and importing it as an inexpensive substitute for alcohol. Jazz musicians and others connected with show business quickly adopted it. Marijuana clubs, or tea pods as they were sometimes called, sprang up in major cities. More than 500 were estimated to be in Harlem alone, outnumbering the speakeasies that dispensed illegal alcohol. Authorities ignored such establishments because marijuana was not illegal, and patrons were not noted for disturbing the peace (Levinthal, 1996).

Although marijuana was not heavily used by the majority of the population, tolerance toward marijuana use changed in the early 1930s. Marijuana became known as the killer weed. It was associated with Mexican immigrants and African Americans who were perceived as competitors for scarce jobs, and who became convenient targets for venting the frustrations produced by a weak economy. By the end of the 1930s, use of marijuana was illegal in the United States.

Heroin, a morphine derivative, was introduced by the Bayer Company in Germany in 1898. The abuse potential of heroin, which is more potent than morphine, was not recognized until about 1910. By 1900, it was conservatively estimated that 250,000 people were dependent on opiates in the United States (Levinthal, 1996). The passage of the Harrison Narcotic Act in 1914 limited opiate use to those with prescriptions. The demographics of opiate use then changed from primarily white female, middle-class, middle-age users to young, white, urban adult males whose drug of choice was intravenous and illegally obtained (Levinthal, 1996).

Use of modern-day cocaine began in the late 1800s and early 1900s when cocaine was widely used in patent medicines and beverages such as Wine Cola (a combination of wine and coca) and Coca-Cola. When its addictive powers were recognized, public outcry led to its inclusion as a controlled substance in the 1914 Harrison Narcotic Act. The use of cocaine among African Americans during this time probably paralleled that of the general public's use of patent medicines and nonalcoholic beverages. Except for a small number of users such as jazz musicians and other members of the avant garde, it virtually disappeared for nearly half a century.

THE 1960S AND 1970S

Flower power, Black power, "Black Is Beautiful," the sexual revolution, and the Vietnam War dominated America in the 1960s and 1970s. Middle- and upper-class people experimented with illegal drugs in unprecedented numbers. Cocaine, heroin, and marijuana were rediscovered and again came to the forefront of America's national concern. The lessons learned about cocaine in the late 1800s had been forgotten. Cocaine regained its image as a glamorous recreational drug and was enthusiastically embraced. Use among the general population, African Americans included, increased (Doweiko, 1998; Ray and Ksir, 1996).

The resurgence of heroin use and dependence during the 1960s and 1970s was influenced by several factors. The 1961 crackdown on heroin smuggling, which reduced supplies on the streets, sent heroin prices soaring, and dosages became more adulterated. The high cost of heroin dependence consequently encouraged new levels of criminal activity and forced a cultural stranglehold on African American and Latino communities in major cities. A second factor influencing increased heroin use and dependence, which affected white Americans more directly, was the counterculture of hippies and flower children who espoused experimentation with mind-altering drugs. In the Vietnam War, American soldiers were introduced to 90 percent to 98 percent pure-grade heroin in Asian markets; however, fewer than 1 percent of those who used heroin maintained use after returning home (Ray and Ksir, 1996). Marijuana was the most commonly used of the illicit drugs during this period. A few puffs on a "joint" was equivalent to the "social martini."

Contemporary Prevalence and Patterns of Tobacco, Alcohol, Marijuana, Cocaine, and Heroin Use Among African Americans

There has been an assumption in the research community that the way to study nonmajority populations in the United States is to compare them to whites of European origin. When this is done, it usually means that the different behaviors, values, and problems within subgroups of populations of non-European origin are ignored. There is also the risk that such comparisons may lead to substantiation of the all-too-common view that difference means deficient. Americans of European origin (as the numerical and cultural majority) have served as the standard to which other (numerically smaller) non-European ethnic groups have been compared (Collins, 1993).

African Americans are seldom surveyed using specific references to cultural values and social practices, family and peer influences, recentness of immigration, country and continent of recent origin, or socioeconomic factors such as family income, education level, or geographic residence (Collins, 1993; Grey, 1996). Studies of cultural context and patterning are not easily accomplished; they go beyond demographic profiles. Most of the data on alcohol, tobacco, and other drug use among African Americans are obtained from large national samples. This research uses traditional epidemiological methodology based on racial, age, and geographic classification categories. This method makes it more useful for comparisons among the various racial groups than for understanding of group variations. To date, this method remains the major approach to national databases. When such broad categories are used, glossing occurs, masking important differences in national origins, cultural traditions, socioeconomic status, and historical experiences in America (Collins, 1993).

When interpreting the prevalence and patterns of alcohol, tobacco, and other drug use data, it is important to acknowledge that the data do not distinguish among the various African American ethnic groups and social classes. In addition, the data are not interpreted in light of the role racism has played and continues to play in the lives of African Americans.

TOBACCO

Smoking is the most common form of tobacco use. In the 1970s, white and African American high school seniors smoked at about the same rates. Until the 1994 National Household Survey on Drug Abuse, the rate of African American seniors who smoked, and that of whites, steadily declined (SAMHSA, 1997). The 1994 survey, using new questionnaire data, revealed that 25.1 percent of black teens (up from 21.2 percent in 1993) had smoked at least once in their lives compared to 42.0 percent of white teens (up from 37.8 percent in 1993). In 1994, questions about tobacco were asked using a self-administered questionnaire that ensured more privacy and thereby improved reporting of tobacco use, particularly for youth. Of those teens who smoked, the rate of frequent smoking (smoking on 20 of the past 30 days) was lower among blacks (3.1 percent) than among their white peers (15.4 percent). These findings were unchanged overall from 1994 to 1995 for both age groupings (SAMHSA, 1997). The percentage of African Americans over 18 years old who have at some point in time smoked and who have smoked within the past month also continues to be lower than that of the general population (SAMHSA, 1997). The number of cigarettes smoked per day by an African American is estimated to be 20 or fewer for 88.4 percent of the males (52.8 percent of whom smoked 10 or less) and 93.6 percent of the females (62.1 percent of whom smoked 10 or less) (Ramirez and Gallion, 1993). Despite consumption rates lower than the general population, African Americans are still less likely to quit smoking than whites (Novotny, Warner, and Remington, 1988). The lower rate of cigarette consumption is offset by the preference for high tar\nicotine (greater than 1.0 mg nicotine) cigarettes and for mentholated cigarettes. Of all blacks, 76 percent smoke menthol brands; Newport, Salem, and Kool represented 60 percent of all cigarettes purchased by blacks (Cummings, Giovina, and Mendicino, 1987). Such cigarette preferences leads to greater dependency on nicotine and potentially to more difficulty in smoking cessation (Orleans et al., 1989). African Americans who smoke fewer than 26 cigarettes per day are 1.6 times more likely to smoke within 10 minutes of awakening compared to whites, a reliable index of high physical dependence (Royce et al., 1993).

The chemical additives in menthol-flavored cigarettes anesthetize the throat and lungs, encouraging deeper and more frequent inhalation and intensifying health risks (Novotny, Warner, and Remington, 1988; Orleans et al., 1989). Wagenknecht and colleagues (1990), in a study of African American smokers, found higher levels of cotinine, a metabolite of nicotine that has no known psychoactive properties, in black smokers than in white smokers. This suggests differences in nicotine metabolism and cotinine excretion, which may explain the lower quitting rates and higher cancer rates among black smokers.

Sociodemographic factors associated with smoking among African Americans, such as low income, education level, occupational status, higher unemployment, male gender, and singleness, are similar to those for the U.S. population. Novotny and colleagues (1988) suggested that when these factors are controlled, blacks are no more likely than whites to become smokers; however, even when these factors are controlled, blacks who smoke are less likely to quit.

ALCOHOL

The considerable variability that exists among African Americans is reflected in their alcohol use patterns as well. Recent research has contradicted the commonly held assumptions that blacks drink more heavily and have more liberal views about alcohol consumption than whites. Research findings are also lessening the often-used justifications for these assumptions—alcohol marketing that has targeted black communities, socioeconomic stress, and racism (Caetano, Clark, and Tam, 1998). According to Caetano and Clark (1998a) and Herd (1993, 1988), blacks are not overly permissive in their attitudes about heavy drinking, have higher abstention rates, and drink less frequently across all socioeconomic classes than whites.

The finding of low rates of alcohol consumption by African American women undermines the assumption that their high number as single parents leads to higher levels of alcohol use than for white women. In a longitudinal study of drinking patterns of blacks and whites from 1984 to 1992, Caetano and Kaskutas (1995) found that higher percentages of black women abstain and drink less frequently than white women. However, for both groups in 1984, frequent heavy drinkers (drinks once per week or more with five or more drinks per occasion) were 4 percent of the sample. This percentage remained fairly stable, with a 1 percent increase for black women and 1 percent decrease for white women from 1984 to 1992.

African American men reported lower alcohol use in 1995 for lifetime, past-year, and past-month use than white men (SAMHSA, 1997). In their study of the drinking patterns of black and white men, Caetano and Kaskutas (1995) also found a higher percentage of black abstainers from 1984 to 1992. However, frequent and heavy drinking remained stable among black males (16 percent in 1984 to 15 percent in 1992) but decreased significantly in white males from 19 percent in 1984 to 12 percent in 1992.

TABLE 5-1 Prevalence of Alcohol Problems Among White and Black Men and Women, 1984 and 1995

Number of Problems[1]	1984		1995	
	Whites (%)	Blacks (%)	Whites (%)	Blacks (%)
Men				
0	75	73	78	75
1	8	7	7	9
2	5	4	4	3
3+	12	16	11	13
Women				
0	86	90	88	89
1	6	5	5	4
2	3	2	3	2
3+	5	3	4	4

[1]Problems were salience of drinking, impaired control, withdrawal, relief drinking, tolerance, binge drinking, belligerence, accidents, health-related problems, work-related problems, financial problems, problems with the police, problems with spouse, and problems with persons other than spouse.

Source: Caetano, R. and Clark, C.L. (1998b). Trends in alcohol-related problems among whites, African Americans, and Hispanics: 1984–1995. Reprinted from *Alcohol, Health and Research World 22*(4), 262.

African American adolescents have higher levels of abstinence and lower levels of heavy drinking than the general teen population (SAMHSA, 1997). The reasons for this are unclear. Prendergast and colleagues (1989), in an extensive study of the research on drinking patterns and African American youth, concluded that the explanation for differences between African American and white youth lay elsewhere than in methodology concerns such as underreporting and unrepresentative samples (failure to include dropouts). They also suggested that these differences extended beyond the explanation that black youth begin drinking later than white youth. Frederick Harper (1991) suggested that researchers do not pay enough attention to positive attributes of African American families, such as the variables associated with nonuse of alcohol and other drugs by African Americans.

At the aggregate level, African Americans who were heavy drinkers had drinking patterns and problems similar to those of the general population. However, important differences emerged when associations of drinking and some social characteristics were examined (Herd, 1988, 1990; Jones-Webb, 1998):

- Heavy drinking among African American men is concentrated in the 30–39 age group, whereas among white males it is highest in the 18–29 age group.
- Low-income status did not significantly differentiate heavier drinkers from other drinkers; African American men of middle-income status are more likely to be heavier drinkers.
- African American men with high incomes are far less likely to be heavier drinkers.
- Younger African American males and those with higher incomes are unlikely to drink heavily.
- Heavy drinking is significantly lower in African American women ages 18 to 39; white women reported drinking larger quantities per occasion.
- White women, regardless of marital status, are more likely to be heavier drinkers than their black counterparts.
- Higher levels of income are associated with increasing rates of drinking in women; however, African Americans in the highest income levels exhibit lower rates of heavy drinking than their white counterparts.
- White and African American women who are unemployed are less likely to be drinkers. African American women who are employed and who do drink are less likely to drink more heavily than their unemployed counterparts who drink.
- Rates of heavy drinking among African American men and women have not declined at the same rate as among white men.

MARIJUANA

Marijuana is the dominant illicit drug used in the United States. In 1995, nearly one-third (31 percent) of the total population over 12 years of age reported smoking marijuana cigarettes (reefers\joints) at least one or more times in their lives, with 4.7 percent reporting use in the past month (SAMHSA, 1997). Among African Americans, 2.8 percent reported use one or more times in their lives, and 5.9 percent reported use in the past month. Among all adult populations, male users outnumber females (SAMHSA, 1997).

Marijuana has been labeled a gateway drug because of its association with other drug use. For example, the likelihood that persons who have never used marijuana will use cocaine is rare (less than half of 1 percent); the likelihood of having used cocaine increases as marijuana use increases. Among those who have used marijuana 200 or more times in their lives, 77.4 percent have tried cocaine (US-DHHS-ADAMHA, 1991). This finding, although not specific to African Americans, does include them and has implications for their drug use and abuse patterns.

COCAINE

Attitudes about cocaine began to change in the 1980s. Deaths of entertainers and sports figures resulting from cocaine use produced a reversal of opinion concerning the drug. The greatest influence was the arrival of crack cocaine in 1985. Cocaine dealers, eager to find better markets in the United States, struggled to find a form of cocaine that could be easily smoked without the elaborate and dangerous equipment involved with freebasing. The result was crack cocaine, which became popular in the 1980s. At $5 to $10 per dose, cocaine was no longer the champagne of drugs available primarily to the rich and famous. Crack cocaine became readily available on the streets of inner cities, the communities of many African Americans. According to the 1995 National Household Survey, 8.1 percent of African Americans have used cocaine one or more times in their lives; past-year and past-month use were 1.9 percent and and 1.1 percent, respectively. Crack use among African Americans is 1.0 percent to 0.5 percent higher than its use in the general population. Crack cocaine use by women is highest among African Americans. African Americans have lower levels of lifetime cocaine use than the general population, but they have higher levels of recent cocaine and crack cocaine use (SAMHSA, 1997).

The numbers of people using all forms of cocaine were lower in the 1990s than in the 1980s when cocaine use reached its peak. Despite this decrease, cocaine emergency room statistics have increased dramatically as measured through DAWN (Drug Alert Warning Network); there has been no decrease in the numbers of heavy users (US-DHHS-ADAMHA, 1991). The implications are that this phenomenon may disproportionally affect African Americans.

HEROIN

In the 1980s, crack cocaine use received most of the media attention, yet heroin use continued in new forms and variations. The risks of overdose death increased dramatically. In the 1990s, there was a decline in cocaine abuse and a resurgence of heroin use. The heroin of the 1990s was 10 times more powerful than the typical street drug of the 1970s. In 1994, a brand of heroin sold in New York City with a purity rate of 90 percent resulted in a number of overdose deaths. Because heroin can be snorted or smoked, the risk from contaminated needles has been reduced, creating an avenue perceived as less dangerous by potential new users.

Household surveys do not adequately measure the prevalence of heroin use and are believed to significantly underestimate current and lifetime use. Nevertheless, the 1994 Household Survey estimates that about 1 percent of the total population has used heroin, with 0.1 percent having used in the past month (SAMHSA, 1995). Rates of lifetime use are higher for Caucasian males (1.0 percent) and for African American males (1.5 percent) (US-DHHS-ADAMHA, 1991).

Medical and Social Consequences of Tobacco, Alcohol, Marijuana, Cocaine, and Heroin Use

The use of both licit and illicit drugs by African Americans is not as pervasive as believed by most Americans (including African Americans themselves). Although actual drug use, except for crack cocaine and heroin, is lower in African Americans, the adverse consequences of drug use on this group may be more serious than for other groups. Even when drugs are used moderately, adverse consequences are intensified by poverty, unemployment, discrimination, poor health, and despair.

Reducing and preventing cigarette smoking could be the most effective means of improving the health status of African Americans (Ramirez and Gallion, 1993). Rates of lung cancer are increasing dramatically. There have been increases in chronic obstructive pulmonary diseases, such as chronic bronchitis and emphysema, and in coronary heart diseases. Smoking also results in infant mortality and low birthweight.

Lifetime alcohol consumption among blacks of all cultural origins is reported as 71.1 percent; this is lower than for whites (86 percent) but slightly higher than for Hispanics (68.9 percent) (SAMHSA, 1997). This varies widely by gender, with only 48 percent of black women having consumed alcohol during the past year as compared with 64.5 percent of white women. Alcoholism results in risks and drinking-associated outcomes, such as cancer, pulmonary disease, malnutrition, liver cirrhosis, and birth defects, that are higher for African Americans than for whites (Jones-Webb, 1998). Heavy use by pregnant women may result in infants born with fetal alcohol syndrome; even moderate use is linked to alcohol-related birth defects (ARBD). Mortality rates from alcohol-related medical problems are also higher (Goddard, 1993). African Americans are at greater risk of being victims of alcohol or illicit drug-related homicides, being arrested for drunkenness or possession of a controlled substance, and being sent to prison rather than to treatment. In a study by Welte and Barnes (1987), African Americans (when compared with other groups) reported the highest number of problems for each ounce of alcohol consumed per day.

How the toxic effects of cocaine affect humans is not completely understood; however, several conditions, including myocardial infarctions, ventricular arrhythmias, and coronary ischemic syndromes, are common in cocaine overdoses. These circulatory abnormalities probably account for most deaths resulting from cocaine-induced heart failure (Doweiko, 1999). Cocaine can also induce increases in blood pressure, which may lead to strokes. Because hypertension and cardiovascular diseases are common among African American populations, the use of cocaine exacerbates these health problems. The use of crack cocaine by women results in problems during pregnancy, including fetal injury and death, and problems in newborns, including growth retardation and neurological impairments. Crack cocaine use over a lifetime is reported by 3.1 percent of black females, as compared to 1.9 percent of white women and 1.6 percent of Hispanic women (SAMHSA, 1997).

Despite the knowledge that narcotics destroy lives, heroin is considered a relatively nontoxic drug to major body organs and systems (Levinthal, 1996). The lifestyle of heroin addicts, however, is linked to serious health problems. Street heroin is not a quality-controlled analgesic, and it possesses serious health risks because of the fillers added by dealers. Heroin users frequently develop HIV; endocarditis; hepatitis A, B, and/or C; liver failure; disorders of the body's blood-clotting mechanisms; malignant hypertension; strokes; and abnormal kidney function and uremia. These effects are largely due to infections contracted through intravenous injection or due to fillers (substances added to the heroin) (Doweiko, 1999). Heroin has lethal potential if the potency of the dosage is increased 15 to 20 times to obtain a better high. Because the potency of street heroin is virtually unknown, the possibility of a lethal dosage exists in any given fix (Levinthal, 1996).

Illicit drug use places African Americans at risk for AIDS and for HIV-positive births. In recent years, the incidence of AIDS has mounted most rapidly in men and women of color. The sharing of contaminated needles and sexual contact with intravenous drug users contribute to approximately 69 percent of the AIDS cases in the United States (Levinthal, 1996).

Importance of Race

When nurses treat clients with alcohol, tobacco, or other drug problems, it is most frequently because these clients have already been diagnosed with related medical problems. For many African Americans, identification of the effects of alcohol, tobacco, and other drug use will take place in physicians' offices, neighborhood clinics, and emergency rooms. The early engagement of these clients as partners in their own treatment is critical to changing problem behaviors. Just as racial injustice supports the plight of African Americans, racial tensions can impede the ability of health professionals to help. African Americans who seek help in health care settings expect the doctors and nurses to be white and to hold preconceived ideas and attitudes about blacks. These expectations do not necessarily correspond to the preference African Americans may have for nurses and doctors of their own race (Davis and Proctor, 1989). **Race** is an issue for health care professionals who work with clients about whom they have little cultural knowledge and with whom they are ill at ease. Professionals may experience an erosion of self-confidence and hide behind a cloak of authority when racial barriers intrude. African Americans often wonder why whites cannot acknowledge the impact of color in society. Cultural shock can occur when skills effective with other groups do not work or when nurses are unable to develop culturally appropriate approaches.

African Americans simultaneously hold views of themselves as racial persons and views of how others perceive them as racial persons. Bell and Evans (1981) labeled this phenomenon double consciousness. Double consciousness cannot be ignored in the treatment of alcohol, tobacco, and other drug problems. Clients will be concerned about the existence or absence of the nurse's goodwill and respect (Davis and Proctor, 1989).

Although negative perceptions of clients with substance abuse problems are not limited to cross-racial encounters, instances of disrespect and lack of caring have special significance for African Americans. Respect and professional courtesy are of particular importance to people who frequently do not receive it. Nurses demonstrate respect by addressing adults with titles rather than by first names, unless given permission, extending warm greetings and salutations, allowing privacy for giving personal information and instructions, speaking directly to the client and family, taking time to clearly explain procedures and directions, and giving permission for questions and clarifications.

A rationale for questions asked while assessing alcohol, tobacco, and other drug use and misuse should be provided. This is particularly important because historically African Americans have had to protect themselves from potential white abuses by engaging in "healthy paranoia" (Grier and Cobb, 1968). Failure to engage across color lines can lead to treatment noncompliance and missed appointments. African Americans are more likely to report certain problems to other African Americans or to whites with more race sensitivity than to whites not attuned to the implication of differences among races (Davis and Proctor, 1989).

TREATMENT

In addition to awareness of the importance of race in encounters with African Americans, nurses need to be informed about other issues that affect the prevention and treatment of alcohol, tobacco, and other drug problems. African Americans rely more on public clinics and emergency rooms, which do not provide preventive health care. Consequently, African Americans have longstanding disparities in knowledge of smoking, alcohol, and other drug risks and in ways to access and successfully obtain health care. They are less likely, for example, to receive cancer prevention information, to associate smoking with cancer and pulmonary disease risks, and to visit physicians' offices (54 percent of blacks versus 70 percent of whites) (Ramirez and Gallion, 1993).

Approaches to treatment should be based on sound concepts about when and how people change behavior, thoughts, and feelings. Prochaska, DiClemente, and Norcross (1992), after extensive research on people who change on their own and those who change with professional help, discovered that people change from problematic to nonproblematic behaviors according to their levels of readiness. These levels of readiness are progressive stages or temporal dimensions when shifts in attitudes, intentions, and behaviors occur. In the simplest form, these stages are:

1. *Precontemplation*—the client is not considering change and does not perceive a problem.
2. *Contemplation*—the client is ambivalent about the need to change.
3. *Preparation*—the client is clear about the need to change and is making plans about which steps are needed.
4. *Action*—the client is actively implementing steps to change.
5. *Maintenance*—the client is sustaining the nonproblematic behaviors achieved.
6. *Relapse* is also included as a normal part of the change process. Not everyone is going to complete the cycle; some recycle in one or more stages of change, never exiting. For a more detailed discussion of the **stages of change** model see Chapter 10.

When clients, for example, have not thought seriously about no longer smoking tobacco or marijuana, rather than viewing this behavior as lack of motivation or as denial, such behavior can be viewed from the stages of change perspective. The nurse's task is to raise the clients' levels of consciousness and to arouse their emotional involvement by providing information about the risks of smoking and its specific effects on health. Precontemplators and contemplators need to understand the risks of not changing; people in both these stages are often demoralized and struggling to understand their problem. Many clients will be in these two stages.

Orleans and colleagues (1989) reported that when given direction and advice from physicians about the effects of tobacco use on their health, African Americans reported it did influence their health-related behaviors. According to Royce and colleagues (1993), African Americans have a stronger desire and readiness to quit smoking than whites. They are more likely to be in the contemplative and action states of smoking cessation and to agree that smoking was harmful to their health. Despite the strong desire to quit and many attempts at quitting, few reported experience with formal treatment programs. Studies such as these suggest treatment programs need to be made more accessible, relevant, and appealing to Africans Americans.

PREVENTION

Cigarette and alcohol marketing targeted at African American communities presents formidable barriers to preventing and quitting alcohol and tobacco use. These pro-smoking and pro-alcohol use pressures should be countered with messages directed to distinctive market segments (various ethnic, socioeconomic, and age groups) within African American communities. Such advertising appeals present subtleties in language and images associated with these various subgroups. Nurses should keep abreast of prevention research that focuses on successful outcomes with African American groups. Research studies have shown that most African American youth, even those in low-income urban areas, do manage to escape the pressures to use alcohol, tobacco, and other drugs. Factors that protect young people are school attendance, strong family ties, adequate coping skills, positive race and self-esteem, and employment. Prevention and treatment approaches should build on the strengths in African American communities.

INTERVENTION IN THE ENVIRONMENT

Drug and social problems are interwoven in African American communities. High unemployment, inadequate education, poor health care, poor nutrition, crime, and inadequate housing are factors that intensify alcohol, tobacco, and illicit drug problems. Nurses should form partnerships with social workers, religious leaders, educators, and others involved in strengthening the social environment of African Americans through political action, community organizing, and advocacy. Special emphasis should be placed on increasing accessible, relevant health care, which includes the intervention and treatment of alcohol, tobacco, and other drug problems.

Latinos and Persons of Hispanic Origin

Currently **Hispanics/Latinos** in the United States number more than 28 million, or 11 percent of the population (U.S. Bureau of Census, 1997). Of these, Mexican Americans account for 60 percent, Puerto Ricans 15 percent, Cubans 5 percent, and Hispanics from Central and South American 22 percent (Chapa and Valencia, 1993). The projected growth of this Hispanic/Latino population will exceed that of other ethnic groups in the twenty-first century. They are younger than members of other ethnic groups, have lower per-capita incomes, and have low educational attainment; for example, 37.6 percent of Hispanic children live below the poverty line. In recent years, the void in research literature concerning alcohol, tobacco, and other drug use among Latino men and women has diminished, and some national statistics are now available that provide general parameters of substance use in these groups. The National Household Survey on Drug Abuse, which refers to groups with this shared cultural background as Hispanic, provides regular statistics that can be used as general estimates of drug use by population. In 1997, of men and women of Hispanic origin living in the United States, the number who reported ever using any illicit drug was 25.9 percent (SAMHSA, 1997), lower than for whites or blacks of all ethnic origins. Use by women was slightly less than half that of men (19.2 percent of females versus 32.4 percent of males). This same group reported ever having used alcohol in 68.9 percent of their total population, although only 55.6 percent used alcohol in the past year. Alcohol consumption among Hispanics is lower than among whites and blacks in all age groups except adolescents (see Table 5-2).

Traditional cultural values shape the use of alcohol among most Latino or Hispanic groups; in many subgroups, these values deter alcohol use by youth and adults, particularly women. Although there is wide variation in alcohol use among groups, there is also some uniformity. Most study findings point out that excessive drinking, as well as drinking and drunkenness, is viewed as predominately a male activity. Abstention rates are high among Hispanic women, and a pattern of both infrequent or light drinking and low rates of alcoholism is prevalent in most groups of Hispanic women. Abstinence for both men and women appears to increase with age. Acculturation, age, cohabitation with an alcohol-consuming partner, and employment status appear to be factors determining use among many Caucasian, black, and Latino/Hispanic women. Several research studies suggest that the rate and degree of acculturation are key factors in substance use. Because acculturation appears to occur as different processes among Cubans, Puerto Ricans, Mexicans, South and Central Americans, and other groups, the level at which it occurs has been linked to use of both alcohol and drugs. Levels of acculturation should therefore be assessed within target populations before planning prevention and treatment interventions.

Central cultural values that have been identified as influencing substance use and the development of addiction in many Latino subcultures include machismo, marianismo, and familialism. These are closely linked to gender differences in alcohol and substance use. Machismo is a concept of manly strength and dominance that includes the attitude that a man should be able to drink without showing the effects. Marianismo describes the traditional view of Latin womanhood and focuses on the Virgin Mary as an ideal of duty, self-sacrifice, passivity, and chastity. Socialization in female role patterns supports behavior to harmonize with, and represent the virtues of, the Virgin Mary. It is critically linked to cultural expectations of women marrying, having children in a heterosexual relationship, and taking care of others in spite of their personal needs and requirements (Reyes, 1998). The notion that drinking or drug use would compromise these ideals and goals has traditionally served to deter use. The other face of marianismo is hembrismo, and it has also been linked to alcohol and drug use. Hembrismo refers to behaviors that indicate toughness, strength, resilience, and independence. Efforts to demonstrate hembrismo in defiance of marianismo have been linked to drug and alcohol use and involvement of young women in the subcultures of drug use, smuggling, and sale. Familism is often cited as a cultural value characteristic of all Latino and/or Hispanic groups. Familism has as its central component the perception of family as a source of support, solver of problems, and source of pride. It refers to the deep identification and attachment of individuals to their nuclear family and involves strong feelings of loyalty, reciprocity, and solidarity. Three aspects of familism have been identified by Sabogal and colleagues (1987) as (1) familial obligations, (2) perceived support from the family, and (3) the family as referent.

TABLE 5-2 Percentage of Persons Age 12 and Older Using Licit and Illicit Drugs by Race/Ethnicity, 1991–1993

Race/Ethnicity	Percentage								
	Cigarette Use (past yr.)	Alcohol Use (past yr.)	Any Illicit Drug Use (past yr.)	Marijuana Use (past yr.)	Cocaine Use (past yr.)	Need Drug Abuse Treatment	Alcohol Dependence	Heavy Cigarette Use (past mo.)	Heavy Alcohol Use (past mo.)
Total surveyed population	30.9%	66.4%	11.9%	9.0%	2.5%	2.7%	3.5%	13.8%	5.1%
Native American	52.7	63.7	19.8	15.0	5.2	7.8	5.6	23.9	4.6
Asian/Pacific Islander	21.7	53.2	6.5	4.7	1.4	1.7	1.8	4.8	0.9
Hispanic—Caribbean	21.2	60.8	7.6	5.6	1.5	1.6	1.9	3.6	2.5
Hispanic—Central American	17.9	51.1	5.7	2.7	1.1	1.5	2.8	2.3	2.2
Hispanic—Cuban	27.3	65.7	8.2	5.9	1.7	2.6	0.9	8.9	2.8
Hispanic—Mexican	29.1	63.7	12.7	9.1	3.9	3.6	5.6	4.7	6.9
Hispanic—Puerto Rican	32.7	59.5	13.3	10.8	3.7	3.7	3.0	11.8	4.0
Hispanic—South American	31.3	74.1	10.7	8.4	2.0	1.7	2.1	6.9	3.0
Hispanic—other	25.9	66.3	10.6	9.1	2.3	3.4	3.1	5.3	4.9
Non-Hispanic black	29.9	55.4	13.1	10.6	3.1	3.9	3.4	9.1	4.7
Non-Hispanic white	31.5	68.9	11.8	8.9	2.4	2.5	3.4	15.5	5.3

Note: Heavy cigarette use is defined as smoking a pack or more per day during the past 30 days. Heavy alcohol use is defined as drinking 5 or more drinks per occasion on 5 or more days during the past 30 days.

Source: Office of Applied Studies, SAMHSA, *National Household Survey on Drug Abuse, 1991–1993.* Rockville, MD: U.S. Department of Health and Human Services.

Observations already noted on gender differences affirm that Hispanic/Latino women generally use fewer drugs, including alcohol and nicotine, but this prevalence varies by geographic region, length of time in the United States, and traditions of the subgroup. In Caetano's work of the late 1980s, Central and South American females were found to have the highest rates of abstention, followed by Mexican American, Cuban, and Puerto Rican women (Caetano, 1985, 1988). Alcohol consumption rates, however, appear to increase with acculturation, employment, higher levels of education, and poverty (Randolph, Stroup-Benham, Black, and Markides, 1998). Alcohol consumption and other drug use are strongly stigmatized among Latino women. Factors that support use tend to be the same as those for men. These include residence in neighborhoods with high levels of both accessibility to illicit drugs and drug-related crime, alienation from family, poverty, and (to some degree) co-occurrence of depression.

Alcohol and drug use among Latino males has been studied in several cultural subgroups. Consumption of alcohol among men self-identified as Hispanic varies by age group, with consumption of alcohol on 51 or more days annually noted as 23.6 percent, lower than for blacks or whites (SAMHSA, 1998). Variations in patterns exist, however. Mexican American and Puerto Rican men have high rates of alcohol dependence, but while they consume greater volumes of alcohol, they appear to do so less frequently than white males (Randolph, Stroup-Benham, Black, and Markides, 1998). Heavier use and the development of alcoholism are attributed to factors such as greater social tolerance of heavy drinking by men and exposure to more risk factors. Additional risk factors related to alcohol consumption for Latino male youth include age, religious preference, education level, income potential, and degree of acculturation to American society (Colon, 1998).

Data on the use of illicit drugs by Hispanics are available in the National Houschold Survey on Drug Abuse (SAMHSA, 1997), although the limitations of self-report and sample selection must be considered for this as for any other group. Findings suggest that patterns of substance use differ significantly among major Hispanic subgroups. For example, Mexican Americans and Puerto Ricans are more likely to be past and/or present drug users than Cubans, with the first two groups using marijuana with twice the frequency of Cubans. Estimates of use by populations published in 1997 indicate that Hispanic males reported using illicit drugs in lower numbers than other groups; 32.4 percent of men had ever used an illicit drug, and 7.15 percent reported use of an illicit drug during the past month. When compared with blacks, 38.8 percent had ever used and 9.3 percent had used during the past month. Use by white men on the same indices is 42.3 percent and 8.7 percent, respectively (SAMHSA, 1998). Although heroin is less frequently used by men across all these ethnic groups than by Caucasians, Hispanic men reported last-year use in a higher percentage (0.6 percent) than that for whites (0.2 percent) or blacks (0.5 percent) (SAMHSA, 1998).

Prevalence patterns of cigarette smoking among Hispanic subgroups parallel demographic patterns observed in the total survey population. Regardless of racial/ethnic group, individuals age 18 or older had relatively higher prevalences of smoking if they resided outside metropolitan areas with populations of more than 1 million, responded to the interview in English versus Spanish, had between 9 and 11 years of schooling, and were unemployed or resided in households receiving welfare (SAMHSA, 1998). Among Hispanic subgroups, women reported smoking in a ratio of about 1 to 3 compared with men, with Puerto Rican groups showing the highest prevalence (30.7 percent of women and 41.1 percent of men). In Cuban, Mexican, and other groups, the prevalence is closer to 22 percent and 35 percent, respectively. The prevalence of use among women is significantly lower than in black or Caucasian groups, with use by men being more comparable (SAMHSA, 1998).

Treatment

There are limited research data available on the involvement in, or effectiveness of, substance abuse treatment by Latinos. The National Household Survey data on the need for treatment for illicit drug use suggest that individuals with the greatest need for substance abuse treatment are more numerous in families with incomes below $42,000, among those who do not have health insurance, and among those with a family member in the household who receives welfare. Of Hispanic subgroups, a percentage ranging from 32 percent to 65 percent earn less than $20,000 annually, 3 percent to 23 percent live with a welfare recipient, and 28 percent to 51 percent lack health insurance. These data suggest that individuals in Hispanic subgroups who need treatment are less likely to receive it for socioeconomic reasons. Research among this population has been done primarily by subgroups, with resulting data specific to these groups. For example, a sample of Mexican Americans in treatment were noted to be mostly male, married, employed (having greater economic stability), and in outpatient treatment rather than in in-patient or detoxification services (Gilbert and Cervantes, 1986). It appears that, when compared with other ethnic groups, Hispanics in treatment are generally younger (below age 45), married, less well educated, and of lower incomes. At the same time, they report drinking heavily for longer periods than whites and having more physical problems than blacks (Cervantes and Pena, 1998).

Humm-Delgado and Delgado (1983) identified five themes to be considered in developing interventions sensitive to the needs of Hispanic/Latino populations:

1. Importance of the family
2. Value attached to cooperation and competition
3. Good relationships with others
4. Role of respect in dealing with individuals
5. Action orientation to problem solving

Asian Americans

There are over 7 million Asians and Pacific Islanders in the United States, according to U.S. Census Reports (1991). The 1990 census identified 30 Asian and 21 Pacific Islander groups with different languages, norms, values, and ethnic histories. Asian Americans include people of Chinese, Japanese, Filipino, and Southeast Asian (Vietnamese, Cambodian, Laotian, Thai, and Malaysian) extraction. Pacific Islanders include Polynesians (Hawaiians, Tongans, and Samoans), Micronesians, and Melanesians. The largest groups are Chinese, Filipino, Japanese, Korean, and Asian Indian.

One prevailing view of Asians is that they are a model minority without substance abuse problems. The dearth of national prevalence data on this issue has furthered this notion and has resulted in sparse information on the needs of this population. Alcohol use has been studied most frequently with regard to Chinese and Japanese peoples, followed by Koreans and Filipinos. Studies on the use and abuse of other substances have largely been limited to Asian Americans or recently emigrated youth in these cultures.

Dominant Asian Beliefs About Substance Use and Abuse

Some dominant beliefs that influence substance use in the Asian community include the importance placed on harmony, a sense of other and a situational orientation greater than among Caucasians, and a traditional belief in the intertwining of soma and psyche (Chun, Eastman, Wang, and Sue, 1998). There is a permissive attitude toward substance use in the elderly because a variety of substances are seen as medicinal and good for many of the disorders that plague older age. Only one reported study focused specifically on the elderly in a male sample (Yamamoto, Lee, Lin, and Cho, 1987). In this group of older Asians, Filipinos were found to have the highest rates of alcohol abuse/dependence (11 percent), followed by Japanese (6 percent) and Chinese (4 percent). Many new immigrants do not understand American attitudes that cigarettes, alcohol, or prescription drugs, which were readily available in their countries and socially acceptable to use, are harmful.

General trends related to alcohol consumption in Asian Americans and Asian Pacific Islanders do not apply across groups. In addition, definitions of drinking and heavy drinking vary, making the comparison of study findings difficult. There are comparatively few prevalence data on substance use in Asians, although limited information is available on larger Asian groups. Those data, however, often lack scientific rigor in that they are anecdotal or based on relatively small community samples. Even less is known about potentially high-risk groups such as Southeast Asian refugees. Results of studies of high school and college-age students conducted in areas with large Asian populations tend to refute the concept of nondrug-using Asians. For example, Hanson and colleagues (1988) reported lifetime alcohol and cigarette use for Asian youth to be comparable to or greater than that for other ethnic groups. Saseo (1987) also reported higher lifetime use of cigarettes, alcohol, and marijuana in this group than for African Americans, whites, or Hispanics. Others have found similar results, refuting the model minority concept (Skager, Fisher, and Maddahian, 1986; Skager, Frith, and Maddahian, 1989). It is problematic, however, that these studies did not differentiate between subgroups of Asians, so the practical significance of these results remains unclear.

Later studies have, to a greater degree, attempted to focus on specific Asian subgroups. McLaughlin and colleagues (1987) conducted a drug use assessment to determine prevalence data for specific population groups. They reported prevalence rates of 29 percent for whites, 19 percent for native Hawaiians, 22 percent for Japanese Americans, 11 percent for Filipino Americans, and 4 percent for Chinese Americans. A later study by Saseo (1991) found that of the Asian groups, Japanese Americans had the highest lifetime use of cigarettes and alcohol (45 percent), followed by Filipinos (38 percent), Vietnamese (36 percent), Koreans (36 percent), Chinese (25 percent), and Chinese Vietnamese (24 percent). Japanese Americans were also highest in lifetime alcohol consumption (69 percent), followed by Koreans (49 percent), Vietnamese (43 percent), Chinese (42 percent), Filipinos (39 percent), and Chinese Vietnamese (36 percent). Most of this drinking appeared to be socially related, and the rates were significantly below national prevalence rates.

A number of social factors that are believed to influence Asian drug use patterns appear repeatedly in study results. More permissive attitudes toward legal and illegal drug use seem to be part and parcel of the process of acculturation. Most studies report few social problems as a result of heavy drinking, although some Asians drink heavily. The emphasis is on drinking at special social occasions; drunkenness, as a habit, is frowned upon. Other differences emerge around what constitutes problematic drinking. Koreans, for example, do not define alcoholism until medical problems are clearly evidenced. Few problems are evidenced in the mainstream legal system because the community asserts its own social controls.

Limited studies indicate that substance use is increasing in this population. For example, Bachman and colleagues (1991) noted that each time Asian Americans were interviewed (about every three years), their reported use almost doubled, even though overall the Asian sample reported the lowest rates of use. Some estimates of illicit drug or alcohol use rank Asians and Pacific Islanders higher than African Americans (Barnes, Welte, and Dintcheff, 1993; Kim, McLead, and Shantzis, 1992; Segal, 1992). Although samples are relatively small, high school senior surveys have reported use rates similar to those of African Americans for cocaine, stimulants, and LSD. Rates were sometimes higher for Asians as compared with African Americans for sedatives, tranquilizers, inhalants, and other opiates (Austin, 1994). There have also been indications that Asians used more nonprescription medications (sleeping pills, cough medicines, cold and allergy medicines) than other ethnic groups. In a 1991 survey, Asians and Pacific Islanders reported the same rate of cocaine use as African Americans, and their inhalant use was higher than for African Americans, although still substantially lower than for whites (Austin, 1994). Kim and colleagues (1992) reported that Asians and Pacific Islanders used inhalants, cocaine, amphetamines, and barbiturates at the same or higher rates than whites and other ethnic groups. Other reports ranked Southeast Asians first in cocaine use and high in amphetamine use (Austin, 1994). It is interesting to note that although most ethnic groups use alcohol first, then marijuana and other illicit drugs, Asians appear to begin with pills and other drugs and later begin to smoke and drink. Comments on surveys have indicated that their motivation for use is less about peer influence and more related to relief of acculturation stress and other social issues.

A key informative survey conducted in Los Angeles, San Diego, and San Francisco asked Asian and Pacific Islander focus groups to identify at-risk groups within their own ethnic groups (Saseo, 1991). Information regarding drugs used, groups identified as at risk, contributing factors, and values or concerns highlighted by drug use are described in Table 5-3.

As is true for most ethnic groups, Asian American females report much less substance use than do males. Asian women also report less substance use than women in other ethnic groups. Austin (1994) indicates that because rates of substance use for Asian women are low, we can expect a rise as these women become more acculturated. Research has reported that as Asian women become more acculturated, the importance of traditional values and the stigma of use may lessen (Chi, Lubben, and Kitano, 1989). Males, however, consistently use alcohol and cigarettes more than females. Annual prevalence rates for males and females are similar in the use of LSD, cocaine, sedatives, barbiturates, stimulants, and inhalants. Asian and Pacific Islander females are at relatively high risk for marijuana, stimulant, and cocaine use. Their reported rates of daily smoking were also alarmingly high—much higher than for African American females and slightly higher than for Hispanic females (Austin, 1994). Betel is commonly used by elderly Cambodian women, Lao women commonly use opium for pain control, and Cambodian women report alcohol and prescription drug use for alleviation of stress, anxiety, and depression (D'Avanzo and Barab, 1997).

TABLE 5-3 Saseo's Key Informant Survey: Results Summary

Ethnic Group	Problematic Use/Abuse	Within-Group At-Risk Populations	Contributing Factors	Values and Concerns Emphasized
Chinese	ETOH Tobacco Prescription drugs	Older adult males Adolescents Immigrants Those with low incomes	Underestimation of health hazards of alcohol, tobacco, and prescription drugs; family and marital issues; juvenile delinquency; gangs; intergenerational conflict	Values: Harmony, filial respect, continuity of generations, welfare of family versus individual
Japanese American	Highest use of ETOH Marijuana	Adolescents Young adults Divorced single adults	Coping with acculturation through substance abuse by newer immigrants	Concerns: Negative parental role modeling
Korean American	Rice wine Whiskey Crack cocaine	Adolescents Young adults Elders (OTC prescription drugs) Males	Drinking and smoking considered gender appropriate for men; delinquency; gangs; truancy; runaways	Concerns: Driving under the influence
Filipino American	ETOH Marijuana Cocaine	Adolescents Young adults Males Recent immigrants	Family and marital problems; problems due to acculturation; juvenile delinquency; gang activity; crime; high school dropouts; unemployment; suicide	Concerns: Driving under the influence (cultural acceptance of smoking and drinking by males supports continuing problems)
Vietnamese	Cigarettes Marijuana	Older and younger males Adolescents Low-income households	Depression; acculturation; loss of traditional male status	Concerns: Juvenile delinquency; gang activity; economic hardship
Cambodian	ETOH Tobacco Crack cocaine Amphetamines	Low-income persons of all ages and genders		Concerns: Same as for Vietnamese
Lao	ETOH Tobacco Marijuana		Peer pressure	Concerns: Same as for Vietnamese
Hmong	Tobacco ETOH Opiates	Adolescents Adults	Stress and peer pressure; chemical "coping"	Concerns: Associated health problems
Thai	ETOH Tobacco Marijuana Amphetamines			Similar to other Southeast Asian groups

Prevention and Screening

Outreach to Asian communities must be through credible community organizations or churches. A service agency may be the least successful place for meeting Asian clients for training and education, community outreach, or provision of services. It is much better to use a familiar and comfortable Asian community environment such as a school, church, or community center.

In Asian cultures, the family is the primary decision-making body and the primary influence on individual family members. Family authority is usually greater than that of individual members, friends, or the community, and families do not conform to Western expectations of their needs. A different focus is recommended; for example, instead of discussing how much substance abuse exists within the Asian community, it is better to emphasize how the family/culture can help prevent substance abuse. Asian families usually avoid seeking help or professional counseling and keep confidential those matters that might bring shame on the family unit. Generational roles within the family must be addressed and honored in order for treatment and referral to be accepted. Elders are respected and revered. The father is generally the authority figure, primary decision maker, and primary economic provider. This strong hierarchy often changes with the first generation born in the United States. Still, roles within the family are subsumed by the overall prosperity and image of the family unit as a whole. The family approach encompasses ancestors and descendants rather than focusing on the individual.

Asian families who appear to be at high risk for developing substance-related problems are those descended from foreign-born parents, those of low economic status and/or with housing problems who experience isolation within a non-Asian community, those who have no communication with family in the homeland, and those who lack citizenship.

It is recommended that health care providers use and create culture-specific resources. Materials, references, and referrals must be specific, not generic. Among first-generation Asians (born and raised in the United States), there may be limited English proficiency because the native language is spoken at home; materials should be bilingual. Illiteracy is not uncommon; for example, Cambodians' educations were interrupted and virtually cancelled during the Pol Pot period. Pictures or videos may be the best primary tools. Because Asian communities place a high value on it, education is a key term in any program presentation to Asian communities and appears to take the edge off taboo subjects such as substance abuse. A program focusing on substance abuse, for example, may draw poor attendance; information embedded in a program on community issues will draw a better response.

Schools and education are viewed as accentuating family teachings, and educators should not attempt to teach values, norms, or culture. Service providers can help in defining the roles of family, school, church, temple, or service agencies to the community so that these institutions are seen as and function as educational resources.

When conducting screening, it is best to:
- Discuss the individual in the third person as he or she rather than using the familiar you.
- Limit confrontation; use indirect information-gathering methods. Do not use a confrontational model because direct, confrontational communication styles are not common in these groups (Amodeo, Robb, Peou, and Tran, 1996).

- Address problems in a community rather than an individual framework. Offer solutions that allow participants to help someone in the community. This approach allows participants not to have to own the shame of the problem. Don't push for verbal participation of individuals in any activity.
- Develop screening questions based on culturally appropriate norms; develop unique approaches.
- Always provide opportunities by which the individual can save face.
- Screening and assessment tools should be based on culturally appropriate norms. Develop or obtain instruments validated with the group with whom you are working.

Treatment

Asian populations are infrequently clients in substance abuse treatment programs, a fact that is perceived as a lack of need for services by these groups. In reality, there is a critical shortage of culturally appropriate treatment and intervention programs as the prevalence of substance abuse increases in these populations. Issues that deter seeking treatment are far greater than language. When more culturally appropriate services were provided, premature terminations among Asians in mental health treatment were found to be reduced to termination levels of white clients (Zane and Saseo, 1992). One study examined parallel services for Asian Americans in Los Angeles (Yeh, Takeuchi, and Sue, 1994). Parallel services mean that programs specifically provide services in a culturally appropriate manner to Asian clients, for example, by matching clients with Asian counselors. These programs produced higher service utilization patterns, and these clients functioned better than those in mainstream programs. In addition, clients stayed in treatment longer in the parallel program. A 1990 study (Atkinson, Jennings, and Liongson) found that students attempting to decide whether or not to seek treatment chose not to use college counseling services because of the lack of ethnically similar or culturally sensitive counselors. Most research on culture/ethnicity focuses on descriptions of ethnic differences in substance use and add little to the theoretical base for prevention or treatment (Collins, 1992; Institute of Medicine, 1990). The need for substance abuse intervention among Asians often appears invisible for a variety of reasons: the stigma, the tendency of these problems to be hidden within the family and community to avoid shame, and the perception that available intervention is not culturally appropriate.

Because expression of emotions is discouraged culturally (based on a need to save face), underreporting is the norm, and stress is frequently expressed in somatic terms (i.e., physical problems for which clients seek medical help). This does not mean that psychological symptoms cannot be described; rather, it is important to use a comprehensive mind/body approach. Somatization is a face-saving mechanism used to gain assistance for emotional problems they dare not express. Because what is spoken is frequently different from the underlying problem, psychological and substance-related problems among Asians are difficult for American health care providers to diagnose. It can be difficult to understand the many differences among Asian groups with respect to language, social systems, and economic status. It is important that the health care provider look closely at the client's culture, not only at ethnicity, when studying counseling relationships (Sue, 1998). Factors such as acculturation may mean that clients of similar ethnicity may be vastly different culturally

(Gordon, 1993; Weibel-Orlando, 1993). Substance abuse professionals who are of the same cultural group appear to be most successful with Asian clients, based on their shared language and culture. It is important for substance abuse counselors to learn as much as possible about the various Asian groups with whom they work. In addition, individuals working in communities should respect and value the heritage and uniqueness of the cultural community and should be visible to community participants. Credibility of treatment services is built using culturally correct routes, which include the use of community groups.

The provider of pharmacotherapeutic treatment of alcohol, psychiatric, and drug problems in the Asian community must consider biophysiological differences in this population. Adverse reactions to some pharmaceuticals can sometimes be explained by the presence or absence of certain enzymes. Asians have fewer problems than Caucasians, for example, metabolizing certain drugs. About 5 percent to 10 percent of Caucasians are poor metabolizers of more than 50 drugs oxidized through a particular enzyme system (CYP2D6). Only 1 percent to 2 percent of Asians have this problem, changing the guidelines for prescription calculation. These drugs include antidepressants, antipsychotics, and cardiovascular drugs, particularly antiarrthymic drugs. Conversely, for another enzyme system (CYP2C19), Asians are more likely to be poor metabolizers, putting them at risk of longer and more concentrated exposure because they clear them less rapidly. Potential difficulties catabolizing diazepam and omeprazole are noteworthy (Lin and Lu, 1997). Another commonly noted problem among Asians is a flushing response on the ingestion of alcohol. Alcohol is broken down in the body by two enzymes: (1) alcohol dehydrogenase, which converts alcohol to acetaldehyde, and (2) aldehyde dehydrogenase (ALDH), which converts acetaldehyde to acetate. ALDH inactivity results in the accumulation of acetaldehyde, which leads to flushing. This reaction is characterized by numerous symptoms, such as facial flushing, nausea, headache, dizziness, and rapid heartbeat (Makimoto, 1998). Genetic predisposition, whereby an individual inherits combinations of the two genes responsible for changes in acetaldehyde metabolism, results in the experience of an unpleasant flushing reaction. Few Caucasians but up to 50 percent of Asians carry a gene combination that results in flushing, with the result that some Asians drink significantly less alcohol and have lower rates of alcoholism. These findings suggest that the presence of an inactive LDH gene may protect, at least partially, from heavy drinking and the risk of alcoholism. Makimoto (1998) further notes that environmental influences also play an important role in determining drinking behaviors. For example, with Asian Pacific Islanders, as drinking norms have become more permissive, alcohol consumption has increased. In Japan, alcohol consumption has increased fourfold since World War II. Asian immigrants, however, appear to have protective factors also. Those who feel a sense of control over their lives, maintain strong commitments to their life activities, and perceive change as an opportunity for personal development are more likely to display positive adjustment to their new American lifestyles and less substance abuse (Chun, Eastman, Wang, and Sue, 1998).

The most accepted and therefore successful substance abuse treatment programs are those that are specifically developed for Asians. Ideally, the staffing patterns for these programs should reflect the cultural and linguistic makeup of the Asian community. The staff should be bicultural and bilingual. A social support model should be used that includes the natural support systems of the client, the extended family, and the temple or church.

Most treatment programs rely on Western treatment approaches and therefore do not address culture-specific needs of Asian clients. Language barriers create a chasm between providers and Asian individuals, and few agencies have trained counselors who speak Asian languages. In many cases, administrative support and funding are lacking for culture-specific programs. Although it is not an ideal solution, Asians who are at least the second generation may successfully use existing infrastructures if they are covered by private or public health insurance.

More recently emigrated Asians, such as Southeast Asians, generally lack financial resources for substance abuse or mental health treatment, and the cultural barriers to treatment may be so great that the few services offered are not used. Substance abuse treatment services must address cultural issues, spiritual beliefs, health care practices, and linguistic barriers in order to be effective; this is especially true for first-generation descendants.

Collaborative service models wherein culture-specific treatment programs team up with Western service models have recently been initiated. Special efforts must be made to ensure that the culture-specific program is not swallowed up in Western treatment strategies.

Programs designed to help Asians with substance abuse problems should incorporate approaches from traditional and cultural perspectives. Treatment may include acupuncture, use of traditional healers, and herbal medicine. Treatment should:

- Have a family focus
- Be flexible in the number and length of sessions
- Maximize existing resources and use them appropriately
- Develop a full continuum of services
- Collect data to capture which specific services are most effective and their cost
- Develop assessment tools to produce outcome data

In doing these things, it is important to include Asians in planning, evaluating, and shaping programs. Funds should be directed to community-based organizations that understand the target population. Groups already working in the community need to receive training in substance abuse. This approach is superior to funding mainstream organizations to enable them to learn to work with Asian populations.

Treatment groups should be organized in a gender-specific fashion, and group members should be clustered based on an optimum and appropriate combination of subcultures (for example, Cambodian female elders, young adult Vietnamese men). Ongoing concrete activities and continued engagement should provide vocational training, for example. Treatment centers should also aid in the development of cultural identity for Asians struggling with intergenerational conflict or personal identity.

Recommendations for the Development of a Treatment Program Model for All Minority Groups

Delgado (1998) articulates nine recommendations for any culturally competent model for prevention and treatment and notes that this model could be broad or group-specific:

1. *Community assets.* A positive approach and use of indigenous resources set a philosophical framework that can influence the development of services and community involvement.

2. *Biculturality.* Staffing, planning, and service delivery should reflect the two cultures involved. Cultural values and expectations should influence choices of procedures, instrumentation, language, and service development.

3. *Community participation.* The identified community should be involved in the planning and delivery of services in the form of advisory committees, task forces, and volunteer activities.

4. *Specificity of services.* A series of factors, such as gender, age, acculturation, income, and sexual orientation, should be used to identify target populations and should be taken into consideration in developing services.

5. *Staff support.* ATOD (alcohol, tobacco, and other drugs) organizations should emphasize staff development approaches, such as supervision, training, and consultation, for both members and nonmembers of staff.

6. *Comprehensive services.* A network of seamless, continuous service resources will be essential to the retention of participants.

7. *Contextualizing of ATOD.* Other social problems must be the context for prevention and treatment education about alcohol, tobacco, and other drug abuse. Social problems such as crime, HIV, and violence interface with substance abuse/dependence and need to be addressed as contributing factors.

8. *Research evaluation.* Research should be both qualitative and quantitative. This combined approach derives from the complexity of factors influencing alcoholism and other drug dependencies.

9. *Multiple target sites.* Settings for prevention and treatment services should include many points of community service delivery, such as schools, health clinics, workplaces, social clubs, and religious meeting places, as well as other settings salient to community members.

CRITICAL THINKING QUESTIONS

1. Consider the influence of ethnic traditions on families' drinking patterns. What are some ways patterns of families more recently emigrated may contrast with groups who arrived earlier in the United States? What are the implications of these differences for health education about substance use?

2. Discuss some ways in which gender differences in substance use patterns can be useful in organizing prevention programs and treatment groups.

3. When implementing a comprehensive assessment, what are some key cultural factors that would indicate the need for an in-depth discussion of alcohol and drug use by the client and his or her significant others?

4. Discuss characteristic patterns of several cultures that influence attitudes about treatment for alcohol and drug problems. Which cultural factors facilitate or deter the client's involvement with self-help groups?

5. Alcohol and drug use cannot be evaluated apart from a sociocultural context. Give five examples of the interaction among educational level, cultural tradition, and religious beliefs that determine patterns of drug use in immigrant groups.

REFERENCES

Abramson, H.J. (1979). Assimilation and pluralism. In S. Thernstrom (ed.), *Harvard Encyclopedia of American Ethnic Groups.* Cambridge, MA: Harvard University Press.

American Academy of Nursing. (1997). *Cultural Diversity in Nursing: Issues, Strategies and Outcomes.* Washington, DC: American Nurses Publishing.

Ames, G.M. (1985). Middle-class Protestants: Alcohol and the family. In L.A. Bennett and G.M. Ames (eds.), *The American Experience with Alcohol: Contrasting Cultural Perspectives.* New York: Plenum Press.

Amodeo, M., Robb, N., Peou, S., and Tran, H. (September 1996). Adapting mainstream substance abuse interventions for Southeast Asian clients. *Families in Society: The Journal of Contemporary Human Services,* 403–412.

Andrews, M.M. (1992). Cultural perspectives on nursing in the 21st century. *Journal of Professional Nursing 8*(1), 7–15.

Asante, M.F. (1987). *Afrocentricity.* Trenton, NJ: African World Press.

Atkinson, D.R., Jennings, R.G., and Liongson, L. (July 1990). Minority students' reasons for not seeking counseling and suggestions for improving services. *Journal of College Student Development 31,* 342–350.

Austin, G. (1994). ATOD use among Asian-American youth. Unpublished manuscript.

Babor, T.F. (1992). Cross-cultural research on alcohol: A quoi bon? In J.E. Helzer and G.J. Canino (eds.), *Alcoholism in North America, Europe, and Asia.* New York: Oxford University Press.

Bachman, J., Wallace, J., Kurth, C., Johnston, L., and O'Malley, P. (1991). *Drug Use Among Black, White, Hispanic, Native American, and Asian American High School Seniors (1976–1989).* Ann Arbor: University of Michigan.

Bales, R. (1944). The "fixation" factor in alcohol addiction: An hypothesis derived from a comparative study of Irish and Jewish racial norms. Unpublished doctoral dissertation, Harvard University.

Barnes, G.M., Welte, J.W., and Dintcheff, B.A. (1993). Decline in alcohol use among 7–12 grade students in New York State, 1983–1990. *Alcoholism: Clinical and Experimental Research 17*(4), 797–801.

Bell, P., and Evans, J. (1981). *Counseling the Black Client: Alcohol Use and Abuse in Black America.* City Center, MN: Hazelden Foundation.

Blane, H.T. (1977). Acculturation and drinking in an Italian-American community. *Journal of Studies on Alcohol 38,* 1324–1346.

Brown, F., and Touley, J. (1989). Alcoholism in the black community. In G.W. Lawson and A.W. Lawson (eds.), *Alcoholism and Substance Abuse.* Rockville, MD: Aspen.

Caetano, R. (1985). Drinking patterns and alcohol problems in a national sample of U.S. Hispanics. In D. Spiegler, D. Tate, S. Aiken, and C. Christian (eds.), *Alcohol Use Among U.S. Ethnic Minorities.* Research Monograph No. 18, National Institute on Alcohol Abuse and Alcoholism. D.H.H.S. Publication No. (ADM) 89-1435. Washington, DC: U.S. Government Printing Office.

Caetano, R. (1988). Alcohol use among Hispanic groups in the United States. *American Journal of Drug and Alcohol Abuse 14*(3), 293–308.

Caetano, R., and Clark, C.L. (1998a). Trends in situational norms and attitudes, toward drinking among whites, blacks and Hispanics, 1984–1995. Berkeley, CA: Alcohol Research Group. Quoted in R. Caetano, C.L. Clark, and T. Tam (1998), Alcohol consumption among racial/ethnic minorities: Theory and research. *Alcohol, Health and Research World 22*(4), 233–243.

Caetano, R., and Clark, C.L. (1998b). Trends in alcohol-related problems among whites, African Americans, and Hispanics: 1984–1995. *Alcohol, Health and Research World 22*(4), 262.

Caetano, R., Clark, C.L., and Tam, T. (1998). Alcohol consumption among racial/ethnic minorities: Theory and research. *Alcohol, Health and Research World 22*(4), 233–243.

Caetano, R., and Kaskutas, L.A. (1995). Changes in drinking patterns among whites, blacks and Hispanics: 1994–1992. *Journal of Studies in Alcohol 56,* 558–562.

Cahalan, D., Cisin, I.H., and Crossley, H.M. (1969). *American Drinking Practices.* New Brunswick, NJ: Rutgers Center of Alcohol Studies.

Campinha-Bacote, J., Yahle, T., and Langenkamp, M. (1996). The challenge of cultural diversity for nurse educators. *Journal of Continuing Education in Nursing 27*(2), 59–64.

Cervantes, R.C., and Pena (1998). *The Hispanic/Latino Evaluation Handbook.* Washington, DC: SAMHSA/CSAP.

Chapa, J., and Valencia, R.R. (1993). Latino population growth, demographic characteristics and educational stagnation: An examination of recent trends. *Hispanic Journal of Behavior Sciences 15,* 165–187.

Chi, I., Lubben, J., and Kitano, H. (1989). Differences in drinking behavior among three Asian-American groups. *Journal of Studies on Alcohol 50,* 15–23.

Christmon, K. (1995). Historical overview of alcohol in the African American community. *Journal of Black Studies 25,* 318.

Chun, K.M., Eastman, K.L., Wang, G.C.S., and Sue, S.S. (1998). Psychopathology. In L.C. Lee and N. Zane (eds.), *Handbook of Asian American Psychology.* Thousand Oaks, CA: Sage.

Collins, R.L. (1992). Sociocultural aspects of alcohol use and abuse: Ethnicity and gender. In J.E. Trimble, C.S. Bolek, and S.J. Niemcryk (eds.), *Ethnic and Multicultural Drug Abuse: Perspectives on Current Research.* Binghamton, NY: Harrington Park.

Collins, R.L. (1993). Sociocultural aspects of alcohol use and abuse: Ethnicity and gender. *Drugs and Society 8,* 89.

Colon, E. (1998). Alcohol use among Latino males: Implication for the development of culturally competent prevention and treatment services. In M. Delgado (ed.), *Alcohol Use and Abuse Among Latinos: Issues and Examples of Culturally Competent Services.* Binghamton, NY: Haworth Press.

Cordiero, P.A., Reagan, T.G., and Martinez, L.P. (1994). *Multiculturalism and TQE.* Thousand Oaks, CA: Corwin Press.

Cummings, K.M., Giovina, G., and Mendicino, A.J. (1987). Cigarette advertising and black-white differences in brand preference. *Public Health Report 102,* 698.

Daniels, D. (1980). *Pioneer Urbanites.* Philadelphia, PA: Temple University Press.

D'Avanzo, C., and Barab, S. (1997). Southeast Asians: Asian Pacific Americans at risk for substance abuse. *Substance Use and Misuse 32*(7 & 8), 829–848.

Davis, L.E., and Proctor, E.K. (1989). *Race, Gender and Class: Guidelines for Practice with Individuals, Families and Groups.* Englewood Cliffs, NJ: Prentice Hall.

Delgado, M. (1998). Summary of key practices, research and policy implications. *Alcohol Use and Abuse Among Latinos: Issues and Examples of Culturally Competent Services.* Binghamton, NY: Haworth Press.

Douglass, F. (1892). *Life and Times of Frederick Douglass.* New York: Collier.

Doweiko, H.E. (1999). *Concepts of Chemical Dependency* (3rd ed.). Pacific Grove, CA: Brooks/Cole.

Franklin, J.H. (1974). *From Slavery to Freedom: A History of Negro Americans* (4th ed.). New York: Alfred Knopf.

Freund, P.J. (1985). Polish-American drinking: Continuity and change. In L.A. Bennett and G.M. Ames (eds.), *The American Experience with Alcohol: Contrasting Cultural Perspectives.* New York: Plenum Press.

Gilbert, M.J., and Cervantes, R.C. (1986). Patterns and practices of alcohol use among Mexican-Americans: A comprehensive review. *Hispanic Journal of Behavioral Sciences 8,* 1–60.

Glassner, B., and Berg, B. (1985). Jewish-Americans and alcohol: Processes of avoidance and definition. In L.A. Bennett and G.M. Ames (eds.), *The American Experience with Alcohol: Contrasting Cultural Perspectives.* New York: Plenum Press.

Glazer, N., and Moynihan, D.P. (1963). *Beyond the Melting Pot.* Cambridge, MA: Harvard University Press.

Gleason, P. (1979). American identity and Americanization. In S. Thernstrom (ed.), *Harvard Encyclopedia of American Ethnic Groups.* Cambridge, MA: Harvard University Press.

Goddard, L. (1993). Background and scope of alcohol and other drug problems. In L. Goddard (ed.), *Center Substance Abuse Prevention, Technical Report 6.* Rockville, MD: U.S. Department of Health and Human Services.

Gordon, J.U. (1993). A culturally specific approach to ethnic minority young adults. In E.M. Freeman (ed.), *Substance Abuse Treatment: A Family Systems Perspective.* Thousand Oaks, CA: Sage.

Gordon, M. (1964). *Assimilation in American Life: The Role of Race, Religion and National Origins.* New York: Oxford University Press.

Greeley, A.M., and McCready, W.C. (1975). The transmission of cultural heritages: The case of the Irish and the Italians. In N. Glazer and D. Moynihan (eds.), *Ethnicity: Theory and Experience.* Cambridge, MA: Harvard University Press.

Greeley, A.M., McCready, W.C., and Theisen, G. (1980). *Ethnic Drinking Subcultures.* New York: Praeger Publishers.

Grey, M. (ed.). (1996). African Americans. In *Cultural Competence for Social Workers: Agenda for Alcohol and Other Drug Abuse Prevention Professionals Working with Ethnic/Racial Communities.* Rockville, MD: U.S. Department of Health and Human Services. Substance Abuse and Mental Health Services Administration (USDHHS-SAMHSA).

Grier, W., and Cobb, P. (1968). *Black Rage.* New York: Bantam Books.

Hanft, S. (1995). English Americans. In J. Galens, A. Sheets, and R.V. Young (eds.), *Gale Encyclopedia of Multicultural America.* New York: Gale Research.

Hanson, D.J. (1995). The United States of America. In D.W. Heath (ed.), *International Handbook on Alcohol and Culture.* Westport, CT: Greenwood Press.

Hanson, W., Johnson, C., Flay, B., Graham, J., and Sobel, J. (1988). Affective and social influence approaches to the prevention of multiple substance abuse among seventh grade students. *Preventative Medicine 17,* 135–154.

Harper, F. (1991). Substance abuse and the black American family. *Urban Review 13,* 1.

Herd, D. (1985a). Ambiguity in black drinking norms: An ethnohistorical interpretation. In L. Bennett and G. Ames (eds.), *The American Experience with Alcohol: Contrasting Cultural Perspectives.* New York: Plenum Press.

Herd, D. (1985b). Migration, cultural transformation and the rise of black liver cirrhosis mortality. *British Journal of Addiction 80,* 397.

Herd, D. (1985c). We cannot stagger to freedom. In L. Brill and C. Winick (eds.), *Yearbook of Substance Use and Abuse* (Vol. 3). New York: Human Services Press.

Herd, D. (1988). Drinking by black and white women: Results of a national survey. *Social Problems 35,* 493.

Herd, D. (1990). Subgroup differences in drinking patterns among black and white men: Results from a national survey. *Journal of Studies on Alcohol 51,* 221.

Herd, D. (1993). Contesting culture: Alcohol-related identity movements in contemporary African American Communities. *Contemporary Drug Problems 20*(4), 739–758.

Hickey, J.V. (1996). Cultural and ethnic diversity: Cultural competence. In *Advanced Nursing Practice: Changing Roles and Clinical Applications.* Philadelphia, PA: Lippincott-Raven Publishers.

Hillstrom, L.C. (1995). French Americans. In J. Galens, A. Sheets, and R.V. Young (eds.), *Gale Encyclopedia of Multicultural America.* New York: Gale Research.

Humm-Delgado, D., and Delgado, M. (1983). Hispanic adolescents and substance abuse: Issues for the 1980's. *Child and Youth Services 6*(1/2), 71–87.

Institute of Medicine. (1990). *Broadening the Base of Treatment for Alcohol Problems.* Report of a study by a committee of the Institute of Medicine: Division of Mental Health and Behavioral Medicine. Washington, DC: National Academy Press.

Jessor, R., Young, H.B., Young, E.B., and Tesi, G. (1970). Perceived opportunity, alienation and drinking behavior among Italian and American youth. *Journal of Personality and Social Psychology 15,* 215–222.

Jones, S. (1995). Polish Americans. In J. Galens, A. Sheets, and R.V. Young (eds.), *Gale Encyclopedia of Multicultural America.* New York: Gale Research.

Jones-Webb, R. (1998). Drinking patterns and problems among African-Americans: Recent findings. *Alcohol Health and Research World 22*(4), 260–264.

Kallen, H.M. (1924). *Culture and Democracy in the United States.* New York: Boni and Liveright.

Kallen, H.M. (1956). *Cultural Pluralism and the American Idea.* Philadelphia, PA: University of Pennsylvania Press.

Kamp, J. (1995). Jewish Americans. In J. Galens, A. Sheets, and R.V. Young (eds.), *Gale Encyclopedia of Multicultural America.* New York: Gale Research.

Kavanaugh, K.H., and Kennedy, P.H. (1992). *Promoting Cultural Diversity: Strategies for Health Care Professionals.* Beverly Hills, CA: Sage.

Kim, S., McLead, J., and Shantzis, C. (1992). Cultural competence for evaluators working with Asian-American communities. In M. Orlandi (ed.), *Cultural Competence for Evaluators.* Rockville, MD: Center for Substance Abuse Prevention.

Kleinman, A. (1978). *Rethinking Psychiatry: From Cultural Category to Personal Experience.* New York: Free Press.

Koren, J. (1899). *Economic Aspects of the Liquor Problem.* Houghton Mifflen.

Leininger, M.M. (ed.). (1978). *Transcultural Nursing: Theories, Concepts and Practices.* New York: John Wiley and Sons.

Leininger, M.M. (1991). Leininger's sunrise model to depict the theory of cultural care, diversity and universality. In *Culture, Care, Diversity and Universality: A Theory of Nursing.* New York: National League for Nursing Press.

Leininger, M.M. (1996). *Transcultural Nursing: Concepts, Theories, Research and Practices* (2nd ed.). Hillard, OH: McGraw-Hill.

Levinthal, C.F. (1996). *Drugs, Behavior and Modern Society.* Boston, MA: Allyn and Bacon.

Lin, I.H., and Lu, A.Y.K. (1997). Role of pharmaco kinetics and metabolism in drug discovery and development. *Pharmacological Review 49*(4), 403–449.

Lolli, G., Serianni, E., Golder, G.M., and Luzzatto-Fegiz (1958). *Alcohol in Italian Culture.* Glucol, IL: Free Press.

Makimoto, K. (1998). Drinking patterns and drinking problems among Asian Americans and Pacific Islanders. *Alcohol, Health and Research World 22*(4), 270–275.

Mann, A. (1992). From immigration to acculturation. In L.S. Luedtke (ed.), *Making America: The Society and Culture of the United States.* Chapel Hill, NC: University of North Carolina Press.

Maquet, J. (1972). *Africanity.* (J. Rayfield, trans.). New York: Oxford Press.

Marcos, L.R. (1979). Effects of interpreters on the evaluation of psychopathology in non-English speaking patients. *American Journal of Psychiatry 136,* 171–174.

McLaughlin, P., Raymond, J., Murakami, S., and Gilbert, D. (1987). Drug use among Asian-Americans in Hawaii. *Journal of Psychoactive Drugs 19,* 85–94.

McNeese, C., and DiNetto, D. (1994). *Chemical Dependency: A Systems Approach.* Englewood Cliffs, NJ: Prentice Hall.

Novak, M. (1972). *Rise of the Unmeltable Ethics.* New York: MacMillan Company.

Novotny, T., Warner, K.E., and Remington, P.L. (1988). Socioeconomic factors and racial smoking differences in the United States. *American Journal of Public Health 78,* 1187.

Orleans, C.T., Schoenback, V.J., Salmon, M.A., Strecher, V.J., Kalsbeek, W., Quade, D., Brooks, E.F., Konrad, T.R., Blackmon, C., and Watts, C.D. (1989). A survey of smoking and quitting patterns among black Americans. *American Journal of Public Health 79*(2), 176.

Pozzetta, G. (1995). Italian Americans. In J. Galens, A. Sheets, and R.V. Young (eds.), *Gale Encyclopedia of Multicultural America*. New York: Gale Research.

Prendergast, M., Maton, K., and Baker, R. (1989). Substance abuse among black youth. *Prevention Research Update 4*. Western Center for Drug Free Schools and Communities.

Prochaska, J.O., DiClemente, C.C., and Norcross, J.C. (1992). In search of how people change: Applications to addictive behaviors. *American Psychologist 49*, 1102.

Ramirez, A.C., and Gallion, K.J. (1993). Nicotine dependence among blacks and Hispanics. In C.T. Orleans and J. Slade (eds.), *Nicotine Addiction Principles and Management*. New York: Oxford Press.

Randolph, W.M., Stroup-Benham, C., Black, S., and Markides, K.S. (1998). Alcohol use among Cuban-Americans, Mexican-Americans, and Puerto-Ricans. *Alcohol, Health and Research World 22*(4), 265–269.

Rapple, B.A. (1995). Irish Americans. In J. Galens, A. Sheets, and R.V. Young (eds.), *Gale Encyclopedia of Multicultural America*. New York: Gale Research.

Ray, O., and Ksir, C. (1996). *Drugs, Society and Human Behavior* (6th ed.). St. Louis, MO: Mosby.

Reyes, M. (1998). Latina lesbians and alcohol and other drugs: Social work implications. In M. Delgado (ed.), *Alcohol Use/Abuse Among Latinos*. Binghamton, NY: Haworth Press.

Room, R. (1985). Forward. In L.A. Bennett and G.M. Ames (eds.), *The American Experience with Alcohol: Contrasting Cultural Perspectives*. New York: Plenum Press.

Royce, J.M., Hymowitz, N., Corbet, K., Hartwell, T., and Orlandi, M. (1993). Smoking cessation factors among African Americans and whites. *American Journal of Public Health 83*, 220.

Sabogal, F., Marin, G, Otero-Sabogal, R. et al. (1987). Hispanic familialism and acculturation: What changes and what doesn't. *Hispanic Journal of Behavioral Sciences 9*(4), 397–412.

Sadoun, R., Lolli, G., and Silverman, M. (1965). *Drinking in French Culture*. New Brunswick, NJ: Rutgers Center of Alcohol Studies.

Saseo, T. (1987). Patterns of drug use and health related practices among Japanese Americans. Unpublished manuscript.

Saseo, T. (1991). *Statewide Asian Drug Service Needs Assessment*. Sacramento, CA: Department of Alcohol and Drug Programs.

Segal, B. (1992). Ethnicity and drug-taking behavior. *Drugs and Society 6*, 269–312.

Simboli, B.J. (1985). Acculturated Italian-American drinking behaviors. In L.A. Bennett and G.M. Ames (eds.), *The American Experience with Alcohol: Contrasting Cultural Perspectives*. New York: Plenum Press.

Skager, R., Fisher, D., and Maddahian, E.A. (1986). *A Statewide Survey of Drug and Alcohol Use Among California Students in Grades 7, 9, and 11*. Sacramento, CA: Office of the Attorney General, Crime Prevention Center.

Skager, R., Frith, S., and Maddahian, E. (1989). *Biennial Survey of Drug and Alcohol Use Among California Students in Grades 7, 9, and 11*. Sacramento, CA: Office of the Attorney General, Crime Prevention Center.

Snyder, D. (1958). *Alcohol and the Jews*. New Haven, CT: Yale University Press.

Spector, R.E. (1996). *Cultural Diversity in Health and Illness*. Norwalk, CT: Appleton and Lange.

Stivers, R. (1976). *A Hair of the Dog: Irish Drinking and American Stereotype*. University Park, PA: Pennsylvania State University Press.

Stivers, R. (1985). Historical meanings of Irish-American drinking. In L.A. Bennett and G.M. Ames (eds.), *The American Experience with Alcohol: Contrasting Cultural Perspectives*. New York: Plenum Press.

Substance Abuse and Mental Health Services Administration, Office of Applied Studies. (1995). *National Household Survey Population Estimates, 1994.* Rockville, MD: U.S. Department of Health and Human Services.

Substance Abuse and Mental Health Services Administration, Office of Applied Studies. (1997). *National Household Survey on Drug Abuse Main Findings 1995.* Rockville, MD: U.S. Department of Health and Human Services.

Substance Abuse and Mental Health Services Administration. (July 6, 1998). SAMHSA News Release.

Substance Abuse and Mental Health Services Administration. (1998). *Prevalence of Substance Use Among Racial and Ethnic Subgroups in the United States 1991–1993.* Rockville, MD: U.S. Department of Health and Human Services.

Sue, S. (1998). Psychotherapeutic services for ethnic minorities: Two decades of research findings. *American Psychologist 43*(4), 301–308.

Sue, D., and Sue, S. (1987). Cultural factors in the assessment of Asian Americans. *Journal of Consulting and Clinical Psychology 55,* 479–487.

Umunna, I. (1967). The drinking culture of a Nigerian community. *Quarterly Journal Studies of Alcohol 28,* 529.

U.S. Bureau of the Census. (1991). *1990 Census.* Washington, DC: U.S. Government Printing Office.

U.S. Bureau of the Census, Population Division. (1997). *Resident Population of the United States: Estimates by Age, Sex, Race, and Hispanic Origin, with Median Age.* (www.gov/population/estimates/nation/infile3-1.tst).

U.S. Department of Health and Human Services. Alcohol, Drug Abuse, and Mental Health Administration—Drug Abuse and Drug Abuse Research (USDHHS-ADAMHA). (1991). *The Third Triennial Report to Congress.* Rockville, MD: USDHHS Public Health Service.

Vaillant, G.E. (1995). *The Natural History of Alcohol Revisited.* Cambridge: Harvard University Press.

Vecoli, R.J. (1995). Introduction. In J. Galens, A. Sheets, and R.V. Young (eds.), *Gale Encyclopedia of Multicultural America.* New York: Gale Research.

Voght, I. (1995). Germany. In D.B. Health (ed.), *International Handbook on Alcohol and Culture.* Westport, CT: Greenwood Press.

von Wormer, K. (1995). *Alcoholism Treatment: A Social Work Perspective.* Chicago, IL: Nelson-Hall.

Wagenknecht, L., Cutter, G., Halley, N., Sidney, S., Manolio, T., Hughes, G., and Jacobs, D. (1990). Racial differences in serum cotinine levels among smokers in the coronary artery risk development in (young) adults study. *American Journal of Public Health 80,* 1053.

Weibel-Orlando, J. (1993). Culture-specific treatment modalities: Assessing client-to-treatment fit in Indian alcoholism programs. In E.M. Freeman (ed.), *Substance Abuse Treatment: A Family Systems Perspective.* Newbury Park, CA: Sage.

Welt, J.W., and Barnes, G.M. (1987). Alcohol use among adolescent minority groups. *Journal of Studies on Alcohol 48,* 329.

Wright, R., Kail, B., and Creecy, R. (1990). Culturally sensitive social work practice with black alcoholics and their families. In S. Logan, E. Freeman, and R. McRay (eds.), *Social Work Practice with Black Families.* White Plains, NY: Longman.

Yamamoto, J., Lee, C., Lin, K., and Cho, K. (1987). Alcohol abuse in Koreans. *American Journal of Social Psychiatry 4,* 210–214.

Yeh, M., Takeuchi, D.T., and Sue, S. (1994). Asian-American children treated in the mental health system: A comparison of parallel and mainstream outpatient service centers. *Journal of Clinical Child Psychology 23*(1), 5–12.

Zane, N., and Huh-Kim, J. (1994). Substance use and abuse among Asian Pacific Americans. In N. Zane, D. Takeuchi, and R.K. Young (eds.), *Cultural Competence for Evaluators* (Vol. 2). Rockville, MD: Substance Abuse Prevention Office.

Zane, N., and Saseo, T. (1992). Research on drug abuse among Asian Pacific Americans. In J.E. Trimble, C. Bolek, and S. Niemcryk (eds.), *Ethnic and Multicultural Drug Abuse.* Binghamton, NY: Harrington Park.

6

Adult Health: Primary Care

Carl A. Kirton, RN, MA, ACRN, ANP-CS

LEARNER OUTCOMES

On completion of this chapter, the learner will be able to:

1. Identify the common health effects of substance use.
2. Identify components of substance use history in the primary care setting.
3. Select an appropriate screening tool for alcohol use in primary care settings.
4. Select an appropriate screening tool for drug use in primary care settings.
5. Screen the client who uses tobacco for nicotine dependence.
6. Identify the key physical and laboratory parameters indicative of substance use.
7. Accurately apply the diagnosis of problem use, abuse, or dependence on alcohol, tobacco, or drugs to clients in a primary care setting.
8. Identify primary care treatments used for clients with substance use problems.

KEY TERMS

alanine aminotransferase (ALT)	gamma-glutamyltransferase (GGT)	rhinophyma
angioma	immunoassay	sensitivity
aspartate aminotransferase (AST)	moderate drinker	specificity
atrophic glossitis	palmar erythema	spider nevi
brief intervention strategies	predictive value	substance misuse

Use of alcohol, tobacco, and illicit substances is linked to major public health problems that directly or indirectly affect the health and welfare of children, adolescents, adults, and elders. The health effects of substance use are enormous and known to be responsible for up to 26 percent of general medical clinic visits (Sullivan and Fleming, 1997) and thought to be responsible for more than 500,000 deaths annually (McGinnis and Foege, 1993). Use also confers significant economic, social, occupational, and recreational burdens on both users and nonusers, all of which affect the health of individuals and society.

Because substance use has an enormous impact on health, screening persons for use, misuse, and abuse is elemental to the provision of primary health care. Unfortunately, not all primary care providers (PCPs) incorporate substance use screening into their practices. According to the 1992 Primary Care Physician Survey, 63 percent of providers routinely screen for alcohol use, and 34 percent routinely inquire about drug use (USDHHS, 1998). A *Healthy People 2000* objective is to increase the proportion of PCPs who screen and counsel for alcohol and other drug use problems. Substance abuse is a preventable illness, and the advanced practice clinician must be skilled at identifying individuals at risk. Practitioners should be equally skilled in creating treatment plans for at-risk individuals and clients with addictive disorders.

Common Health Problems Related to Substance Use

The health effects of substance use are numerous and affect many body systems. In primary care, clients often seek treatment for signs and symptoms of **substance misuse** and abuse; unless screening is adequate, the clinician will not link these problems to a pattern of use or interpret such links to clients. As a result, the client remains ignorant about the implications of substance use. This reinforces denial and may lead to an eventual problem that adversely affects the client's health (see Table 6-1). This situation is increasingly problematic inasmuch as advanced practice curricula are often taught from a problem-oriented approach and include little education in prevention, assessment, and treatment of substance-related health problems.

Because of the importance of substance use in primary care practice, a discussion of the screening and treatment of substance use in the primary care setting follows. Mechanisms and rationale for the referral of clients to other providers who can assist in the treatment of substance use disorders are also addressed.

Primary Care Substance-Related Assessment, Prevention, and Interventions

Screening and History Taking

Second to the client-provider interaction, the client history is the most meaningful component of the primary care encounter. The history is used to collect data about the client for the purposes of making diagnoses about health problems. The history also helps the clinician to

TABLE 6-1 Signs and Symptoms of Substance Misuse and Abuse.*

Narcotics	Stimulants
Dilated pupils	Decreased fatigue
Runny nose	Alertness
Yawning	Increased initiative
Drowsiness	Talkativeness
Nausea	Wakefulness
Watery eyes	Mood elevation
Anorexia	Tachypnea
Restlessness	Tremors
Insomnia	Vasomotor center stimulation
Tachypnea	Loss of appetite
Elevated or lowered blood pressure	Weight loss
Hyperactive bowel sounds	Increased gastrointestinal motility
Euphoria	Increased heart rate and blood pressure
Insensitivity to pain	Pale and diaphoretic skin
Cold moist skin	Restlessness
Piloerection	Dizziness
	Tremors
	Hyperactivity
	Confusion
Depressants	**Cocaine**
Sedation	Feeling of well-being followed by depression
Drowsiness	Brief intense euphoria
Dizziness	Excitement
Dry mouth	Restlessness
Increased or decreased heart rate	Increased heart rate and blood pressure
Dilated pupils	Runny nose
Depressed breathing	Dry sniffles
Uncoordinated movements	
Confused behavior	
Difficulty in operating equipment	
Hallucinogens	**Alcohol**
Nystagmus	Slurred speech
Hypertension	Impaired coordination
Tachycardia	Slowed reflexes
Bizarre behavior	Unsteady gait
Agitation	Relaxed inhibition
Hallucinations	Alcohol smell on breath
Delusions	Glazed eyes
Altered mood and perceptions	Frequently used in combination with depressants,
Detail focused	antidepressants, and stimulants
Anxiety attacks	
Violent without apparent cause	

*These are general signs and symptoms, and the list is not all inclusive. Mixtures of substances may also present differently.

Source: From Kemp, D. (1989). Evaluating chemical dependency in critical care nurses. In S. Cardin and C.R. Ward (eds.), *Personnel Management in Critical Care Nursing,* p. 181. Baltimore: Williams & Wilkins.

determine if emotional, behavioral, cognitive, and environmental stimuli are contributing factors in substance use.

Standard health histories often include simple questions that ask if the client uses alcohol, drugs, or tobacco. Unfortunately, when all categories are addressed with only one or two questions, few data are obtained. Clients should be asked about substance use at the initial health intake visit and then periodically thereafter. Adolescents and older adults should be asked about substance use every time they seek medical treatment (Sullivan and Fleming, 1997). Adolescence is a common time of experimentation with alcohol and drugs (particularly marijuana). Older adults are prescribed drugs more frequently than persons in any other age group; although their drinking patterns fluctuate from light to moderate, approximately 8 percent of them have drinking problems.

Because both alcohol and drug use have negative social connotations, clients may feel embarrassed or ashamed about acknowledging use of illicit substances. Clients who are **moderate drinkers** (defined by the National Institute on Alcohol Abuse and Alcoholism as 9 drinks or less per week for women and 14 drinks or less per week for men) or recreational drug users may not disclose use because they do not believe that their drinking or drug use is problematic and that it is therefore inconsequential to their health.

When questioning clients about their substance use, the examiner must be sensitive to the meaning of the question, as the manner in which it is asked may influence the client's response. For example, asking the client, "Do you drink or do drugs?" may convey a tone that is judgmental and paternalistic. A direct question such as "How much do you drink?" or "How often do you use a drug [over-the-counter, prescription, or street drug]?" is more matter-of-fact and may convey to the client that the provider acknowledges that people use alcohol, tobacco, and other drugs. A client who denies currently using any drugs should be asked about a previous history of substance use, as this information may be important to assessing the client's chief complaint. Similarly, clients should be asked about the number of and frequency with which cigarettes are smoked.

An appropriate screening tool should be used to further classify a positive response to any one of these questions. These tools are not diagnostic instruments; rather, they assist the advanced practice clinician to better clarify if problem or excessive drinking or drug use exists. Screening tools for substance-related problems are widely available, but not all screening tools are valid and reliable for use with all groups. When the clinician is knowledgeable about available tools and their use in appropriate client populations, the **sensitivity** (ability of a test to detect disease), accuracy, and relevance to the assessment increase.

SCREENING FOR ALCOHOL USE

The screening instrument most widely used in primary care settings is the CAGE, a four-item questionnaire used to screen for the presence of alcohol abuse or dependence (Table 6-2). Although the tool is popular, it does not perform consistently with respect to age, gender, and ethnicity, making it less sensitive than other longer instruments such as the Alcohol Use Disorders Identification Test (AUDIT). It appeals to providers because of its brevity.

The tool is designed to estimate the magnitude of a drinking problem. A single positive response to a question on the CAGE tool indicates that drinking patterns warrant further investigation. Two or more positive responses to the questionnaire strongly suggest the probability that problem drinking or alcohol dependence is present.

TABLE 6-2 CAGE Screening Tool.

C: Have you ever felt you ought to **Cut down** on your drinking?

A: Have people **Annoyed** you by criticizing your drinking?

G: Have you ever felt bad or **Guilty** about your drinking?

E: Have you ever had a drink first thing in the morning (an **Eye-opener**) to steady your nerves or get rid of a hangover?

Scoring: 1 positive response warrants further investigation by the health care provider; 2 positive responses suggest alcohol dependence; and 4 positive responses indicate alcohol dependence.

Source: Reprinted by permission of the American Psychiatric Association. From Mayfield, D., McLeod, G., and Hall, P. (1974). The CAGE questionnaire: Validation of a new alcoholism instrument. *American Journal of Psychiatry 131,* 1121–1123.

The advanced practice nurse (APN) should know that although the CAGE is widely used, its ability to detect problem drinking in individuals in certain groups is highly variable. In the older adult, a single positive response warrants further investigation. This is because the physical changes that occur with aging cause the older adult to develop severe intoxication with less alcohol consumption than the younger adult. Debate continues about valid tools for problem drinking in this population. In tool comparison studies, investigators have identified the CAGE as being significantly more effective than the Michigan Alcoholism Screening Test (MAST) with elderly clients (Jones et al., 1993; Maisto, 1995). To screen an elderly client, the clinician may consider using the Michigan Alcoholism Screening Test— Geriatrics version (MAST-G), which was specifically designed for this population (see Table 6-3). This tool is a simple yes/no questionnaire with 24 items. With a score of 5 or greater, the MAST-G has a sensitivity of 70 percent and a **specificity** (ability to rule out the presence of a disease) of 81 percent in detecting problem drinking in the older adult (Morton, Jones, and Managaro, 1996). The number of questions ($N = 24$) limits the tool's use in the primary care setting because the administration time may often exceed 10 minutes.

Several researchers have demonstrated that the CAGE is a relatively weak predictor of alcohol-related problems in adolescents, young adults, and women (Heck and Williams, 1995; O'Hare and Tran, 1997). The CAGE questionnaire has also been shown to be an inconsistent indicator of alcohol use disorders when used in male and female primary care clients of different racial and ethnic backgrounds (Volk, Cantor, Steinbauer, and Cass, 1997). To screen the adolescent client, the RAFFT tool has been devised (Gerchufsky, 1996) (see Table 6-4). It, like the CAGE, is appealing because of its brevity.

Because of social stigma, women are more likely to feel guilty about their drinking; this may result in a false-positive on the "guilt" part of the CAGE test. The T-ACE, which uses three of the questions on the CAGE test, adapts to this possibility (Gerchufsky, 1996) (see Table 6-5). Like its counterpart, the T-ACE can be administered in approximately one minute. Unlike the CAGE, this tool has only been widely tested in age groups considered to be of childbearing potential and not general medical populations. Therefore, the **predictive value** (number of true positives) is limited in primary care populations, and its applicability must be carefully considered.

To overcome some of the limitations of the CAGE or to more fully evaluate a problem suggested by other data, the provider may consider using the AUDIT (see Table 6-6). This

TABLE 6-3 Michigan Alcoholism Screening Test–Geriatrics Version (MAST-G).

Directions: The following is a list of questions about your past and present drinking habits. Please answer yes or no to each question by marking the line next to the question. When you are finished answering the questions, please add up how many "yes" responses you checked and put that number in the space provided at the end.

	YES (1)	NO (2)
After drinking, have you ever noticed an increase in your heart rate or a beating in your chest?		
When talking with others, do you ever underestimate how much you actually drink?		
Does alcohol make you sleepy so that you often fall asleep in your chair?		
After a few drinks, have you sometimes not eaten or been able to skip a meal because you didn't feel hungry?		
Does having a few drinks help decrease your shakiness or tremors?		
Does alcohol sometimes make it hard for you to remember parts of the day or night?		
Do you have rules for yourself that you won't drink before a certain time of the day?		
Have you lost interest in hobbies or activities you used to enjoy?		
When you wake up in the morning, do you ever have trouble remembering part of the night before?		
Does having a drink help you sleep?		
Do you hide your alcohol bottles from family members?		
After a social gathering, have you ever felt embarrassed because you drank too much?		
Have you ever been concerned that drinking might be harmful to your health?		
Do you like to end an evening with a nightcap?		
Did you find your drinking increased after someone close to you died?		
In general, would you prefer to have a few drinks at home rather than go out to social events?		
Are you drinking more now than in the past?		
Do you usually take a drink to relax or calm your nerves?		
Do you drink to take your mind off your problems?		
Have you ever increased your drinking after experiencing a loss in your life?		
Do you sometimes drive when you have had too much to drink?		
Has a doctor or nurse ever said he or she was worried or concerned about your drinking?		
Have you ever made rules to manage your drinking?		
When you feel lonely, does having a drink help?		
TOTAL "YES" response		

Scoring: 5 or more "yes" responses is indicative of an alcohol problem.

Source: Blow, F.C., Brower, K.J., Schulenberg, J.E., Demo-Dananberg, L.M., Young, J.P., and Beresford, T.P. (1992). The Michigan Alcoholism Screening Test—Geriatric Version (MAST-G): A new specific screening instrument. *Alcoholism: Clinical and Experimental Research 16,* 372.

TABLE 6-4 RAFFT Screening Tool.

R: Do you drink to **relax**, to feel better about yourself, or to fit in?

A: Do you drink **alone**?

F: Do any of your close **friends** drink?

F: Does anyone in your **family** have an alcohol problem?

T: Have you ever gotten into **trouble** for drinking?

Scoring: 1 positive response warrants further investigation by the health care provider; 2 positive responses suggest alcohol dependence; and 4 positive responses indicate alcohol dependence.

Source: Reprinted by permission from Riggs, S.R., and Alario, A. (1989). Adolescent substance use instructor's guide. In C. Dube, M. Goldstein, D. Lewis, E. Meyers, and W. Zwick (eds.), *Project ADEPT Curriculum for Primary Care Physician Training,* Vol. II, pp. 1–57. Providence, RI: Brown University.

TABLE 6-5 T-ACE Screening Tool.

T: How many drinks does it **take** to make you feel drunk?

A: Have people **annoyed** you by criticizing your drinking?

C: Have you ever considered **cutting** down on your drinking?

E: Have you ever used alcohol as an **eye-opener**?

Scoring: 1 positive response warrants further investigation by the health care provider; 2 positive responses suggest alcohol dependence; and 4 positive responses indicate alcohol dependence.

Source: Sokol, R.J., Martier, S.S., and Ager, J.W. (1989). The T-ACE questions: Practical prenatal detection of risk drinking. *American Journal of Obstetrics and Gynecology 60,* 863–870.

tool has been tested in primary care settings in several different countries and has validity across cultural backgrounds, age, and gender (Babor, de la Fuente, Saunders, and Grant, 1992). Clay (1997) compared the CAGE tool to the AUDIT and found that the AUDIT identified more clients with problem drinking. The AUDIT is a 10-item instrument; on completion, a score is obtained. A score of zero is indicative of a nondrinker, whereas a score of 8 or more suggests problem drinking. The maximum score that can be obtained on the AUDIT is 40 points. With a score of 8 points, the sensitivity of this test is 61 percent and specificity is 90 percent (O'Conner, 1996).

SCREENING FOR DRUG ABUSE

Very few instruments are felt to be valid screening tools for clients who abuse drugs. One tool is the Drug Abuse Screening Test (DAST) (see Table 6-7), which is a 28-item tool originally designed to quantify the extent of an individual's drug use (O'Conner, 1996). The DAST is lengthy and therefore limited in use in high-volume clinical settings. Clinicians may prefer to use a tool that is similar to the CAGE for alcohol screening that has been adapted to screen for drugs; it is called the CAGE—AID (see Table 6-8). This tool has been tested in primary care populations (Brown and Rounds, 1995). However, Sullivan and Fleming (1997) point out that this tool is more effective in identifying drug use and may not be sensitive enough to detect a problem in clients who have not experienced any negative effects, such as health problems, legal difficulties, and family disruption from their drug use.

TABLE 6-6 Alcohol Use Disorders Identification Test (AUDIT).

1. How often do you have a drink containing alcohol?

	(Score)
[ ] Never	(0)
[ ] Monthly or less	(1)
[ ] Two to four times a month	(2)
[ ] Two to three times a week	(3)
[ ] Four or more times a week	(4)

2. How many drinks containing alcohol do you have on a typical day when you are drinking?

	(Score)
[ ] 1 or 2	(0)
[ ] 3 or 4	(1)
[ ] 5 or 6	(2)
[ ] 7 to 9	(3)
[ ] 10 or more	(4)

3. How often do you have six or more drinks on one occasion?

	(Score)
[ ] Never	(0)
[ ] Less than monthly	(1)
[ ] Monthly	(2)
[ ] Weekly	(3)
[ ] Daily or almost daily	(4)

4. How often during the last year have you not been able to stop drinking once you had started?

	(Score)
[ ] Never	(0)
[ ] Less than monthly	(1)
[ ] Monthly	(2)
[ ] Weekly	(3)
[ ] Daily or almost daily	(4)

5. How often during the last year have you failed to do what was normally expected from you because of drinking?

	(Score)
[ ] Never	(0)
[ ] Less than monthly	(1)
[ ] Monthly	(2)
[ ] Weekly	(3)
[ ] Daily or almost daily	(4)

6. How often during the last year have you needed a first drink in the morning to get yourself going after a heavy drinking session?

	(Score)
[ ] Never	(0)
[ ] Less than monthly	(1)
[ ] Monthly	(2)
[ ] Weekly	(3)
[ ] Daily or almost daily	(4)

7. How often during the last year have you had a feeling of guilt or remorse after a drink?

	(Score)
[ ] Never	(0)
[ ] Less than monthly	(1)
[ ] Monthly	(2)
[ ] Weekly	(3)
[ ] Daily or almost daily	(4)

8. How often during the last year have you been unable to remember what happened the night before because you had been drinking?

	(Score)
[ ] Never	(0)
[ ] Less than monthly	(1)
[ ] Monthly	(2)
[ ] Weekly	(3)
[ ] Daily or almost daily	(4)

9. Have you or someone else been injured as a result of your drinking?

	(Score)
[ ] No	(0)
[ ] Yes, but not in the last year	(2)
[ ] Yes, during the last year	(4)

10. Has a relative or friend, or a doctor or other health worker, been concerned about your drinking or suggested you cut down?

	(Score)
[ ] No	(0)
[ ] Yes, but not in the last year	(2)
[ ] Yes, during the last year	(4)

Procedure for Scoring AUDIT

Questions 1–8 are scored 0, 1, 2, 3, or 4. Questions 9 and 10 are scored 0, 2, or 4 only. The minimum score (for nondrinkers) is 0, and the maximum possible score is 40. A score of 8 or more indicates a strong likelihood of hazardous or harmful alcohol consumption.

Source: Babor, T.F., de la fuente, J.R., Saunders, J., and Grant, M. AUDIT: The Alcohol Use Disorders Test: Guidelines for Use in Primary Health Care. Geneva: World Health Organization (1992).

TABLE 6-7 Drug Abuse Screening Test (DAST).

1. Have you used drugs other than those required for medical reasons?

2. Have you abused prescription drugs?

3. Do you abuse more than one drug at a time?

4. Can you get through the week without using drugs (other than those required for medical reasons)?*

5. Are you always able to stop using drugs when you want to?*

6. Do you abuse drugs on a continuous basis?

7. Do you try to limit your drug use to certain situations?*

8. Have you had "blackouts" or "flashbacks" as a result of drug use?

9. Do you ever feel bad about your drug abuse?

10. Does your spouse (or parents) ever complain about your involvement with drugs?

11. Do your friends or relatives know or suspect you abuse drugs?

12. Has drug abuse ever created problems between you and your spouse?

13. Has any family member ever sought help for problems related to your drug use?

14. Have you ever lost friends because of your use of drugs?

15. Have you ever neglected your family or missed work because of your use of drugs?

16. Have you ever been in trouble at work because of drug abuse?

17. Have you ever lost a job because of drug abuse?

18. Have you gotten into fights when under the influence of drugs?

19. Have you ever been arrested because of unusual behavior while under the influence of drugs?

20. Have you ever been arrested for driving while under the influence of drugs?

21. Have you engaged in illegal activities to obtain drugs?

22. Have you ever been arrested for possession of illegal drugs?

23. Have you ever experienced withdrawal symptoms as a result of heavy drug intake?

24. Have you had medical problems as a result of your drug use (e.g., memory loss, hepatitis, convulsions, or bleeding)?

25. Have you ever gone to anyone for help for a drug problem?

26. Have you ever been in a hospital for medical problems related to your drug use?

27. Have you ever been involved in a treatment program specifically related to drug use?

28. Have you been treated as an outpatient for problems related to drug abuse?

Scoring: A score of greater than 5 requires further evaluation for substance abuse problems.

*Items 4, 5, and 7 are scored in the "no" or false direction.

Source: Reprinted from Skinner, H.A. (1982). The Drug Abuse Screening Test. *Addictive Behavior 7*(4), 363–371 with permission from Elsevier Science.

TABLE 6-8 CAGE-AID Screening Tool.

C: Have you ever felt you ought to **cut down** on your drug use?

A: Have people **annoyed** you by criticizing your drug use?

G: Have you ever felt bad or **guilty** about your drug use?

E: Have you ever used drugs first thing in the morning (an **eye-opener**) to steady your nerves or get rid of a hangover?

Scoring: 1 positive response warrants further investigation by the health care provider; 2 positive responses suggest drug dependence; and 4 positive responses indicate drug dependence.

Source: Reproduced by permission. From Brown, R.L., and Rounds, L.A. (1995). Conjoint screening questionnaires for alcohol and drug abuse. *Wisconsin Medical Journal 94*, 135–140.

SCREENING FOR TOBACCO USE

Clients who smoke cigarettes or use tobacco products, such as chewing tobacco or snuff, often readily acknowledge this when asked; therefore, screening tools are generally not necessary. However, clients often minimize their use when reporting it with statements such as "I only smoke a little," or "I only smoke on weekends," or "I only have a cigarette or two." The negative effects of these substances on health are well known to some clients and most providers. The advanced practice clinician must know that no level of tobacco use has been determined to be safe.

Smoking as few as one to four cigarettes a day increases the risk of coronary artery disease and nonfatal myocardial infarction by a factor of 2.5 over nonsmokers (Andrews, 1998). Addiction to nicotine, the reason people smoke, can occur as a result of smoking as little as four cigarettes (Plantz and Adler, 1998). The APN needs to understand the physiological dependence (nicotine addiction) and psychological models (learned behaviors) that seek to explain smoking behaviors. Knowledge of these models facilitates choices about selecting and evaluating appropriate treatment strategies for tobacco-addicted clients. It is noteworthy that one tenet of psychological theories is based on evidence that demonstrates a strong association between depression and smoking. Depression is twice as common among those who smoke than in people who have never smoked and has been linked to increased smoking initiation and to failures in smoking cessation efforts (Andrews, 1998). Providers must be certain to screen all smokers for symptoms of depression as well as to obtain an accurate history of tobacco use (Rigotti, 1995) (see Table 6-9).

OBTAINING HISTORY OF SUBSTANCE USE

Positive outcomes of screening tests warrant further investigation. The history should provide the clinician with information about the type, pattern of use, and frequency of substance use as well as the presence of mild, moderate, or severe addiction. Treatment plans can then be developed for the client. Inquiries into the types, amount, frequency, and patterns of use help the clinician understand the client's knowledge and insight into his or her substance use. Key areas to be explored in the health history are outlined in Table 6-9.

Physical Examination and Laboratory Assessment

The physical examination is an adjunct to the client's history in the detection of alcohol- and drug-related problems. It cannot be used as a diagnostic measure because few physical signs are pathognomonic of early difficulties, problem drinking, or other substance use. Signs suggestive of substance abuse or dependence are detailed in Chapter 7. A few of these signs are briefly discussed here.

When assessing the skin, be alert to "red facies," which may be seen in the lightly pigmented person who drinks excessively or who smokes. The palms of the hands may be flushed as well **(palmar erythema). Spider nevi** and **angiomas** on the face are characteristic of excessive alcohol consumption but are not specific to this disorder. **Rhinophyma,** a bulbous nose or a "strawberry appearance" of the nose, has a statistical association with alcoholism, but not all clients with this finding are alcoholics. The clinician should assess the skin over the entire body for track marks that may indicate injection drug use.

TABLE 6-9 Substance Health History.

Pattern of use	• Frequency
	• Amount per occasion
	• Number of occasions per week
	• Circumstances of use
	• Amount required to feel desired effect
	• Presence of binges
	Tobacco use
	• The number of cigarettes smoked per day
	• The time of the first cigarette
Preoccupation and efforts to control	• Use when decided not to or used more than intended
	• Changes in the circumstances of use
	• Periods of abstinence or attempts to decrease amount
	• Feeling of loss of control over drinking or drug use
	Tobacco use
	• Periods of abstinence or attempts to decrease the number of cigarettes smoked
	• Ability to refrain from smoking in places where it is forbidden
Concern by self or others	• If yes, note who is the concerned individual and the reasons for concern
Problems resulting from use	• Briefly describe problems: social, medical, and legal
Family history	• Positive or negative for alcoholism or abuse
	• Positive or negative for other substance dependence or abuse
Prior treatment experiences	• If yes, when, where, and status after treatment. If tobacco, identify the type(s) of cessation strategy used

Source: Adapted from O'Conner, P.G. (1996). Routine screening and initial assessment. In J. Kinney (ed.), *Clinical Manual of Substance Assessment* (2nd ed.), pp. 40–56. St. Louis, MO: Mosby.

The nose and its internal structures should be carefully examined as inhalation of cocaine and heroin results in inflammation. Long-term use of these substances damages nasal structures. Nasal perforation or erosion of the anterior nares or vestibule is evidence of drug use by the intranasal route.

Chronic gingivitis and periodontitis may be seen in the client who drinks immoderately. Burns on the inside of the lip may be incurred from smoking crack or heroin. A smooth tongue (**atrophic glossitis**) often indicates a nutritional deficiency as a result of alcohol use.

The nail beds of the hand should be examined carefully. Clients who smoke cigarettes and marijuana often have staining of the nails and fingertips. Burns on the hand and fingers may also be seen as a result of injury that occurs when preparing substances such as crack cocaine. Long-term smoking results in clubbing of the fingers.

In the intravenous drug user, a heart murmur suggests that heart valves have accumulated a vegetative lesion transmitted by drug solutions or needles contaminated with skin flora, the latter being the most common source of infection. Other organisms can be implicated as well.

Evidence of drug use in the examination of the musculoskeletal system includes muscle wasting as a result of poor nutrition related to alcohol and drug use. Tremors may be evident.

The neurological exam of a heavy drug user indicates recent or remote memory loss, pupillary changes, and signs of cerebellar abnormalities.

Laboratory tests, when combined with a comprehensive health history and physical examination, can be used as adjuncts to identify clients who use or abuse alcohol or drugs. The most widely available tests to detect alcohol consumption are of limited use because they are only moderately specific and valid in establishing chronic alcohol intake. Recent alcohol intake is measurable only by direct alcohol measurement, such as a Breathalyzer test. Direct alcohol measurement is rarely necessary in the primary care setting, but the APN should be aware of simple signs such as alcohol on the breath that indicate the need for further investigation.

Using Laboratory Markers of Alcohol Ingestion

Several laboratory markers can be used to detect alcohol ingestion; however, most are only available to research and specialty labs. Laboratory markers used to detect alcohol consumption are listed in Table 6-10. The most common laboratory parameters used in the clinical setting are discussed here.

The mean corpuscular volume (MCV) is elevated in 31 percent to 96 percent of alcoholics (Ciraulo and Shader, 1991). However, it can also be elevated in certain types of anemias, menopause, elderly clients, and smokers, as well as a result of ingestion of certain drugs. The advanced practice clinician should evaluate an elevated MCV using a wide differential diagnostic list that includes problem drinking.

Gamma-glutamyltransferase (GGT) is a hepatic enzyme bound to liver cell membranes. It is elevated in alcoholics before the noticeable development of liver disease and correlates in magnitude with the quantity of alcohol consumed (Ciraulo and Shader, 1991). It is elevated in 34 percent to 85 percent of alcoholics or heavy drinkers. Women produce lower values of GGT than men; thus, the upper limit of normal range for women is lower than that for men (Allen, 1995). Women alcoholics have been observed to manifest pathologic changes earlier and at lower doses of alcohol than men.

The **aspartate aminotransferase (AST)** and **alanine aminotransferase (ALT)** can also be used to assess for evidence of chronic alcohol ingestion. These are less valid than other markers because the specificity of these tests is low. The AST/ALT ratio improves the usefulness of these tests. An AST/ALT ratio greater than 2 is suggestive of alcoholic liver disease and is highly sensitive but moderately specific.

Using Laboratory Markers of Drug Ingestion

Metabolites of drugs can be detected in the urine, feces, sweat, hair, and nails. When the PCP uses a laboratory method for the detection of drug use, the urinalysis is the most common method. Unlike other methods, examination of the urine is noninvasive, the specimen is easy to collect, and the cost of testing is relatively low.

Employees whose performance is impaired can have a significant impact on workplace and public safety. Screening employees for drug use is designed to reduce these effects and assist the employee in reducing and eliminating substance abuse problems. The designation of urine toxicologies for drug screening for federal employees was enacted in 1988 and revised in 1994 (USDHHS, 1988). Since then, the federal government has required drug screening of all workers, and it is estimated that more than half and as high as 75 percent of

TABLE 6-10 Biological Tests Used to Detect Alcohol Consumption over Various Ingestion Periods.

Test	Sensitivity[a]	Specificity[b]	Detection Limits[c] Amount	Time	Ease of Use[d]	Result Time[e]	Cost[f]	Availability[g]
Recent Intake (Direct alcohol measurement)								
Breath	High	High	Any	min/hr	Easy	min	Low	Wide
Blood	High	High	Any	min/hr	Easy	hr	Moderate	Clinical lab
Urine	High	High	Any	hr	Easy	hr	Moderate	Clinical lab
Saliva	High	Moderate	Any	min/hr	Easy	min	Low	Easy to get
Sweat	Moderate	High	Low	hr/days	Difficult	days	High	Research lab
Acute Intake								
5-hydroxytryptophol	High	Moderate	Low	hr/day	Very difficult	days/wk	High	Research lab
Beta-hexosaminidase	Moderate	Moderate	?Moderate	hr/day	Difficult	days/wk	Moderate	Research lab
Subacute Intake								
Carbohydrate-deficient transferrin	Moderate/ high	High	High	days/wk	Difficult	days	High	Reference lab
Acetaldehyde adducts	Moderate	?	High	days/wk	Very difficult	days/wk	High	Research lab
Chronic Intake (Liver tests)								
Gamma glutamyl-transferase	Moderate	Moderate/ high	High	wk/mo	Easy	hr/day	Moderate	Clinical lab
AST/ALT	Low	Low/ moderate	High	mo/yr	Easy	hr/day	Moderate	Clinical lab
Red blood cell mean corpuscular volume	Low	Low/ moderate	High	mo/yr	Easy	hr/day	Low	Clinical lab

[a] *Sensitivity* is the rate of detection of alcohol intake at the level indicated in column 1: low, <40%; moderate, 40–60%; high, 60–100%.

[b] *Specificity* is the ability of the test to indicate only alcohol consumption: low, <40%; moderate, 40–60%; high, 60–100%.

[c] *Detection limits* refer to the amount of alcohol over time possibly detected by that test: any, any amount; low, one or two drinks; moderate, <5 drinks/day; high, >5 drinks/day.

[d] *Ease of use* refers to the technical complexity required for performing the test.

[e] *Result time* alludes to the time it would take to obtain a result under normal circumstances.

[f] *Cost* of the test is given in relative terms. Low implies cost generally less than $10, moderate implies cost less than $50, and high suggests cost greater than $50. Some research tests have not had a commercial price established and therefore would be considered "high" based on the present technology. Note that although Breathalyzers have an initial cost of over $500, cost per administration is quite low.

[g] *Availability* identifies the type of facility in which the tests are performed routinely at this time. Except by special arrangements made with research laboratories, most tests need to be available in at least a reference laboratory to be easily accessible to most clinicians.

U.S. companies have employee drug-testing programs. Federal agencies or private establishments may contract with PCPs to conduct routine or pre-employment drug screening. The advanced practice clinician who assists with urine toxicology screening must be aware of collection procedures. Specific guidelines for workplace drug-testing programs are available in

Mandatory Guidelines for Federal Workplace Drug Testing Programs as published in the Federal Register on January 25, 1993 (58 FR 6062). The guidelines are also available online at www.health.org/GDLNS-94.htm.

Drug use can also be detected by analysis of the client's serum for drug metabolites. Basic drug screen panels are designed to detect the most commonly abused illicit drugs. Expanded drug screens that include other illicit drugs are available if required by the client's employer or contracting agencies. All screening tests are determined by a method called **immunoassay,** which is a laboratory technique using antibodies capable of recognizing and binding to drugs.

Specimens that test negative contain no drug or are below the cutoff level (see Table 6-11). All specimens identified as positive are confirmed using different analytical methods such as gas chromotography/mass spectrometry. Table 6-11 lists the classes of drugs detected in a basic drug screen level. The screening cutoff and confirmation cutoff are also listed. To accurately screen and use test information, the provider must also be cognizant of the optimal time of testing. False-positive drug tests can occur when the client either is using prescribed, therapeutic medications or ingests certain foods (see Table 6-12). A careful history helps to eliminate the possibility of false-positives.

TABLE 6-11 Basic Urine Screen for Illicit Drug Use.

Class	Screening Cutoff	Confirmation Cutoff
Amphetamines	1,000 ng/mL	Amphetamines, 500 ng/mL Methamphetamines, 500 ng/mL
Cannabinoids	50 ng/mL	THC-COOH, 15 ng/mL
Cocaine	300 ng/mL	Benzoyl ecgonine, 150 ng/mL
Opiates	300 ng/mL	Codeine, 300 ng/mL Morphine, 300 ng/mL
Phencyclidine	25 ng/mL	Phencyclidine, 25 ng/mL

TABLE 6-12 Drug Detection Time and False-Positive Results in a Basic Drug Screen.

Class	Length of Time Drug Can Be Detected in Days	May Cause False-Positive Results
Amphetamines	1–2 days	Chlorpromazine Excessive Nutra-Sweet® Pseudoephedrine ranitidine
Cannabinoids	Social use: 2–5 days Chronic use: 14–21 days	None known
Cocaine	2–4 days	None known
Opiates	2–3 days	Poppy seeds Dextromethorphan
Phencyclidine	Up to 14 days	Dextromethorphan Trihexyphenidyl

Using Laboratory Markers of Smoking Addiction

There are no specific laboratory tests that indicate excessive smoking. Findings in the arterial blood gas (ABG), such as hypoxemia or hypercarbia, occur as a result of the health effects of chronic tobacco use. There may be increases in the hematocrit, total white high-density lipoproteins, vitamin C levels, and albumin in the chronic smoker.

Diagnosis

The history, physical examination, and laboratory data are combined to determine the likelihood of a substance use disorder. Diagnostic criteria allow PCPs to plan treatment and monitor progress; make communication possible between clinicians and researchers; enable public health planners to ensure availability of treatment facilities; help health care insurers to decide whether treatment will be reimbursed; and allow clients access to medical insurance coverage (National Institute on Alcohol Abuse and Dependence, 1995). The most widely used criteria for accurate substance abuse or substance dependence diagnoses are detailed in *The Diagnostic and Statistical Manual of Psychiatric Disorders,* Fourth Edition (DSM-IV). Other diagnostic schemas exist. The World Health Organization (WHO) publishes the International Classification of Diseases (ICD) that includes criteria for all causes of death and illness. The ICD criteria for a substance abuse diagnosis are listed in Table 6-13. The PCP should be familiar with ICD coding criteria, as this schema is the classification system required by most fiscal agencies for reimbursement purposes.

TABLE 6-13 International Classification of Diseases (ICD-10) Criteria for a Substance-Related Diagnosis.

Criteria for a Substance Dependence Diagnosis

Three or more of the following must have been experienced or exhibited by the client at some time during the previous year:

- Difficulties in controlling substance-taking behavior in terms of its onset, termination, or levels of use
- A strong desire or sense of compulsion to take the substance
- Progressive neglect of alternate pleasures or interests because of psychoactive substance use; increase in amount of time necessary to obtain or take the substance or to recover from its effects
- Persisting with substance use despite clear evidence of overtly harmful consequences, depressive mood states consequent to heavy use, drug-related impairment of cognitive functioning, or familial or legal problems
- Evidence of tolerance, such as increased doses of the psychoactive substances are required in order to achieve desired effects originally produced by lower doses
- A physiological withdrawal state when substance use has ceased or been reduced, as evidenced by the characteristic withdrawal syndrome for the substance or use of the same (or a closely related) substance with the intention of relieving or avoiding withdrawal symptoms

Other Terms That May Be Used
Hazardous use: Use that places the person at risk for adverse consequences
Harmful use: Use resulting in physical or psychological harm

Source: Reproduced with permission from the World Health Organization.

Accuracy in the diagnosis of abuse or dependence is limited by the fact that a diagnosis is generally made after frequent long-term encounters with clients. In the general medical population, the infrequency of medical visits by individuals most at risk, such as adolescents, compromises the ability of the clinician to diagnose accurately. Intermittent use of substances and periods of abstinence further complicate the ability to arrive at an accurate diagnosis. To improve diagnostic accuracy, the clinician should always inquire about potential social complications that occur in the client's life as a result of substance use. The substance-abusing client often experiences repetitive negative social consequences as a result of this use. These include, but are not limited to, problems in relationships with family and friends; inability to fulfill school or work-related obligations; repetitive automobile, industrial, or personal injuries and accidents; arrest or traffic violations; and frequent health problems in a client who otherwise should be healthy.

The roles of the client's family members or significant others have been well established in identifying individuals at risk. Because early symptoms are often behavioral, family members are usually the first to notice changes in the client's behavior as a result of substance use. Whenever possible, the family should be included as part of the assessment. This is not, however, always feasible, especially when the client is seeking health care for other reasons. Family members who want to help a client often respond by being available for provider visits and giving a collateral history.

Treatment of Clients with Substance Use Problems

Treatment begins by informing the client of the diagnosis derived from the assessment. Clients who are low-risk drinkers should be counseled about continuing to drink in moderation. Table 6-14 lists practical advice that health care providers can convey to the low-risk drinker in order to avoid medical complications of alcohol. No safe limit of other drugs or cigarette smoking has been determined.

Clients with a substance use problem should be told of the assessment of their substance use in a straightforward but empathetic manner. Avoid language such as "I think you *may* have a problem with drugs or alcohol" or "You *might* have a problem with drugs or alcohol." Direct statements such as "You have signs that indicate you are alcohol-dependent" or "Your history indicates that you are addicted to drugs" convey certainty in the diagnosis. Use follow-up such as "I want to help you with your problem. The data from my examination suggest that there is a problem related to your use of _____ ." This imparts to the client that the caregiver has carefully considered the data and will assist the client in obtaining con-

TABLE 6-14 Recommendations for Low-Risk Alcohol Consumption.

A standard drink contains 12 grams of pure alcohol. A standard drink equals one 12-ounce bottle of beer or wine cooler, one 5-ounce glass of wine, or 1.5 ounces of distilled spirits.

Levels of Consumption with Lowest Risk for Health Outcomes

Men: no more than 2 drinks per day, or 14 drinks per week

Women: no more than 1 drink per day, or 7 drinks per week

Men and women over 65: no more than 1 drink per day and modified in relation to prescription drug intake

Source: Adapted from U.S. Department of Health and Human Services, Public Health Service, National Institutes of Health, National Institute on Alcohol Abuse and Alcoholism. (1995). *The Physicians Guide To Helping Patients With Alcohol Problems.* Washington, DC: Author.

trol over his or her addiction. When appropriate, the client should be provided with education or instruction about the data, such as an elevated GGT or a positive finding of urine testing, that support the diagnosis.

Undoubtedly, the client will respond to this type of direct statement. He or she may respond with surprise, anger, or denial. This response is important and should be carefully noted as it may help the clinician determine where the client is in acknowledging the problem. Prochaska and Goldstein (1991) provide a framework of readiness for changing behaviors that can be linked to the client's response (see Table 6-15). With knowledge of the client's readiness to change, the clinician can begin to contemplate an appropriate treatment plan for the client. The newly diagnosed client is likely to be in the precontemplation, contemplation, or preparation/determination stage. If the client is seeking care for substance use, the client is more likely to be in the latter stages of action: action, maintenance, and perhaps relapse.

Treatment strategies are designed after careful consideration of the client's clinical and social data. Treatment strategies and settings must be carefully matched to the client's level of substance use. Treatment strategies fall into three categories: (1) clients at risk for use problems (see Table 6-16); (2) clients with a substance abuse diagnosis; and (3) clients with a substance dependence diagnosis.

TABLE 6-15 Stages of Behavioral Change.

Precontemplation	The client does not see the behavior as a problem or does not want to change the behavior. This stage is sometimes characterized as "denial."
Contemplation	The client is beginning to understand that the behavior is causing difficulties in living or taking a toll in health or quality of life.
Preparation/Determination	The client is considering various options for change.
Action	The client is taking concrete steps to change the behavior in specific ways.
Maintenance	The client avoids relapsing to problem behaviors.
Relapse	The client slips back into problematic use or abuse.

Source: Adapted from Prochaska, J., DiClemente, C., and Norcross, J. (1992). In search of how people change. *American Psychologist 47*(9), 1102–1114.

TABLE 6-16 Risk Factors for Acute Alcohol Problems.

- Solitary drinking
- Lack of specific drinking norms
- Tolerance of drunkenness
- Social tolerance of negative behavior when drinking
- "Medicinal" use of alcohol to reduce tension
- Lack of ritualized and/or ceremonial use of alcohol
- Separation of alcohol use from overall eating patterns
- Lack of childhood socialization into drinking patterns
- Drinking with strangers
- Drinking pursued as recreation
- Drinking concentrated among young males
- Belief in a cultural milieu that stresses individualism, self-reliance, and high achievement

Source: O'Conner, P.G. (1996). Routine screening and initial assessment. In J. Kinney (ed.), *Clinical Manual of Substance Assessment* (2nd ed.), p. 49. St. Louis, MO: Mosby.

TREATING THE CLIENT WHO IS AT RISK FOR OR HAS PROBLEM DRINKING

Research findings suggest that treatment for the client at risk for problem drinking in the primary care setting can consist simply of an approach called **brief intervention strategies** (Sullivan and Fleming, 1997). This approach is a structured treatment strategy that focuses on informing and advising the client about the effects of substance use on his or her health status and linking consumption with evidence of negative health outcomes. The provider negotiates with the client about the need for change and monitors the client to evaluate the effectiveness of the intervention as indicated by behavioral change.

Over the past decade, research TIP has consistently demonstrated the effectiveness of the brief intervention as a treatment strategy (Sullivan and Fleming, 1997). It has been observed to be effective with a variety of drugs, settings, and client populations (Kinney and West, 1996). Finfgeld (1997) found that nurses were effective in facilitating resolution of problem drinking through brief intervention strategies. Senft and colleagues (1997) evaluated the effectiveness of brief interventions in a busy health maintenance organization (HMO) primary setting, and the interventions were found to result in a modest reduction in the frequency of alcohol consumption. In general, clients with recurrent and significant alcohol- or other drug-related problems that have interfered with role performance within the past 12 months; who have caused legal, social, or interpersonal problems; or who pose danger to themselves and others are less likely to respond to brief interventions (Sullivan and Fleming, 1997). Critical elements of brief intervention strategies used by the PCP are described in Table 6-17.

TABLE 6-17 Critical Elements of Brief Intervention Strategies.

Initial Visit

- Review findings of the laboratory and/or physical assessment with the client.

- Inform the client about the effects that alcohol may have on the client's current health status. For example, "Given your diabetes, obesity, smoking, high cholesterol, and drinking, your risk for developing heart disease far exceeds that of other clients your age."

- Advise clients with alcohol-related problems, medical problems, or medical problems that are exacerbated by alcohol consumption (e.g., hypertension, obesity, diabetes, hyperlipidemia) to eliminate alcohol from their diet.

- Counsel clients without comorbidities affected by alcohol ingestion about low-risk consumption (see Table 6-14).

- Talk with the client about a plan for change to reduce alcohol consumption. The plan should be direct and simple, with measurable outcomes. For example, "The client will reduce his daily intake of beer by two beers daily." Provide the client with a written plan and prepared educational materials.

- Provide a follow-up appointment; request that the client record consumption patterns.

Follow-up Visit

- Determine the client's ability to adhere to the proposed plan to reduce consumption. Consider verification or collaborative history (e.g., urine test, GGT, family interview) when and if appropriate.

- Provide clients who meet treatment goals with positive acknowledgment for their work and realistic support for the efforts involved. Work with the client to modify the plan to encourage further reduction in substance use.

Source: Adapted from Sullivan, E.F., and Fleming, M. (1997). A guide to substance abuse services for primary care clinicians. *Treatment Improvement Protocol (TIP) Series 24.* Substance Abuse and Mental Health Services Administration (SAMHSA), Center for Substance Abuse Treatment. Rockville, MD: U.S. Department of Health and Human Services.

Behavior change, even with brief intervention treatment, is difficult, and the provider should expect the client to have difficulty, at least initially, acting on the original, agreed-upon plan. Support in the form of self-help or support groups and individual or couples counseling may increase client compliance.

TREATING THE CLIENT WHO ABUSES ALCOHOL

The client with an alcohol abuse diagnosis should initially be provided with brief intervention strategies as described in Table 6-17. Repeated failures of brief intervention strategies as evidenced by continued abuse of drugs, including alcohol, warrant specialized treatment strategies and consultation with an expert in addictions care. The PCP, however, remains essential in coordinating, monitoring, and providing follow-up for the physical and psychological care of the client.

Depending on the evident effects of substance use on the client's health and well-being, initial intervention goals may only focus on reducing alcohol ingestion to acceptable levels (see Table 6-14), thereby anticipating a reduction in related abusive behaviors. The actual tasks agreed upon by the client and provider should be established in a written treatment plan.

A client who abuses alcohol has treatment needs of many dimensions, such as learning about the problem, recognizing the consequences of the problem, gaining alternate coping skills, and receiving family, financial, and vocational counseling and strategies to prevent relapse. It is unreasonable to expect that the PCP can provide all components of treatment. To assist in meeting the treatment goals, adjunctive therapies or expert addictions care is often warranted. The PCP should consider referring the client with a substance abuse diagnosis to self-help groups or centers that provide individual or group therapy. The type of referral depends on the client's willingness to accept treatment, coverage or lack thereof by the client's health insurer or managed care provider, client availability, and the numbers and types of community resources. The Substance Abuse and Mental Health Services Administration (SAMHSA) distributes a *National Directory of Drug Abuse and Alcoholism Treatment and Prevention Programs* that can be obtained by calling 1-800-729-6686. This resource provides information about resources available by region.

The PCP commonly uses self-help groups as a supplement to care. Alcoholics' Anonymous (AA) is the single most often recommended "treatment" for alcoholism (Bena-Bayon, 1991). For clients without health care insurance or whose coverage does not include substance abuse treatment, this remains a viable alternative as participation in AA requires no dues or fees, although participants may make a small donation. Another added benefit of this self-help group is that attendance and participation are informal. Meetings are diverse and tailored to the individual needs of the client. For example, there are groups for women, homosexuals, adolescents, and elders. Other groups that address abuse and addiction include Rational Recovery and Women for Sobriety.

The PCP should assess clients at regular intervals to evaluate the success of the treatment plan and monitor clients for symptoms of decreased intake and/or alcohol withdrawal. Nausea, vomiting, tremors, paroxysmal sweats, anxiety, and agitation, as well as visual, auditory, or tactile hallucinations, suggest a sudden shift to abstinence, which may precipitate potential dangerous withdrawal syndromes (see Chapter 7).

The provider should consider verifying the client's progress by such measures as evaluating laboratory findings (e.g., the level of GGT). The provider should ensure that the client knows that diagnostic tests or other measures are part of the comprehensive treatment plan. Clients who demonstrate improvement in their consumption should be encouraged to continue reduction, with goals of controlled drinking or a long-term goal of abstinence.

Clients who continue to use alcohol despite repeated attempts to abstain may experience better control with the use of drugs that deter alcohol consumption. The PCP needs to recognize pharmacotherapy in alcoholic disease as a bridge to recovery. Drugs used to deter alcohol use should never be used unless the client is engaged in treatment services that assist with recovery. Disulfiram (Antabuse) is one drug used to discourage alcohol use. Table 6-18 describes considerations for prescription of disulfiram as therapy in alcoholic disease. Naltrexone (ReVia) has also been approved for use in maintenance therapy in the alcohol-abusing client after a period of total cessation of drinking. Before prescribing this medication, the PCP should ensure that the client's withdrawal symptoms have stopped, as this medication competitively binds to opioid receptors and may worsen symptoms. The initial starting dose is one-half tablet (25 mg) daily with food. If the client tolerates this dose, the dosage is increased to the full dose of one tablet, or 50 mg, daily. The client's liver function should be evaluated prior to prescribing naltrexone because the liver extensively metabolizes the medication. Clients with any liver function test elevations five times normal or any factors in personal or family history indicating liver abnormalities should not be started on this medication. Studies indicate that naltrexone reduces alcohol craving when used as part of a comprehensive treatment program (Eisendarth, 1997).

TABLE 6-18 Disulfiram (Antabuse).

Dosage: 250–500 mg HS

Description: A form of aversion therapy that reduces the urge to drink by allowing acetaldehyde, the metabolite of alcohol, to accumulate after alcohol ingestion. This results in several unpleasant side effects. This drug should **not** be used in the alcohol-dependent client.

Considerations:

- The client must have a comprehensive history and physical examination before using disulfiram. Psychiatric evaluation should be included to rule out mood disorder or schizophrenia.
- The client should have a history with the PCP. It is essential that the client return for monthly evaluation while on this medication.
- Disulfiram is contraindicated in patients with:
  — Cardiovascular disease (marked hypotension and cardiac arrhythmia can occur)
  — Depression (it exacerbates condition)
  — Schizophrenia (it exacerbates condition)
- Disulfiram is considered a short-term treatment. The client must be in a treatment program while using this drug.
- Teach the client that drinking causes the client to experience palpitations, flushing, tachycardia, tachypnea, and shortness of breath.
- Teach the client about hidden sources of alcohol (e.g., cold and flu remedies, alcohol-enriched desserts).
- Never prescribe more than a 30-day treatment program of this drug.

TREATING THE CLIENT WHO IS ALCOHOL-DEPENDENT

The most desirable goal for the client who is psychologically and physically dependent on alcohol is abstinence. Sudden abstinence, however, will result in withdrawal symptoms that could compromise the client's health. The provider must consider the validity of the client's self-report and previous history of withdrawal symptoms as a basis for determining the most appropriate setting for alcohol withdrawal. Individuals with histories of seizures and delirium tremors, for example, must be closely monitored, preferably in in-patient settings.

Three types of treatment settings are used for alcohol withdrawal. The type of services extended to the client is often determined in collaboration with members of other health care disciplines and after extensive medical and psychosocial assessment. In facilities without the services of a physician or APN, the client's PCP may be called on to assess and monitor the client's health status. Regardless of the extent of the PCP's involvement in this kind of situation, it is essential that he or she develop networks with the agency working with the client in order to provide ongoing support to the client.

Care in in-patient treatment centers is required for clients at risk for severe withdrawal symptoms that require 24-hour medical and nursing care, who have a high relapse potential, and who must be removed from an environment that allows access to the drug of choice. In-patient treatment should also be considered as a treatment option based on the amount of alcohol consumed by the client. For example, men consuming 16 ounces or more of alcohol daily for 10 to 14 days or more and women consuming 8 ounces or more daily for 10 to 14 days or more should be considered for in-patient treatment. In-patient management, including detoxification, is extensively discussed in Chapter 7.

Management of the client in withdrawal is optimally handled in consultation with an expert in addictions care. Residential treatment facilities may be appropriate for the client who requires 24-hour supervision but does not necessarily need the 24-hour care required for medical detoxification. The client who requires social support to maintain abstinence is most appropriate for this type of facility. Some residential treatment facilities have the capabilities and staff to provide detoxification services. The PCP has an essential role in the care of the client in this type of facility, as primary care services are almost never available in these settings.

Outpatient treatment is fast becoming the treatment of choice for clients dependent on alcohol who require detoxification. Clients with minimal withdrawal risk (see Table 6-19) can

---

TABLE 6-19 Candidates for Whom Outpatient Detoxification Is a Safe Procedure.

- Clients with a strong psychosocial support system
- Clients with no history of severe withdrawal symptoms and not currently alcohol-dependent or concurrently abusing other drugs
- Clients who are currently attending day treatment or intensive outpatient treatment programs
- Clients who contract not to drive automobiles or operate hazardous machinery during detoxification
- Clients without organic or psychiatric cognitive impairment

Source: Adapted from Nagey, M.D. (1994). *Intensive Outpatient Treatment for Alcohol and Other Drug Abuse (TIP) Series 8.* Substance Abuse and Mental Health Services Administration (SAMHSA), Center for Substance Abuse Treatment. Washington, DC: U.S. Department of Health and Human Services.

be adequately managed with appropriate medical resources. Outpatient treatment exists on two levels, described in Table 6-20. Fundamentally, outpatient treatment requires that the client attend up to nine hours weekly in individual therapy, group therapy or a combination of both. Individual therapy uses psychodynamic principles with modifications such as limit setting and explicit advice or suggestions to help clients address difficulties in interpersonal functioning that may have contributed to substance use (Sullivan and Fleming, 1997). Group therapy is one of the most frequently used techniques. It offers the experience of providing closeness, sharing painful experiences, communicating feelings, and helping others who are struggling with control over substance abuse (Sullivan and Fleming, 1997). Intensive outpatient therapy requires that the client attend the program a minimum of nine hours a week. In this setting, the client may be required to enter a day treatment program, which requires attendance at the facility for approximately eight hours a day; it has the client engaged in a variety of treatment strategies. Some programs have evening hours for employed clients.

Once the client has completed therapy and has been successfully detoxified, he or she should continue therapy that focuses on relapse prevention. Relapse prevention is discussed in Chapter 7.

Treating the Client Who Has a Drug Abuse or Dependence Diagnosis

Treatment goals for the client with a drug abuse or dependence diagnosis are generally directed toward the goal of complete abstinence. Drug-addicted clients can be safely treated in the outpatient setting under the care of the PCP; however, the anticipated severity of the client's withdrawal symptoms should guide the health care provider's selection of the most appropriate treatment setting. Table 6-21 gives a brief synopsis of treatment settings and outpatient treatment guidelines for clients with a diagnosis of abuse or dependence of selected illicit drugs.

Treating the Client Who Has a Nicotine Addiction

Nicotine addition has received a great deal of attention recently in response to the landmark settlement between the tobacco industry and 46 states that requires cigarette makers to compensate states for the medical cost of treating smoking-related diseases (Nasar, 1998).

The health effects of tobacco smoke are well known (see Table 6-22). Incorporating smoking cessation interventions into the clinician's daily practice is imperative, not only to maintain and improve the health of smokers but also to promote the health of nonsmokers (Andrews, 1998). The reasons why people smoke are very complex and beyond the discussion of this review.

When clients are motivated to quit tobacco use, brief intervention strategies are successful and can be used to assist the client in smoking cessation. According to the Agency for Health Care Policy and Research (1996), simple supportive strategies are beneficial in encouraging smoking cessation (see Table 6-23). Other authors have concluded that simple interventions such as brief counseling and follow-up supportive telephone calls have been successful in smoking reduction when used by APNs (Reeve, 1998).

Clients who smoke more than 10 cigarettes a day, smoke within 60 minutes of awakening, and give a history of withdrawal symptoms with past attempts to quit are nicotine-dependent.

TABLE 6-20 American Society of Addiction Medicine: Adult Patient Placement Criteria for the Treatment of Psychoactive Substance Use Disorders.

Criteria Dimensions	Level I Outpatient Treatment	Level II Intensive Outpatient Treatment	Level III Medically Monitored Intensive Inpatient Treatment	Level IV Medically Managed Intensive Inpatient Treatment
1 Acute Intoxication and/or Withdrawal Potential	No withdrawal risk	Minimal withdrawal risk	Severe withdrawal risk but manageable in Level III	Severe withdrawal risk
2 Biomedical Conditions and Complications	None or very stable	None or nondistracting from addiction treatment and manageable in Level II	Requires medical monitoring but not intensive treatment	Requires 24-hour medical nursing care
3 Emotional and Behavioral Conditions and Complications	None or very stable	Mild severity with potential to distract from recovery	Moderate severity needing a 24-hour structured setting	Severe problems requiring 24-hour psychiatric care with concomitant addiction treatment
4 Treatment Acceptance and Resistance	Willing to cooperate but needs motivating and monitoring strategies	Resistance high enough to require structured program, but not so high as to render outpatient treatment ineffective	Resistance high despite negative consequences and needs intensive motivating strategies in 24-hour structure	Problems in this dimension do not qualify client for Level IV treatment
5 Relapse Potential	Able to maintain abstinence and recovery goals with minimal support	Intensification of addiction symptoms and high likelihood of relapse without close monitoring and support	Unable to control use despite active participation in less intensive care and needs 24-hour structure	Problems in this dimension do not qualify client for Level IV treatment
6 Recovery Environment	Supportive recovery environment and/or client has skills to cope	Environment unsupportive, but with structure or support, the client can cope	Environment dangerous for recovery necessitating removal from the environment; logistical impediments to outpatient treatment	Problems in this dimension do not qualify client for Level IV treatment

Source: Reproduced with permission from the American Society of Addiction Medicine. (1991). *Adult Patient Placement Criteria for the Treatment of Psychoactive Substance Use Disorders* (1st ed.). Chevy Chase, MD: ASAM.

TABLE 6-21 Selected Treatment Options for a Client with Drug Abuse or Dependence.

Drugs	Treatment Settings	Outpatient Treatment Guidelines
Benzodiazepines and other sedative-hypnotics	Consider hospitalization if the client is 65 years of age or older. Clients who abuse benzodiazepines and who frequently have addictive behaviors should be hospitalized. Clients who are polysubstance users should be hospitalized.	Slowly taper the use of these drugs for clients who have been using long-acting forms of the drugs for medical purposes. Consider switching clients who have been using a short-acting drug to a long-acting drug, and then slowly taper use. Once the client has been tapered to the lowest dose tolerable, start valproate 125 mg TID. Increase the dose to 750–1,200 mg daily. The short-acting benzodiazepine is stopped abruptly. Valproate should be continued for 30 days and then gradually discontinued. Consider prescribing antidepressants for the depressed client.
Marijuana	Outpatient treatment is sufficient. No withdrawal symptoms are expected.	Pharmacological therapy is not indicated.
Hallucinogens	Outpatient treatment is sufficient. No withdrawal symptoms are expected.	Pharmacological therapy is not indicated.
Phencyclidine	Clients with acute overdose require hospitalization. Outpatient treatment is sufficient. No withdrawal symptoms are expected.	Pharmacological therapy is not indicated.
Amphetamines, cocaine, and crack cocaine	Outpatient treatment is sufficient. No withdrawal symptoms are expected. Following abstinence, clients may be agitated, depressed, and/or have insomnia.	Pharmacological therapy is not indicated. Use chlordiazepoxide (Librium) 10–25 mg for insomnia.
Opioids	Outpatient detoxification is feasible in designated clinics. Brief or rapid detoxification can occur in hospitalized settings, although this method is not widely advocated.	Management is dependent on symptomatology: Grade 1: yawning, sweating, lacrimation, rhinorrhea Grade 2: mydriasis, piloerection, muscle twitching, anorexia Grade 3: insomnia, tachycardia, tachypnea, hypertension, abdominal cramps, vomiting, weakness Grade 1 or 2 symptoms are treated with clonidine 0.1–0.2 mg daily. Methadone or levo-alpha-acetylmethadol (LAAM) is the most commonly used drug to treat outpatient detoxification symptoms. For a complete discussion of detoxification and methadone maintenance, see Chapter 7.

TABLE 6-22 Smoking-Related Mortality Rates.

Disease	Men	Women	Overall
Cancers			
Lung	81,179	35,741	116,920
Lung from environmental tobacco smoke	1,055	1,945	3,000
Other	21,659	9,743	31,402
Total	**103,893**	**47,429**	**151,322**
Cardiovascular Diseases			
Hypertension	3,233	2,151	5,384
Heart disease	88,644	45,591	134,235
Stroke	14,978	8,303	23,281
Other	11,682	5,172	16,854
Total	**118,537**	**61,217**	**179,754**
Respiratory Diseases			
Pneumonia	11,292	7,881	19,173
Bronchitis/emphysema	9,234	5,541	14,775
Chronic airway obstruction	30,385	18,579	48,964
Other	787	668	1,455
Total	**51,698**	**32,669**	**84,367**
Diseases among infants	1,006	705	1,711
Burn deaths	863	499	1,362
All Causes	**275,997**	**142,519**	**418,624**

Sources: Centers for Disease Control and Prevention (1993); Centers for Disease Control and Prevention (1994); American Cancer Society (1996); U.S. Environmental Protection Agency (1992).

The Fagerstrom Test for Nicotine Dependence is frequently used in primary care practice to test for nicotine dependence (see Table 6-24).

Clients determined to be addicted to nicotine are candidates for pharmacological adjuncts to assist with smoking cessation. Pharmacologic agents are divided into two major categories: nicotine and nonnicotine therapies (see Table 6-25). Nicotine therapies focus on replacing enough nicotine to decrease the withdrawal symptoms associated with nicotine withdrawal. These include nicotine gums, transdermal patches, and nasal sprays. The oral drug bupropion hydrochloride (Zyban) is approved as an adjunct to smoking cessation. Although this drug is an antidepressant, its effectiveness is unrelated to its antidepressant properties. The drug's mechanisms involved in smoking cessation are not well understood. The protocol for prescribing Zyban and follow-up of clients using this drug are described in Table 6-26.

Prior to prescribing nicotine-containing therapies to clients, a careful review of the medical history is made. Clients with severe coronary artery disease and myocardial infarction should be prescribed these drugs with caution. Table 6-25 lists the common adverse reactions and the precautions to be taken with each of the currently available drugs used in smoking cessation.

TABLE 6-23 Common Elements of Supportive Smoking Cessation Treatments.

Supportive Treatment Component	Examples
Encourage the client in the quit attempt.	• Note that effective cessation treatments are now available. • Note that half of all people who have ever smoked have now quit. • Communicate a belief in the client's ability to quit.
Communicate care and concern.	• Ask how the client feels about quitting. • Directly express concern and willingness to help. • Be open to the client's expression of fears of quitting, difficulties experienced, and ambivalent feelings.
Encourage the client to talk about the quitting process.	Ask about: • Reasons the client wants to quit • Difficulties encountered while quitting • Success the client has achieved • Concerns or worries about quitting
Provide basic information about smoking and quitting.	Explain: • The nature/time course of withdrawal • The addictive nature of smoking • The fact that any smoking (even a single puff) increases the successful likelihood of full relapse

Source: Fiore, M.C., Bailey, W.C., Cohen, S.J., et al. (1996). *Smoking Cessation.* Clinical Practice Guideline No. 18. Rockville, MD: U.S. Department of Health and Human Services, Public Health Service, Agency for Health Care Policy and Research. AHCPR Publication No. 96-0692.

TABLE 6-24 Items and Scoring for Fagerstrom Test for Nicotine Dependence.

Questions	Answers	Points
1. How soon after you wake up do you smoke your first cigarette?	Within 5 minutes 6–30 minutes 31–60 minutes After 60 minutes	3 2 1 0
2. Do you find it difficult to refrain from smoking in places where it is forbidden (e.g., in church, at the library, in the cinema)?	Yes No	1 0
3. Which cigarette would you hate most to give up?	The first one in the morning All others	1 0
4. How many cigarettes/day do you smoke?	10 or less 11–20 21–30 31 or more	0 1 2 3
5. Do you smoke more frequently during the first hours after waking than during the rest of the day?	Yes No	1 0
6. Do you smoke if you are so ill that you are in bed most of the day?	Yes No	1 0

Proposed scoring cutoffs: 0–2, very low; 3–4, low; 5, medium; 6–7, high (heavy); and 8–10, very high.

Source: Adapted from Fagerstrom, K.O., Heatherton. T.F., and Kozlowski, L.T. (1992). Nicotine addiction and its assessment. *Ear, Nose, and Throat Journal 69*(11), 763–767.

TABLE 6-25 Pharmacological Aids for Smoking Cessation.

Brand Name/ Manufacturer	Length of Daily Dosage	Treatment	Comments/Adverse Reactions
Transdermal Nicotine Patch Habitrol (Norvartis Consumer) 21 mg 14 mg 7 mg	21 mg/24 hr 14 mg/24 hr 7 mg/24 hr	4–8 weeks 2–4 weeks 2–4 weeks	24-hr patch. Adverse reactions: local erythema, GI upset, arthralgia, myalgia, tachycardia. Precaution: post-MI, arrhythmia or severe angina or HTN, renal or hepatic disease, hyperthyroidism, pheochromocytoma, diabetes, PUD. Apply to clean, dry, nonhairy site on trunk or upper outer arm.
Nicoderm CQ (SK Beecham) 21 mg (OTC) 14 mg 7 mg	21 mg/24 hr 14 mg/24 hr 7 mg/24 hr	4–8 weeks 2–4 weeks 2–4 weeks	Remove patch after 16 or 24 hours. Adverse reactions: local erythema, tachycardia, tobacco withdrawal symptoms, GI upset, arthralgia, myalgia, tachycardia. Precaution: post-MI, arrhythmia or severe angina or HTN, renal and hepatic disease, hyperthyroidism, pheochromocytoma, diabetes, PUD. Apply to clean, dry, nonhairy site on trunk or upper outer arm.
Nicotrol (McNeil) (OTC) 15 mg	15 mg/16 hr	2–6 weeks	Remove patch at bedtime; rotate sites; avoid use post-MI, severe angina, or HTN. Adverse reactions: local erythema, tachycardia, withdrawal symptoms. Apply to clean, dry, nonhairy site on trunk or upper outer arm.
ProStep (Lederle) 22 mg 11 mg	22 mg/24 hr 11 mg/24 hr	4–8 weeks 2–4 weeks	Contraindicated post-MI, serious arrhythmia, or severe angina. Precaution: increased HTN, arrhythmias, renal hepatic impairment, hypothyroidism, DM, PUD. Adverse reactions: local erythema.
Nicotine Gum Nicorette 2 mg & 4 mg (SK Beecham)	9–12 pieces/day (maximum 30)	2–3 months (maximum 6)	Chew 30 min. 1 piece every 1–2 hours while awake; chew and park on buccal mucosa. Do not eat or drink during 15 min. prior to use; avoid using with acidic food or drink. Adverse reactions: trauma to oral mucosa, teeth, and dental work; GI symptoms.
Nasal Spray/Inhaler Nicotrol NS (McNeil) Aqueous nasal spray	1–2/hr max. 5/hr, 40 doses/day	variable max./3 mo.	One spray each nostril = 1 dose. Adverse reactions: nasopharyngeal and ocular irritation. Do not use post-MI, serious arrhythmias, angina, or HTN.
Nicotrol inhaler (McNeil)	6–16 cartridges/day, not exceed 16/day	3–12 weeks	Device consists of 2 parts: a mouthpiece and a cartridge with 42 in a pack. Adverse reactions: coughing and nose and throat irritation; dyspepsia.
Oral Agents Clonidine HCL Cataress (Boehringer Ingelheim)	0.1 BID	variable	Also dispensed in patch form. Precaution: severe CAD, recent MI, CVA, renal failure. Avoid abrupt cessation, potential CNS depressants. Adverse reactions: dry mouth, sedation, rash, constipation, insomnia, agitation, orthostatic hypotension.
Zyban (Glaxo Wellcome) Bupropion	150 mg daily for 3 days, then 150 mg BID at least 8 hrs apart	7–12 weeks	Contraindicated in seizure disorders, bulimia, anorexia nervosa. Monitor for HTN if used with nicotine replacement. Used with caution in bipolar disease, psychosis, recent MI, CHF, suicidal tendencies. Monitor for hypotension if used with nicotine replacement.

BID: twice a day; CAD: coronary artery disease; CHF: congestive heart failure; CNS: central nervous system; CVA: cerebrovascular accident; DM: diabetes mellitus; HTN: hypertension; MI: myocardial infarction; OTC: over-the-counter; PUD: peptic ulcer disease.

Source: Modified with permission from Nurse Practitioners' Prescribing Reference. (1998). *Smoking Cessation.* Rockville, MD: National Institutes of Health.

TABLE 6-26 Bupropion Hydrochloride (Zyban).

Dosage: 150 mg BID

Description: A weak inhibitor of the neuronal uptake of norepinephrine, serotonin, and dopamine. It does not inhibit monoamine oxidase. The drug's effectiveness in smoking cessation does not appear to be related to its antidepressant properties, but its mechanism of action for smoking cessation is unknown. It is presumed that its action is mediated by noradrenergic and dopaminergic responses.

Considerations:

- The client must have a comprehensive history and physical examination. Psychiatric evaluation should be included to rule out anorexia nervosa, bulimia, and concurrent use of monoamine oxidase inhibitors.
- Bupropion hydrochloride is contraindicated in clients with a history of seizure disorders.
- Bupropion hydrochloride is initiated one week prior to the date contracted for smoking cessation.
- Teach the client that potential side effects include rash, nausea, agitation, and migraines.
- Therapy is initiated with 150 mg for 3 days to monitor side effects; then it is increased to 150 mg BID.
- The length of therapy is 7 to 12 weeks.
- Arrange follow-up to assist the client in efforts with smoking cessation.

Summary

The explosive growth of managed care has forced PCPs into the role of gatekeepers of client management. Because of the prevalence of substance-related disorders, it is likely that all PCPs will encounter clients with these problems and will treat them within the primary care environment. Increasingly, PCPs will be prepared to initiate and oversee withdrawal and abstinence care of alcohol, drug, and nicotine dependence.

Routine assessment for substance-related disorders should be commonplace in primary care practice. Brief intervention strategies by the provider are successful in helping clients reduce substance use. For those with abuse and dependence disorders for whom brief interventions have failed, the PCP can consult with nursing and medical addictions experts to obtain the information necessary to assist in the care of these clients.

Case Study

Mr. Morse is a 36-year-old African American male who is a chief operating officer of Draxto Industries. He comes to your office because of redness in his left eye. This symptom began approximately 2 days ago. He denies trauma to the left or right eye. The associated symptoms are that of excessive lacrimation and pruritis. The right eye is unaffected. Mr. Morse's past medical history is positive for a questionable history of hypertension; he is not currently on any treatment for this condition. He denies any surgical or psychiatric history. He drinks wine on social occasions; he has smoked one pack of cigarettes daily since he was 17 years old and denies any illicit drug use. He states that he has attempted to quit smoking several times. His longest cigarette-free period was 1 year after he was told about the slight elevation in his blood pressure. The review of systems is positive for aphthous ulcers in the mouth approximately 2 to 3 years ago and hemorrhoids, which are relieved with the use of over-the-counter preparations. His family history is significant for coronary artery disease. One sister died from complications associated with HIV. He has four children; all are alive and well. His last tuberculosis test was performed more than 5 years ago. He does not recall specifically having a chest x-ray, although he does remember having some type of x-ray.

Physical Examination
BP: 152/90; P: 88 BPM; R: 16; T: 98°F, oral; weight: 192 lbs.

HEENT:	Right red conjunctiva. Excessive lacrimation present. The pupils are equal, round, and reactive to light and accommodation (PERRLA). The extraocular movements are intact. The fundus is not well visualized. The visual acuity is grossly normal.
Cardiac:	S1 and S2 are normal. No murmurs, rubs, or gallops.
Chest:	Lungs are clear in the anterior and posterior chest wall.
Abdomen:	Soft, nontender, nondistended; positive bowel sounds; no organomegaly.
Musculoskeletal:	No clubbing, cyanosis, or edema.
CNS:	Motor and sensory examinations are grossly normal.

1. Based on the history and physical examination, what is the mostly likely diagnosis for Mr. Morse?
2. How should Mr. Morse's primary care provider manage his chief complaint?
3. What should Mr. Morse be told concerning his cigarette smoking?
4. What should Mr. Morse be told about the effect of his smoking on others?
5. Mr. Morse tells his provider that he will stop smoking cold turkey. Is this strategy recommended?
6. Mr. Morse has tried smoking cessation gums and patches in the past without success. What other treatment options should his primary care provider consider at this time?

CRITICAL THINKING QUESTIONS

1. The new advanced practice nurse is working in a women's program at a substance abuse treatment agency that primarily services African American women. Discuss some of the appropriate tools that could be used in screening for alcohol use in this population. Which tool is most suited to the patterns of alcohol use in this population? Discuss the limitations of the tool that you have selected.
2. During a routine physical examination including a substance abuse screening, a client reports that he has one to two glasses of wine each evening. Occasionally, he may have a martini. His score on the CAGE is zero. The client now expresses concern that he may be drinking too much based on your questioning. What client education points could you make to assist this client in assessing whether he has a drinking problem?

3. You are an advanced practice nurse in charge of three school-based high school clinics staffed by registered professional nurses. Discuss screening tools specific to the adolescent that you would recommend be used by the registered nurses in the clinic. Describe and analyze several primary prevention strategies for alcohol, drug, and tobacco use that could be effective in this client population.

4. You are hired as an advanced practice nurse to provide episodic health care to clients in a grassroots harm reduction program for injection drug users. It includes a needle exchange program. Assess your views and values about harm reduction and your feelings about working in such a program. Discuss how primary care interventions can be incorporated into such a program.

5. A client in your clinical practice has expressed interest in treatment for nicotine addiction. Analyze the client's history and risk factors that can detract from his successful completion of treatment. Discuss which of the currently available therapies, or combinations thereof, would be most appropriate for this client. Discuss outcome measures that would indicate compliance.

REFERENCES

Agency for Health Care Policy and Research. (1996). *Smoking Cessation: A Clinical Guideline from AHCPR*. Washington, DC: Author.

Allen, J.P. (1995). Assessing alcohol problems: A guide for clinicians and researchers. In *Alcoholism and Treatment Handbook Series 4*. Bethesda, MD: National Institute on Alcohol Abuse and Alcoholism.

American Cancer Society. (1996). *Cancer Facts and Figures—1996*. Atlanta, GA: Author.

American Psychiatric Association. (1994). *Diagnostic and Statistical Manual of Mental Disorders* (4th ed.). Washington, DC: 194–204.

Andrews, J. (1998). Optimizing smoking cessation strategies. *The Nurse Practitioner 23*(8), 47–67.

Babor, T.F., de la Fuente, J.R., Saunders, J., and Grant, M. (1992). *AUDIT: The Alcohol Use Disorders Identification Test: Guidelines for Use in Primary Health Care*. Geneva: World Health Organization.

Bena-Bayon, M. (1991). Alcoholic Anonymous. In D. Ciraulo and R. Shader (eds.), *Clinical Manual of Chemical Dependence*. Washington, DC: American Psychiatric Press.

Brown, R.L., and Rounds, L.A. (1995). Conjoint screening questionnaire for alcohol and other drug abuse: Criterion validity in a primary care practice. *Wisconsin Medical Journal 94*(3), 135–140.

Centers for Disease Control and Prevention. (1993). Smoking-attributable mortality and years of potential life lost—United States, 1990. *Morbidity and Mortality Weekly Report 42*(33), 645–648.

Centers for Disease Control and Prevention. (1993). Mortality trends for selected smoking-related and breast cancer—United States, 1950–1990. *Morbidity and Mortality Weekly Report 42*(44), 863–866.

Centers for Disease Control and Prevention, Office on Smoking and Health. (1994). Unpublished data.

Ciraulo, D.M., and Shader, R.I. (1991). *Clinical Manual of Chemical Dependence*. Washington, DC: American Psychiatric Press.

Clay, S.W. (1997). Comparison of AUDIT and CAGE questionnaires in screening for alcohol use disorders in elderly primary care outpatients. *Journal of the American Osteopathic Association 97*(10), 588–592.

Eisendarth, S.J. (1997). Psychiatric disorders. In L. Tierney, S.J. McPhee, and M.A. Papadakis (eds.), *Current Medical Diagnosis and Treatment* (36th ed.). Stamford, CT: Appleton and Lange.

Finfgeld, D.L. (1997). Resolution of drinking problems without formal treatment. *Perspectives in Psychiatric Care: The Journal for Nurse Psychotherapist 33*(3),14–23.

Gerchufsky, G. (1996). Making screening part of your routine. *Advance for Nurse Practitioner 4*(11), 29–50.

Heck, E.J., and Williams, M.D. (1995). Using the CAGE to screen for drinking-related problems in college students. *Journal of Studies on Alcohol 56*(3), 282–286.

Jones, T.V., Lindsey, B.A., Yount, P., Soltys, R., and Farani-Enayat, B. (1993). Alcoholism screening questionnaires: Are they valid in elderly medical outpatients? *Journal of General Internal Medicine 8*(12), 674–678.

Kinney, J., and West, D. (1996). Substance use treatment. In J. Kinney (ed.), *Clinical Manual of Substance Use*. St. Louis, MO: Mosby.

Maisto, S.A. (1995). Contrasting self-report screens for alcohol problems: A review. *Alcoholism Clinical and Experimental Research 19*(6), 1510–1516.

McGinnis, J.M., and Foege, W.H. (1993). Actual causes of death in the United States. *Journal of the American Medical Association 270*(18), 2207–2212.

Morton, J.L., Jones, T.V., and Managaro, M.A. (1996). Performance of alcoholism screening questionnaires in elderly veterans. *American Journal of Medicine 101*(2), 153–159.

Nasar, S. (1998). The ifs and buts of the tobacco settlement. *The New York Times,* November 29, XX.

National Institute on Alcohol Abuse and Dependence. (1995). Diagnostic criteria for alcohol abuse and dependence. *Alcohol Alert,* No. 30 PH 359.

O'Connor, P.G. (1996). Routine screening and initial assessment. In J. Kinney (ed.), *Clinical Manual of Substance Assessment* (2nd ed.). St. Louis, MO: Mosby.

O'Hare, T., and Tran, T.V. (1997). Predicting problem drinking in college students: Gender differences and the CAGE questionnaire. *Addictive Behaviors 22*(1), 13–21.

Plantz, S.H., and Adler, J. (1998). Nicotine addiction. www.emedicine.com/med/topic1642.htm.

Prochaska, J.O., and Goldstein, M.G. (1991). Process of smoking cessation: Implications for clinicians. *Clinical Chest Medicine 12*(4), 727–735.

Reeve, K.D. (1998). Tobacco use cessation intervention in a nurse practitioner managed clinic. *Journal of the American Academy of Nurse Practitioners 10*(10), 445.

Rigotti, N.A. (1995). Smoking cessation. In A. Gorell, L. May, and A. Mulley (eds.), *Primary Care Medicine*. Philadelphia: Lippincott.

Senft, R.A., Polen, M.R., Freeborn, D.K., and Hollis, J.F. (1997). Brief intervention in a primary care setting for hazardous drinkers. *American Journal of Preventative Medicine 13*(6), 464–470.

Sullivan, E.F., and Fleming, M. (1997). A guide to substance abuse services for primary care clinicians. *Treatment Improvement Protocol (TIP) Series 24*. Substance Abuse and Mental Health Services Administration (SAMHSA), Center for Substance Abuse Treatment. Rockville, MD: U.S. Department of Health and Human Services.

U.S. Department of Health and Human Services. (1988). *Mandatory Guidelines for Federal Workplace Testing Programs*. Federal Register 53: 11970. Washington, DC: Author.

U.S. Department of Health and Human Services. (1998). *Healthy People 2000: Midcourse Review and 1995 Revision*. Washington, DC: Author.

U.S. Environmental Protection Agency. (1992). *Respiratory Health Effects of Passive Smoking: Lung Cancer and Other Disorders*. Office of Health and Environmental Assessment, Office of Research and Development. EPA/600/6-90/006F. Washington, DC: Author.

Volk, R.J., Cantor, S.B., Steinbauer, J.R., and Cass, A.R. (1997). Item bias in the CAGE screening test for alcohol use disorders. *Journal of General Internal Medicine 12*(12), 763–769.

7

Adult Health: Acute Care

Phyllis Lisanti, RN, PhD

LEARNER OUTCOMES

On completion of this chapter, the learner will be able to:

1. Examine the physiological and psychological effects of specific substance abuse such as alcohol, cocaine, heroin, marijuana, sedative-hypnotic, and inhalant use.
2. Discuss the long-term health implications of drug abuse.
3. Formulate the acute and chronic care nursing interventions for substance-abusing clients.
4. Discuss the physiological mechanisms of intoxication, toxicity, and withdrawal from drugs of abuse.
5. Differentiate signs and symptoms of the various categories of drugs of abuse.
6. Formulate advanced practice interventions in acute care patient management during intoxication, toxicity, and withdrawal from substances.
7. Discuss the role of the advanced practice acute care nurse in the pharmacologic management of detoxification.
8. Analyze the issues of pain management in the substance-abusing client.

KEY TERMS

acute interventions	overdose	toxicity
delirium tremens	substance abuse	withdrawal
intoxication		

Epidemiology

Individuals who abuse substances typically use the health care system more than nonsubstance-abusing individuals; hence, alcohol and tobacco abusers have a disproportionate impact on hospital costs. It has been demonstrated that the substance-using group (13 percent) incurs costs that equal those incurred by the remaining (87 percent) client population (Kinney, 1996).

These high health care costs derive from the fact that alcohol plays a major role in intentional and unintentional injuries. It is believed that 50 percent of all trauma fatalities involve alcohol, 30 percent of motor vehicle crashes, 40 percent to 56 percent of falls, 40 percent of near drownings, 12 percent to 61 percent of burns, and 56 percent of assaults (Bennett and Thomas, 1998). Alcohol is also related to 30 percent of suicides, 50 percent of homicides, and 36 percent of pedestrian fatalities (Kinney, 1996).

The rates of **substance abuse** and dependence are high in individuals with human immunodeficiency virus/acquired immunodeficiency syndrome (HIV/AIDS). Approximately one-half of all new diagnoses of HIV infection are substance abuse–related (Muma, Lyons, Borucki, and Pollard, 1997). With coexisting physical problems associated with HIV, continued substance use results in complex illness phenomena. Other infectious diseases that are directly linked to injection drug use include hepatitis B, hepatitis C, tuberculosis, and multidrug-resistant tuberculosis.

Additional infectious diseases commonly encountered in substance-abusing populations are endocarditis, bacteremia, fungal infections, body lice/scabies, venereal warts, and sexually transmitted diseases (including syphilis, gonorrhea, chlamydia, herpes simplex, and chancroid) (USDHHS, 1993).

Damage to organ systems by substance abuse presents an astounding array of infections such as cellulitis, abscesses, and septic thrombophlebitis. Diseases include pneumonia, lung abscess, osteomyelitis, and arthritis, all of which are common in this population.

Alcohol. Examples of the widespread long-term effects of chronic alcohol abuse on body systems are highlighted in Table 7-1. All drugs that produce euphoria have acute effects on the nervous system during **intoxication;** with chronic use, neuroadaptive changes occur that are the basis for tolerance and dependence. Table 7-2 demonstrates major alcohol-related neurological syndromes. Other neurological consequences include nerve trauma, Saturday Night Palsy (Geller, 1994), stroke, and seizures.

Cocaine. Cocaine use and intoxication can lead to a variety of neurological problems. Cocaine is a potent sympathomimetic, and its neurological effects are related to those properties (see Table 7-3).

Heroin. Conflicting evidence exists regarding heroin's specific damage. Health problems related to heroin/opioid use are most commonly related to routes of administration or other external variables (Geller, 1994).

Marijuana. Data on the long-term health effects of marijuana use are inconclusive. There have been reports of memory impairment, short-term memory deficits, decreased capacity for sustained attention, decreased rates of processing, and perceptual motor impairment.

TABLE 7-1 Effects of Chronic Alcohol Abuse.

Body Systems	Effects
Central nervous system	Alcoholic dementia; Wernicke's encephalopathy (confusion, nystagmus, paralysis of ocular muscles, ataxia); Korsakoff's psychosis (confabulation, amnesic disorder); impairment of cognitive function, psychomotor skills, abstract thinking, and memory; depression, attention deficit, labile moods, seizures, sleep disturbances
Peripheral nervous system	Peripheral neuropathy including pain, paresthesias, weakness
Immune system	Increased risk for tuberculosis and viral infections; increased risk for cancer of oral cavity, pharynx, esophagus, liver, colon, rectum, and possibly breast
Hematologic system	Bone marrow depression, anemia, leukopenia, thrombocytopenia, blood-clotting abnormalities
Musculoskeletal system	Painful, tender swelling of large muscle groups; painless progressive muscle weakness and wasting; osteoporosis
Cardiovascular system	Elevated pulse and BP; decreased exercise tolerance; cardiomyopathy (irreversible); increased risk for hemorrhagic stroke, coronary artery disease, hypertension, sudden cardiac death
Hepatic system	Steatosis (reversible)—nausea, vomiting, hepatomegaly, alcoholic hepatitis (reversible)—anorexia, nausea, vomiting, fever, chills, abdominal pain; cirrhosis; cancer
Gastrointestinal system	Gastritis, peptic ulcer, esophagitis, esophageal varices, enteritis, colitis, Mallory-Weiss syndrome, pancreatitis; decreased appetite, indigestion, malabsorption, vitamin deficiencies
Renal system	Diuretic effect from inhibition of antidiuretic hormone
Endocrine and reproductive system	Altered gonadal function, testicular atrophy, decreased beard growth, decreased libido, diminished sperm count, gynecomastia, glucose intolerance
Integumentary system	Palmar erythema, spider angiomas, rosacea, rhinophyma

Source: Reproduced with permission from Lisanti, P., and Duphorne, P. (1996). Substance abuse and dependence. In S. Lewis, I. Collier, and M. Heitkemper (eds.), *Medical-Surgical Nursing: Assessment and Management of Clinical Problems* (4th ed.). Philadelphia: W.B. Saunders/Mosby, p. 159.

SEDATIVE-HYPNOTICS. There are little data on the long-term effects of sedative-hypnotics, but data available indicate deficits of a neuropsychological nature similar to those seen in alcoholics (Geller, 1994).

VOLATILE INHALANTS. This abuse is rare outside the preadolescent and adolescent populations; however, abuse is associated with permanent central nervous system (CNS) damage (see Table 7-4).

Tables 7-1, 7-2, and 7-3 highlight organ system damage by alcohol and other substance use. It is not the purpose of this chapter to provide comprehensive information on this damage; however, it is clear that all body systems are adversely affected by use of alcohol and other substances (Geller, 1994).

TABLE 7-2 Major Alcohol-Related Neurological Syndromes.

Syndrome	Clinical Findings	Lesion/Etiology
Intermediate brain syndrome	Some difficulty in new learning, some concreteness, lack in mental flexibility Impairment on neuropsychological testing	Occurs in alcoholics with normal nutritional status. Could be result of subclinical nutritional deficiency and direct neurotoxic effect of alcohol.
Wernicke's encephalopathy	Disorientation Confusion Nystagmus Ocular palsies Ataxia	Midbrain punctate hemorrhages. Nutritional (thiamine) deficiency with or without additional genetically determined enzyme deficiency.
Korsakoff's psychosis	Profound deficit in new learning (recent memory) Some deficits in remote memory Intelligence and verbal abilities usually preserved May confabulate	Midbrain gliosis. Basal forebrain frequently follows Wernicke's encephalopathy. Can occur alone. Permanent syndrome not seen in uncomplicated thiamine deficiency. Only partially responsive to thiamine. Possible neurotoxic component.
Alcoholic dementia	Global decline in intellectual functions; memory affected but not predominantly Apathy, irritability, emotional lability	Etiology unclear. Direct neurotoxic effect of alcohol and possible subclinical nutritional deficiencies, trauma, or metabolic components.
Central pontine myelinolysis	Rapid-onset paraparesis or quadriparesis Dysarthria Dysphagia	Edema of the pons 2° electrolyte disturbance. Hyponatremia.
Marchiafava-Bignami	Gradual-onset dementia with psychosis Convulsions Focal symptom aphasia	Degeneration of corpus callosum related to alcohol. Etiology unknown.
Alcoholic cerebellar degeneration	Acute onset with Wernicke's encephalopathy Subacute onset alone Marked gait ataxia Little arm ataxia or dysarthria	Degeneration of Purkinje cells in cerebellar vermis. Possibly mainly due to thiamine deficit. Possibly a direct neurotoxic effect of alcohol. Not dose-related. Possible genetic susceptibility.
Alcoholic polyneuropathy	Gradual onset of symmetrical loss of sensation in toes, fingers Symmetrical motor loss, beginning distally Loss of reflexes	Degeneration of myelin sheaths of peripheral nerves. Thiamine deficiency.
Optic neuropathy (tobacco-alcohol amblyopia)	Acute or subacute onset of impaired vision Central scotomata	Thiamine deficiency.

Source: Reproduced with permission from Miller, N.S. (1994). *Principles of Addiction Medicine.* Chevy Chase, MD: American Society of Addiction Medicine, Chapter 6, p. 3.

TABLE 7-3 Acute and Chronic Neurological Effects of Cocaine.

Condition	Timing	Observation
Stroke	Intoxication	Intracerebral hemorrhage: 49% frequency associated Cerebral infarction: 22% A-V malformations
Seizures	Intoxication	Single Multiple Status epilepticus associated with high blood levels
Transient neurological symptoms	Intoxication	Dizziness Blurred vision Ataxia Tinnitus Transient hemiparesis
Headache	Intoxication Withdrawal Early abstinence	Can be de novo migraine
Dystonia	Withdrawal	

Source: Reproduced with permission from Miller, N.S. (1994). *Principles of Addiction Medicine.* Chevy Chase, MD: American Society of Addiction Medicine, Chapter 6, p. 11.

TABLE 7-4 Effects of Chronic Inhalant Abuse.

Substance	Source	Symptoms
Gasoline	Fuel	Tremor, ataxia, myoclonus, chorea, encephalopathy
Halogenated hydrocarbons	Degreasers Spot removers Typewriter correction fluid	CNS edema, hemorrhage
h-Hexane	Glues, cements	Blurred vision, photophobia, blindness, basal ganglia hemorrhage
Methyl-n-butyl ketone	Paints, inks, resins	Can be de novo migraine
Nitrous oxide		Sensory disturbances, ataxia, impotence, multiple sclerosis–like syndrome
Toluene	Solvents: paint thinners, glues, lacquers	Peripheral neuropathy, optic neuropathy, ataxia, severe muscle weakness, encephalopathy
Tricholorethane	Typewriter correction fluid	Diffuse CNS damage

CNS, central nervous system.

Source: Reproduced with permission from Miller, N.S. (1994). *Principles of Addiction Medicine.* Chevy Chase, MD: American Society of Addiction Medicine, Chapter 6, p. 13.

Immunosuppressant Effects of Psychoactive Drugs

It is hypothesized that opiates may modulate immune function. Recent research indicates that chronic opiate use has immunosuppressant effects that may be indirectly related to opiate-induced alterations of neuroendocrine function. High levels of alcohol and/or metabolites have the potential to alter cellular immune responses during retroviral infection. Opiates, alcohol, and cocaine share the ability to modulate surface molecules on T-cells and thereby affect immune function adversely. The immune function modulation is different for each of these drugs and should be explored based on the nurse's area of specialty function (Kinney, 1996).

On behavioral grounds alone, there is a recognized link between substance intoxication and increased risk of HIV infection. Sexual activity is more likely to be casual and risky when the individual is using, or intoxicated with, a psychoactive drug.

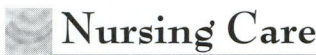 # Nursing Care

Acute Care Interventions

Common problems secondary to the abuse of drugs are **intoxication, overdose,** and **withdrawal,** as described in Table 7-5. Management of drug overdose derives from the properties of the substance used. Drug overdose can be accidental or intentional. Accidental overdose usually involves only one substance, whereas intentional overdose is likely to involve multiple substances and results in a complex and potentially confusing clinical picture. The first priority of care in overdose is always the client's airway/breathing/circulation (ABC) (see Table 7-6). After implementing **acute interventions** to stabilize the client, a thorough history and physical examination are completed. When the client is unwilling or unable to participate in obtaining a history, a collateral history should be obtained from family members and close friends.

A client who intentionally overdoses should not be discharged from a treatment facility until seen by an addictions and/or psychiatric professional and appropriate plans made for follow-up. The acute medical-surgical problem must be managed first and the client safely detoxified. When an acute condition exists, rehabilitation and treatment for problems with substance abuse are not realistic goals.

Withdrawal syndromes from all classes of drugs are similar inasmuch as they produce symptoms of acute anxiety and protracted depression. Withdrawal from CNS depressants, of which alcohol is one, produce the most dangerous withdrawal situations. Abrupt withdrawal brought about by sudden cessation of drug intake may be life-threatening unless appropriately managed. Medical management is directed toward decreasing symptoms and includes a gradual reduction in dosage achieved by the substitution of medications (e.g., benzodiazepines) that have similar effects on the central nervous system.

Although withdrawal from narcotics is the least life-threatening, symptoms are dramatic, temporarily disabling, and painful. Methadone is often recommended for treating withdrawal, although any opiate may be administered. Symptoms of withdrawal may be reduced by administering the drug of choice in decreasing amounts over two weeks. Nonopiates may also be administered to produce detoxification and include clonidine (Catapres) and various benzodiazepines.

TABLE 7-5 Effects of Frequently Abused Drugs.

Drug	Psychological Effects	Physiologic Effects	Effects of Overdose	Withdrawal Syndrome
Stimulants Cocaine, amphetamines, methylphenidate, phenmetrazine, other stimulants	Elation, psychomotor agitation, grandiosity, talkativeness, ↑ alertness, mood swings	Dilated pupils, ↑ blood pressure, ↑ TPR, diaphoresis, nausea, vomiting, insomnia, loss of appetite	Agitation, ↑ body temperature, hallucinations, convulsions, possible death	Severely depressed mood, prolonged sleep, apathy, irritability, disorientation
Depressants Chloral hydrate, barbiturates, methaqualone, benzodiazepines, alcohol	Disorientation, euphoria, emotional lability, ↑ sexual and aggressive drives with intoxication (↓ with increased doses), talkativeness	Slurred speech, staggering, constricted pupils, ↓ respirations, sedation, nausea	Shallow respirations, cold and clammy skin, weak and rapid pulse, coma, possible death	Anxiety, insomnia, tremors, delirium, convulsions, possible death
Narcotics Opium, morphine, codeine, heroin, methadone, other narcotics	Euphoria, ↓ sexual and aggressive drives	↓ respiratory rate, nausea, "nodding out," insensitivity to pain, constricted pupils	Slow and shallow breathing, clammy skin, constricted pupils, coma, possible death	Watery eyes, runny nose, yawning, loss of appetite, tremors, panic, chills and sweating, cramps, nausea
Hallucinogens LSD, psilocybin, mescaline, peyote, amphetamine variants, phencyclidine	Hallucinations, illusions, altered body and time perception, mood swings, suspiciousness, confusion, anxiety, panic, intense emotions, depersonalization	Lack of coordination, dilated pupils, ↑ blood pressure, tremors, blurred vision, nausea, dizziness, weakness, ↓ response to pain	More prolonged episodes, possibly resembling psychotic states	NA
Cannabis Marijuana, tetrahydro-cannabinol, hashish	Euphoria, impaired memory and attention, relaxation, poor judgment, apathy, abrupt mood changes, slowed time sensation	↑ appetite, tachycardia, reddened eyes	Fatigue, paranoia, hallucinogen-like psychotic state (at very high doses)	Insomnia, hyperactivity (rare syndrome)
Inhalants Glues, aerosols, cleaning solutions, nail polish removers, lighter fluids, paints and paint thinners, other petroleum products, halothane, nitrous oxide, amyl nitrite, butyl nitrite	Giddiness, lightheadedness, decreased inhibitions, floating sensation, illusions, clouding of thoughts, drowsiness, amnesia	Eye irritation, sensitivity to light, double vision, ringing in ears, irritation in lining of nose and mouth, cough, nausea, vomiting, diarrhea, faint heartbeat, cardiac irregularities or dysrhythmias	Anxiety, mental impairment, depressed respiration, cardiac dysrhythmias, sudden death	No clinically relevant syndrome; development of tolerance likely at high doses

LSD, Lysergic acid diethylamide; NA, no data available; TPR, temperature, pulse, respirations.

Source: Reproduced with permission from Lisanti, P., and Duphorne, P. (1996). Substance abuse and dependence. In S. Lewis, I. Collier, and M. Heitkemper (eds.), *Medical-Surgical Nursing: Assessment and Management of Clinical Problems* (4th ed.). Philadelphia: W.B. Saunders/Mosby, p. 151.

TABLE 7-6 Emergency Management: Drug Overdose.

Possible Etiology	Possible Assessment Findings	Management
Ingestion, inhalation, or injection of drugs, either accidentally or intentionally	Aggressive behavior Agitation Disorientation Lethargy Stupor Hallucinations Depression Slurred speech Pinpoint pupils Seizures Needle tracks Cold, clammy skin Rapid, weak pulse Slow or rapid shallow respirations Cardiac or respiratory arrest	Establish and maintain an airway. Anticipate need for intubation if respiratory distress is evident. Establish IV access. Obtain information about substance: name, route, when taken, period of time taken, amount taken. Obtain a health history, including drug use and allergies. Assess level of consciousness. Monitor vital signs, including temperature. Perform a 12-lead ECG and then continue to monitor with ECG. Use measures to decrease systemic absorption (if appropriate), including: • Gastric lavage • Induced emesis (e.g., syrup of ipecac) • Absorbents (e.g., activated charcoal) • Induced diarrhea (e.g., magnesium) • Antidote

ECG, Electrocardiogram; IV, intravenous.

Source: Reproduced with permission from Lisanti, P., and Duphorne, P. (1996). Substance abuse and dependence. In S. Lewis, I. Collier, and M. Heitkemper (eds.), *Medical-Surgical Nursing: Assessment and Management of Clinical Problems* (4th ed.). Philadelphia: W.B. Saunders/Mosby, p. 152.

Chronic Care and Home Management

Before rehabilitation is considered, all acute medical-surgical problems must be resolved. The client must recognize and show initial understanding of the substance-related problem and be willing to accept long-term treatment. Outcomes are more positive when the nurse can work closely with the family, significant others, and the client in evaluating the need for inpatient treatment or long-term care.

Rehabilitation may be available for the client in private or public psychiatric hospitals or in facilities specifically designed to meet the health care needs of the substance-abusing client. It is important that a multidisciplinary team of nurses, physicians, social workers, and recreational therapists collaborate with the client and family in planning care and in creating a therapeutic environment. The client can progress from hospitalization to halfway houses, therapeutic communities, or other community-based programs.

Complete abstinence from drugs is optimal to restoration of health. The use of other drugs triggers craving for the abused substance and results in relapse because paired associations occur at the midbrain level. Relapse prevention is an essential component of any recovery program and includes behavioral, cognitive, educational, and self-control techniques.

The advanced practice acute care nurse (APACN) needs to identify behaviors suggesting the likelihood of relapse, such as:

- Feelings of powerlessness, helplessness, and depression
- Loneliness and isolation
- Irregular eating and sleeping habits
- Periods of confusion, restlessness, anger, defensiveness, and denial
- Loss of daily structure

The APACN must work with the individual to identify risk situations that are likely to lead to drug use and to practice ways to avoid or deal with these situations. Conditioned urges and drug cravings should be consistently extinguished by substituting other activities for drug use. When medical conditions exist, negative consequences of drug use should be recalled to counteract distorted memories of the drug euphoria. To achieve this objective, the APACN states factually and nonjudgmentally the relationship between use and negative health outcomes. The nurse can guide the client in learning stress management techniques for promoting a healthy lifestyle.

Healthy lifestyle behaviors include appropriate exercise, rest, nutrition, work, and recreation. The APACN promotes these behaviors through nonjudgmental education and counseling, as well as role modeling.

Major Components of Acute Care for Substance-Abusing Clients

Early recognition and identification of the client with substance-related problems are central to successful treatment outcomes. The nurse must be aware of a wide range of signs and symptoms of substance abuse and dependence in order to prevent health problems and reduce risk. A rapid assessment for possible substance-related emergency conditions is essential, regardless of age or condition, and particularly for clients involved in motor vehicle and other accidents or trauma, burns, falls, and assaults.

Assessment for substance use should be considered within the context of all comprehensive client evaluations. All clients should be screened for substance abuse as part of an initial evaluation. Screening needs to be followed by a more thorough comprehensive assessment to formulate diagnoses and to assess severity of the health care problem.

A wide variety of screening tools is available to determine substance abuse and use; however, screening tools for alcohol have been used more consistently in a range of populations, and their reliability and validity are well established.

Alcohol Screening Tools

The CAGE is a four-item questionnaire recognized as a moderately effective and easily used alcohol screening device. It takes only minutes to administer, and two to three yes responses are highly suggestive of alcoholism and would trigger further evaluation for substance abuse (see Table 6-2).

Beginning the assessment with a focus on alcohol is indicated for several reasons. Alcohol is the most commonly used substance, and its use is socially acceptable. Questions and discussion about alcohol use can serve as an introduction to the more comprehensive assessment of substance use.

Other alcohol screening tools include:
- Michigan Alcoholism Screening Test (MAST) (24-item yes/no questionnaire) (see Table 6-3)
- Brief MAST (10-item yes/no questionnaire) (Table 7-7)
- Trauma Scale (5-item questionnaire) (Table 7-8)
- Alcohol Use Disorders Identification Test (AUDIT) (10-item questionnaire), a newer tool developed through the World Health Organization that appears promising as an effective instrument to detect problem drinking. (see Table 6-6)

Substance abuse screening may be accomplished with the Drug Abuse Screening Test (DAST). The DAST is a 28-item questionnaire designed to explore the extent of drug abuse (see Table 6-7). When rapid screening is positive for substance use, the following questions may be used to gather additional information about the individual's involvement with substances (see Table 7-9).

The screening interview is an important way to detect substance abuse problems. The physical examination and laboratory tests are important in evaluating medical complications of substance abuse/use that the client may be experiencing. Toxicology blood screening identifies the types of drugs used and the levels present in the client's system.

The nurse is responsible for all phases of client care related to substance use including initial contact, prevention activities, risk reduction activities, early intervention, follow-up

TABLE 7-7 Brief MAST.

Points	Questions
(2)	1. Do you feel you are a normal drinker?*
(2)	2. Do friends or relatives think you are a normal drinker?*
(5)	3. Have you ever attended a meeting of Alcoholics Anonymous?
(2)	4. Have you ever lost friends or girlfriends/boyfriends because of your drinking?
(2)	5. Have you ever gotten into trouble at work because of drinking?
(2)	6. Have you ever neglected your obligations, your family, or your work for 2 or more days in a row because you were drinking?
(2)	7. Have you ever had delirium tremens (DTs), had severe shaking, heard voices, or seen things that weren't there after heavy drinking?
(5)	8. Have you ever gone to anyone for help about your drinking?
(5)	9. Have you ever been in a hospital because of drinking?
(2)	10. Have you ever been arrested for drunk driving or driving after drinking?

Scoring: <3 points indicate nonalcoholic; 4 points suggest alcoholism; 5 or more points indicate alcoholism.

*Negative responses are alcoholic responses.

Sources: Selzer, M.L. (1971). The Michigan Alcoholism Screening Test: The quest for a new diagnostic instrument. *American Journal of Psychiatry 27*(12), 1653–1658; and Pokorny, A.D., Miller, B.A., and Kaplan, H.B. (1972). The Brief MAST: A shortened version of the Michigan Alcoholism Screening Test. *American Journal of Psychiatry 129*(3), 342–345.

TABLE 7-8 Trauma Scale.

Since your 18th birthday:

- Have you had any fractures or dislocations to your bones or joints?
- Have you been injured in a road traffic accident?
- Have you injured your head?
- Have you been injured in an assault or fight (excluding injuries during sports)?
- Have you been injured after drinking?

Two or more positive answers are the criteria for a positive test.

Source: Skinner, H.A., Holt, S., Schuller, R., Roy, J., and Israel, Y. (1984). Identification of alcohol abuse using laboratory tests and a history of trauma. *Annals of Internal Medicine 101*(6), 847–851.

TABLE 7-9 HALT/BUMP.

Question	Response
Do you usually use drugs/drink to get	**H**igh?
Do you sometimes drink or use drugs	**A**lone?
Have you found yourself	**L**ooking forward to drinking/using drugs?
Have you noticed an increased	**T**olerance?
Do you have memory lapses—	**B**lackouts that occurred while drinking?
Do you find yourself using/drinking in	**U**nplanned ways?
Do you use/drink when you feel anxious, stressed, or depressed for	**M**edicinal reasons
Do you work at	**P**rotecting your supply, having drugs or alcohol available at all times?

The mnemonics for these questions are HALT and BUMP.

Source: Kinney, J. (1996). *Clinical Manual of Substance Abuse.* (2nd ed.). St. Louis: Mosby, p. 46.

care, and rehabilitation. Following screening and/or assessment in acute care settings, initial treatment is directed at detoxification and stabilization of the client's condition.

The National Nurses' Society on Addictions (NNSA) delineates five major professional activities in the role of the nurse regarding substances. The five major activities include (Kinney, 1996):

1. Identify the problem with any substance of abuse.
2. Communicate about the problems related to substances of abuse.
3. Educate about substance use, abuse, addiction, and dependence.
4. Counsel the client's family and significant others about substance abuse, addiction, and related health problems.
5. Refer for definite treatment of the substance problem and continuing care.

NNSA's role expectations for professional nurses in this field are consistent with the expectations for the APACN.

Management Approaches by the Advanced Practice Acute Care Nurse

Acute care interventions related to substance abuse involve the areas of intoxication, overdose, and withdrawal (see Table 7-5). The APACN must be knowledgeable about the signs, symptoms, behaviors, and management of intoxication, overdose, and withdrawal.

Toxic reactions occur as a result of combining alcohol with other drugs or excessive/high use of any substance. Toxic reactions may lead to respiratory and circulatory arrest if adequate interventions are not provided. Naloxone (Narcan), an opiate antagonist, may be given if opiates have been used with alcohol or in excess.

Acute Intoxication*

DEFINITION OF INTOXICATION

Intoxication responses, usually less than 24 hours, are related directly to the ingestion of psychoactive drugs. Specific effects and duration of intoxication will vary among drugs, individual users, and settings in which drug use takes place. All psychoactive drugs produce a disinhibition, euphoria, or feeling of well-being. Physiological effects are most commonly evident in the central nervous and cardiopulmonary systems.

Intoxication effects are typically dose-related, and toxic or overdose responses can be manifested at larger doses. Common psychological toxic effects of most drugs of abuse include psychotic symptoms.

CENTRAL NERVOUS SYSTEM DEPRESSANTS (ETOH, BARBITURATES, SEDATIVE-HYPNOTICS)

Actions

These substances cause a descending depression of CNS functioning via enhancement of the action of inhibitory neurotransmitters, beginning at the level of the cerebral hemispheres, progressing to the limbic and cerebellar sites, and finally to the brainstem. They also inhibit ascending conduction from the reticular activating system. Depressants used concurrently produce extreme synergistic effects and are commonly used in conjunction with CNS stimulants. The continued use of CNS depressants results in the development of tolerance. The withdrawal response is evident upon cessation of use.

Effects

INTOXICATION RESPONSES

> *Frequently observed intoxication responses include:*
> - General slowing of mental functions; poor comprehension, memory disturbances, reduced judgment, drowsiness, limited attention span
> - Impaired motor coordination; slurred speech, ataxia, increased reaction time, hyper-reflexia

---

*The discussion of acute intoxication is adapted, with permission, from Compton, M. (1991). Nursing care in acute withdrawal. *Substance Abuse Education in Nursing 22,* 349–508.

- Euphoric mood; labile mood; decreased anxiety
- Disinhibition
- Cranial nerve dysfunction; nystagmus, diplopia
- Decreased heart rate, blood pressure, and respirations

TOXIC/OVERDOSE RESPONSES

These toxic/overdose effects include:
- Depressed level of consciousness (confusion to obtunded to comatose)
- Decreased/absent response to painful stimuli
- Marked respiratory depression; slow and noisy respirations, apnea, respiratory arrest; pulmonary edema, aspiration pneumonia, atelectasis
- Amnesic disorder
- Specific to ETOH overdose: fluid and electrolyte imbalances; hepatic encephalopathy; acute upper GI hemorrhage

CENTRAL NERVOUS SYSTEM STIMULANTS

Actions

CNS stimulants create euphoria by increasing the extracellular concentration of catecholamines within the central and autonomic nervous systems. These substances produce direct cardiovascular actions that act as potent cardiac stimulators and vasoconstrictors. In addition, cocaine acts as a local anesthetic. The continued use of CNS stimulants results in the development of tolerance. The withdrawal response is evident with cessation of drug use.

Effects

INTOXICATION RESPONSES

Frequently observed intoxication responses include:
- Psychological disinhibition; decreased anxiety, impaired judgment, impulsivity, hypersexuality
- Clear sensorium without confusion/hallucinations, decreased fatigue, heightened curiosity, increased interest in environment, increased self-esteem
- Psychomotor activation, tremulousness
- Increase in heart rate and blood pressure
- Decreased appetite
- Mydriasis

TOXIC/OVERDOSE RESPONSES

These toxic/overdose effects include:
- Hyperactivity
- Anxiety, confusion, hallucinations, paranoia (can progress to acute psychotic reactions including delirium, panic attacks, extreme paranoid delusions with violent and assaultive behaviors)
- Seizures and coma
- Diaphoresis, hyperpyrexia
- Tachycardia with cardiac arrhythmia, pulmonary edema, cardiac arrest

- Hypertensive crisis with extreme vasoconstriction (can lead to myocardial infarction, cerebral stroke, placental infarction, spontaneous abortion, fetal cerebrovascular accident)

Narcotics

Actions

These substances bind to opiate receptors in various areas of the central and autonomic nervous systems, resulting in euphoria and analgesia. The use of narcotics also results in brainstem depression, peripheral vasodilation, and decreased gastrointestinal motility. The continued use of narcotics results in the development of tolerance. The withdrawal response is evident upon cessation of use.

Effects

Intoxication Responses
Frequently observed intoxication responses include:
- Euphoria with altered sensory perception, poor comprehension, memory disturbances
- Drowsiness, decreased social interaction
- Miosis/abnormal contraction of pupils
- Mild hypotension with tachycardia, decreased respirations

Toxic/Overdose Responses
These toxic/overdose effects include:
- Depressed level of consciousness (obtunded to comatose)
- Depressed respirations leading to apnea and respiratory arrest (pulmonary edema, aspiration pneumonia, or atelectasis may also develop)
- Bradycardia, marked hypotension, shock
- Gastrointestinal atony

Hallucinogens: LSD, Mescaline, and Psilocybin

Actions

These substances act at multiple receptor sites within the CNS, resulting in CNS stimulation and depression. They also induce euphoria and perceptual alterations. General sympathetic effects are noted on the cardiovascular system. Continued hallucinogen use does not result in tolerance.

Effects

Intoxication Responses
Frequently observed intoxication responses include:
- Euphoria with transcendent experience qualities; perceptual alterations (primarily visual), increased sensory sensitivity, synesthesias; altered thought associations, hypersuggestibility; distractibility, labile mood; body image changes, sense of depersonalization; altered judgment
- Increased heart rate, mild hypertension, mild temperature increases, flushed face

- Pupil dilation
- Mild incoordination, hyperreflexia, fine tremor, restlessness
- Nausea

Toxic/Overdose Responses
These toxic/overdose effects include:
- Acute dysphoric reaction with anxiety, panic, hypervigilance, and paranoid delusions

Hallucinogen: Phencyclidine (PCP)

Actions

This substance is similar in action to that of other hallucinogens. It acts upon multiple CNS receptor sites with general sympathomimetic actions on body systems. PCP produces symptoms of CNS depression at high doses.

Effects

Intoxication Responses
Frequently observed intoxication responses include:
- Mild agitation, excitement, poor judgment
- Increase in heart rate and blood pressure
- Decreased response to painful stimuli
- Ataxia, dysarthria, hyperreflexia
- Diaphoresis
- Pupillary constriction with blank, staring appearance

Toxic/Overdose Responses
These toxic/overdose effects include:
- Muscle rigidity; tonic-clonic movements, seizures, status epilepticus
- Tachycardia with cardiac arrhythmias
- Tachypnea, Cheyne-Stokes respirations
- Hyperthermia
- Nystagmus
- Late toxic responses: delirium, psychosis with alterations in body image, aggressive/bizarre behavior, auditory and visual hallucinations, violence, hostility; CNS depression, coma, catatonic syndrome, absent corneal and gag reflexes; respiratory depression, apnea

Volatile Inhalants (Aerosols, Paint Thinner, Gasoline, Plastic/Model Cement)

Actions

These substances act as CNS depressants by inhibiting neuronal firing. The continued use of inhalants results in the development of tolerance. The withdrawal response is not consistent upon cessation of use.

Effects

INTOXICATION RESPONSES

Frequently observed intoxication responses include:

- Euphoria, dizziness, excitation, pleasant exhilaration, visual and auditory hallucinations
- Sneezing (most likely due to local effects of inhaling drug)
- Nausea and vomiting

TOXIC/OVERDOSE RESPONSES

These toxic/overdose effects include:

- Confusion, loss of self-control, loss of consciousness, seizures
- Headache, tinnitus, blurred vision, diplopia, nystagmus
- Muscle incoordination, slurred speech, decreased reflexes
- Cardiac arrhythmias, pulmonary edema
- Suicide attempts

MARIJUANA

Actions

The specific site of action is unknown, although specific THC receptors have been theorized to exist within the CNS to produce euphoria. Marijuana has been shown to have antiemetic properties, and it aids in decreasing intraocular pressure. The continued use of marijuana results in the development of tolerance. The withdrawal response is not evident upon cessation of use.

Effects

INTOXICATION RESPONSES

Frequently observed intoxication responses include:

- Altered time sense, decreased inability to concentrate, passivity, lassitude, impaired short-term memory, drowsiness or hyperactivity, altered sensory perception
- Tachycardia with orthostatic hypotension
- Conjunctival infection, nystagmus
- Increased appetite
- Dry mouth

TOXIC/OVERDOSE RESPONSES

These toxic/overdose effects include:

- Anxiety or panic reactions (especially in first time users)
- Depersonalization
- Paranoid delusions

ASSESSMENT

Assessing a client for drug intoxication includes evaluation of specific body systems, mental status, drug intake, and data from laboratory tests.

Body Systems Approach

The APACN should focus the physical examination of a client at risk for intoxication on the cardiovascular, respiratory, and neurological systems.

CARDIOVASCULAR SYSTEM

The APACN assesses the following conditions:

- Heart rate and rhythm, heart sounds, presence or periodic episodes of murmurs; presence of arrhythmias on ECG
- Peripheral pulses (strength and regularity)
- Blood pressure, orthostatic changes
- Jugular distension
- Skin color and temperature

RESPIRATORY SYSTEM

The following functions are assessed:

- Respiration rate and rhythm
- Chest sounds
- Adventitious or decreased breath sounds
- Secretions, cough
- Presence of cyanosis, evidence of hypoxia

NEUROLOGICAL SYSTEM

Areas examined include:

- Rapid eye movement
- Level of consciousness
- Cranial nerve exam, including presence of corneal and gag reflexes
- Deep tendon and stretch reflexes
- Cerebellar exam, including gait, coordination, presence of tremor
- Sensory exam and response to painful stimuli
- Autonomic evidence of sympathetic stimulation

Brief Mental Status Examination

Eight components of this examination include:

1. General appearance and behavior
2. Level of consciousness and orientation
3. Emotional status
4. Attention level
5. Language/speech
6. Memory
7. Content of thought; presence of hallucinations or delusions
8. Suicidal, homicidal, or violent ideation

Brief History of Drug Intake

Ascertain drug(s), amount, route, and time used:

- Ensure confidentiality; promote atmosphere to maximize honest communication.
- Utilize reports of others (e.g., those who brought the client to medical attention).

- Utilize alternate sources of information (e.g., mental exam, physical assessment, urine/blood toxicology reports, collateral histories from family and/or friends) to enhance veracity of self-reports.

Data Collection

This aspect of assessment includes the evaluation of urine/blood toxicology reports.

NURSING INTERVENTIONS

Nursing interventions are implemented to address physiological needs and safety of the client. The APACN should:

- Perform cardiovascular, respiratory, and neurological nursing assessments as appropriate; watch for patterns of change over time.
- Monitor vital signs.
- Monitor toxicology reports.
- Implement seizure precautions.
- Monitor intake and output.
- Administer pharmacological agents as ordered to counteract toxic effects of drugs (e.g., Narcan) and monitor effects.
- Implement nursing interventions to enhance removal of drug from body (e.g., gastric lavage, urinary excretion).

Nursing interventions are also developed to address the psychological needs and safety of the client at risk for intoxication. The APACN should:

- Orient the client to reality as necessary.
- Stay with the client as much as possible.
- Create an accepting and supportive environment; attempt to be nonjudgmental in all interactions.
- Restrain the client only as necessary.
- Administer pharmacological agents as ordered and monitor effects.
- Assess for potential for violence and take actions to avoid escalation in levels of agitation and anxiety.
- Implement suicide precautions as necessary.

The APACN should also evaluate the potential for long-term care:

- Assess the severity of the client's drug use problem.
- Assess the client's potential for accepting referrals.
- Involve family/significant others in the plan of care.
- Obtain consultation as necessary.
- Assess for the presence of concomitant health problems, and provide appropriate health teaching.
- Refer to community or institutional resources as necessary.
- Prepare/monitor for withdrawal syndrome as necessary.

Withdrawal Syndrome*

DEFINITION OF WITHDRAWAL

Withdrawal consists of a constellation of physiological and psychological responses that follow abrupt cessation or reduced intake of a substance upon which an individual is dependent. Physiologically, withdrawal represents a homeostatic response to the physiological changes induced by chronic use of a substance. Because substances are psychoactive, changes are consistently noted in neurophysiological systems.

Withdrawal symptoms vary greatly across classes of substances. Marked physiological signs are common with opiates and CNS depressants. Such signs are less obvious or less well documented with CNS stimulants and hallucinogens, as well as nicotine, but intense subjective symptoms can occur upon withdrawal from heavy use of these substances.

Withdrawal is also characterized by the following four traits:
1. Morbidity associated with withdrawal or the likelihood of relapse does not directly relate to the intensity of physical withdrawal.
2. Typically, withdrawal symptoms are somewhat opposite in nature from the direct effects of the substance.
3. Withdrawals from all classes of substances are similar in producing symptoms of acute anxiety and protracted depression.
4. Polydrug use—the use of more than one drug—is increasingly the norm rather than the exception; as a result, any withdrawal syndrome may be accompanied by a second set of symptoms or can be masked by intoxication of another substance.

The substance abuser is frequently found to be self-medicating, a behavioral disorder that antedates drug exposure. The withdrawal syndrome evokes evidence of a previously masked set of psychiatric symptoms, such as phobias, anxiety, neurosis, or borderline personality.

WITHDRAWAL FROM CENTRAL NERVOUS SYSTEM DEPRESSANTS (ETOH, BARBITURATES, SEDATIVE-HYPNOTICS)

Withdrawal from CNS depressants produces the most dangerous types of withdrawal syndrome. Abrupt withdrawal is *never* advocated or therapeutically indicated. In contrast to the CNS depression caused by depressant ingestion, abstinence is associated with systemic adrenergic hyperactivity manifested at the levels of the cerebral cortex, limbic system, and brainstem.

It has been hypothesized that chronic depressant intake results in rebound increased CNS stimulation without the depressant effects of the drug. Uncontrolled CNS overstimulation predominates.

Physiological Mechanisms

Physiological effects of withdrawal include the following:
- The degree of mild to severe symptoms depends on the chronicity of depressant dependence and the degree of tolerance established.

---

*The discussion of withdrawal syndrome is adapted, with permission, from Compton, M. (1991). Nursing care in acute withdrawal. *Substance Abuse Education in Nursing 15-2463*(2), 412–419.

- Onset of withdrawal syndrome varies with the half-life of depressant (e.g., within 6–8 hours for ETOH; 24–36 hours for phenobarbital).
- Symptoms do not follow a specific sequence but commonly progress in severity as follows:
  - Tremulousness, tachycardia, headache, irritability, anxiety, postural hypotension, insomnia, moderate diaphoresis, hyperreflexic deep tendon reflexes (DTRs), disorientation. These symptoms are usually the extent of a mild withdrawal syndrome. Approximately 10 percent of clients will progress to symptoms of extreme autonomic excess (e.g., extreme sympathetic nervous stimulation).
  - Multiple generalized seizures are most common within the first 72 hours of a withdrawal syndrome. They are more likely to progress to status epilepticus in barbiturate withdrawal.
  - Myoclonic contractions may occur.
  - Hallucinosis, usually auditory as a third-person voice, occurs while sensorium is clear and memory is intact; patient may recognize these as hallucinations.
  - Withdrawal delirium (referred to as **delirium tremens** or DTs in ETOH withdrawal) may occur. They are characterized by impaired recent and remote memory; disorientation; and terrifying visual, auditory, or tactile hallucinations.
  - Extreme hypertension is possible.
  - Profuse diarrhea may be present.
  - Hyperpyrexia with profound diaphoresis may occur.
  - Vascular collapse and death may occur.

Common Concomitant Medical Problems Complicating Physiological State

Concomitant medical problems include:
- Malnutrition
- Opportunistic infections (e.g., *Pneumocystis carinii* pneumonia, cytomegalovirus)
- Liver disease
- Trauma, burns
- Aspiration pneumonia
- Pressure necrosis, skin breakdown

WITHDRAWAL FROM CNS STIMULANTS (AMPHETAMINE, COCAINE)

Physiological Mechanisms

Physiological effects of withdrawal include the following:
- Stimulants act at the neurotransmitter level to provide subjective feelings of euphoria, activation, disinhibition, well-being, and alertness. Withdrawal symptoms are subtle and not obviously manifested systemically and are best documented and understood within the psychological realm.
- Onset of withdrawal symptoms varies with half-life of the stimulant (e.g., cocaine, 30–60 minutes; amphetamine, 4–6 hours).
- Two recently reported physiological sequelae of stimulant withdrawal theoretically relate to alterations in systemic neurotransmitter systems:

1. Myocardial ischemia was noted up to four weeks post–cocaine abstinence, perhaps due to cocaine-mediated chronic dopamine depletion that increases risk for coronary artery vasospasm.
2. Acute dystonia was reported during acute cocaine withdrawal, perhaps due to cocaine-mediated chronic dopamine and norepinephrine depletion that lowers the threshold for dystonia responses.

Common Concomitant Medical Problems Complicating Physiological State

These concomitant medical problems include:
1. Malnutrition
2. Opportunistic infections
3. Trauma

WITHDRAWAL FROM NARCOTICS

Physiological Mechanisms

Physiological effects of withdrawal include the following:
- Narcotics bind to endogenous *mu* opiate receptors in the CNS and produce responses of euphoria, analgesia, and respiratory depression. Withdrawal is characterized by rebound excitability in those organs whose functions were previously depressed.
- Withdrawal syndrome results in moderate discomfort; it never leads to life-threatening illness.
- Great individual variation is noted in withdrawal syndrome intensity; it depends on chronicity of opiate use, tolerance, and rate at which drug is removed from receptors.
- Withdrawal syndrome onset varies with the half-life of opiate (e.g., heroin and morphine, 10–12 hours; methadone, 24–36 hours).
- Nine physiological manifestations include:
  1. Stomach cramps, nausea, and vomiting
  2. Diaphoresis
  3. Hypertension
  4. Backaches or muscle aches
  5. Lacrimation and rhinorrhea
  6. Gooseflesh
  7. Yawning
  8. Mydriasis
  9. Diarrhea

Common Concomitant Medical Problems Complicating Physiological State

Six concomitant medical problems include:
1. HIV, hepatitis, tuberculosis
2. Opportunistic infections
3. Cellulitis
4. Bacterial endocarditis
5. Aspiration pneumonia
6. Pressure necrosis

Psychological States Associated with Withdrawal

CNS Depressants

In a mild withdrawal, acute anxiety, irritability, and nervousness, which may be manifested as demanding or annoying behavior, are evident. The client may complain of difficulty concentrating. Insomnia and nightmares are also common. In a more severe withdrawal, psychological responses related to disorientation and delirium, including paranoia, violence, fear, and depersonalization, are evident. A protracted withdrawal syndrome lasting at least three weeks post–depressant abstinence can occur, evidenced by complaints of spontaneous anxiety, depressive episodes, transient psychotic reactions, impaired cognitive performance, increased irritability and impatience, fatigue, low stress tolerance, emotional lability, and distractibility.

CNS Stimulants

A withdrawal syndrome accompanying stimulant abstinence is believed to be related to central neurotransmitter derangements secondary to chronic stimulant use. Psychological states associated with withdrawal are best described as occurring in three temporally related phases, best described with cocaine abstinence:

1. The crash phase, usually occurring between 9 and 96 hours post–cocaine use, is manifested by early symptoms of depression, agitation, and high drug craving. This phase proceeds to feelings of increased depression, fatigue with desire for sleep, and absence of drug craving. Depressant use is common during this phase. Late in the crash phase, client behaviors include hypersomnolence and hyperphagia.
2. The withdrawal phase, occurring for the next 8 to 10 weeks after cocaine abstinence (similar temporally to the protracted withdrawal syndrome described with depressant withdrawal), results in marked anhedonia, anergia, anxiety, and high cocaine craving.
3. If relapse is not experienced during the withdrawal phase, the client enters indefinite extinction phases, characterized by a return to normal moods and hedonic response with episodic craving.

Narcotics

Distinct psychological sequelae of opiate withdrawal are not evident. Psychological states are similar to those experienced during mild depressant withdrawal; generalized anxiety, restlessness, and dysphoria are common. Inconclusive evidence exists that a protracted withdrawal syndrome may also occur, with subtle disturbances of mood and sleep persisting for weeks to months.

Assessment

Assessing a client for acute withdrawal syndrome includes obtaining a nursing history, collecting data on the drug history, and conducting a physical examination.

Nursing History

Components of the history should include:
- Drug of choice or substance primarily used
- Other types of drugs used and possible interactions

- Frequency, amount, and duration of drug use
- Half-life of substance(s) ingested
- Minutes/hours since last use of substance(s)
- Past history of and response to withdrawal
- Client's acceptance/knowledge of dependence and desired outcome

Data on Drug History

While the client is in acute withdrawal, obtaining a complete drug history may be impossible. Focus on the information that is important to determining withdrawal response.

Physical Examination

The physical examination should include eight components:
1. Mental status, including level of consciousness, orientation, memory, mood, affect, and reality testing
2. Presence of anxiety, restlessness, and drug-seeking behaviors
3. Vital signs
4. Plasma or urine toxicology reports
5. Presenting symptoms
6. Hydration status
7. Nutritional status
8. Skin assessment and integrity

NURSING INTERVENTIONS

The APACN should address the acute physiological state of the client experiencing the withdrawal syndrome by:

- Obtaining vital signs frequently
- Recording accurate intake and output; initiating aggressive intravenous fluid replacement; watching for signs of fluid overload
- Monitoring laboratory values
- Administering vitamin supplements as ordered
- Administering pharmacological treatments as ordered and evaluating response; watching for oversedation and respiratory depression
- Placing client on seizure precautions with suction available
- Providing comfort measures
- Maintaining skin integrity
- Ensuring adequate nutritional intake
- Promoting pulmonary hygiene
- Monitoring client responses and behaviors after guest visits

The APACN should also assess the psychological state of the client by performing a mental status examination (an instrument such as the Mini-Mental State Exam is helpful). Seven specific areas to be evaluated are:

1. Level of consciousness
2. Affect and mood (presence of anxiety, depression, and mood swings)

3. Suicidal or homicidal thoughts
4. Memory
5. Judgment
6. Reality testing
7. Coping and defining mechanisms

It is also important that the APACN establishes effective communication patterns with the client. In order to establish a short-term trusting relationship, the nurse should:

- Attempt to be nonjudgmental in interactions.
- Examine personal opinions/feelings about substance use and personal pattern of substance use; appreciate how these affect interactions with a substance-abusing client.
- Be honest and clear in interactions.
- Anticipate anger, denial, and defensiveness from the client; accept these responses as part of the disease.
- Treat the client with respect and in ways that enhance self-esteem.

The following eight interventions can be used to care for clients experiencing behavioral disturbances due to withdrawal:

1. Offer emotional and psychological support.
2. Provide a safe, nonthreatening environment. A private, well-lit, quiet room is ideal. Avoid placing clients in an intensive care unit as much as possible.
3. Provide frequent reorientation cues as appropriate. Avoid the use of physical restraints. Ambulate the client, with assistance as appropriate, to decrease anxiety and to allow environmental exploration.
4. Provide the client with short-term alternative ways to deal with anxiety and dysphoria.
5. Administer pharmacological agents and antidotes as appropriate. Evaluate effects.
6. Utilize interpersonal supports as indicated.
7. Utilize methods for interpersonal security.
8. Do not attempt to address and change substance use behavior while the client is experiencing acute withdrawal.

Following crisis intervention, the APACN should evaluate the need and potential for referral of the client by:

- Assessing the client's readiness and desire to change substance use behavior
- Discussing potential referrals with the client
- Obtaining consultation as necessary
- Becoming familiar with and referring the client to institutions and/or community agencies

Tables 7-6 and 7-10 describe emergency management of drug overdose and cocaine toxicity, respectively, and Table 7-11 describes the effects (early and long-term) of cocaine use.

TABLE 7-10 Emergency Management: Acute Cocaine Toxicity.

Possible Etiology	Possible Assessment Findings	Management
Intranasal Parenteral Oral Vaginal Rectal Sublingual	Cardiovascular manifestations: cardiac palpitations with feelings of impending doom, tachycardia, hypertension, dysrhythmias, myocardial ischemia or infarction Euphoria, agitation, combativeness Seizures Hallucinations, confusion, paranoia Fever	Establish and maintain airway. Anticipate need for intubation if respiratory distress is evident. Establish IV access and give IV fluid replacement. Administer: • Lidocaine or propranolol IV for ventricular dysrhythmias • Midazolam IV for agitation • Haloperidol IV for psychosis • Diazepam or lorazepam IV for seizures • Naloxone IV for CNS depression • Propranolol or labetalol for hypertension and tachycardia Do a 12-lead ECG, and maintain ECG monitoring. Be prepared to perform CPR or defibrillation. Monitor vital signs, including level of consciousness. Obtain medical history, including drug use.

Source: Reproduced with permission from Lisanti, P., and Duphorne, P. (1996). Substance abuse and dependence. In S. Lewis, I. Collier, and M. Heitkemper (eds.), *Medical-Surgical Nursing: Assessment and Management of Clinical Problems* (4th ed.). Philadelphia: W.B. Saunders/Mosby, p. 154.

TABLE 7-11 Effects of Cocaine Use.

System/Function	Early Effects	Long-Term Effects
Central nervous system	Excitation, euphoria, restlessness, talkativeness	Depression, hallucinations, tremors, visual disturbances, dysarthria, seizure activity, headaches, insomnia, stroke
Cardiovascular system	Tachycardia, hypertension, angina, dysrhythmias, palpitations	Ventricular dysrhythmias, hypotension, congestive heart failure, myocardial infarction, cardiomyopathy
Respiratory system	Increased respiratory rate, dyspnea, chest pain, epistaxis	Chronic cough, inflamed throat, congestion of lungs, brown or black sputum production, pneumonia, respiratory distress or arrest, pulmonary edema, rhinorrhea, rhinitis, erosion and perforation of the nasal septum
Emotions	Behavior changes or mood swings	Depression or suicidal thoughts
Gastrointestinal system	Decreased appetite	Dehydration, weight loss, nausea; intestinal ischemia may cause gangrene
Sexuality	Heightened sexual desire, delayed ejaculation and orgasm (women may have difficulty achieving orgasm)	Difficulty in maintaining erection and ejaculation, loss of interest in sexual activity (women may develop aberrant sexual behavior)

Source: Reproduced with permission from Lisanti, P., and Duphorne, P. (1996). Substance abuse and dependence. In S. Lewis, I. Collier, and M. Heitkemper (eds.), *Medical-Surgical Nursing: Assessment and Management of Clinical Problems* (4th ed.). Philadelphia: W.B. Saunders/Mosby, p. 153.

Kindling in Alcohol Withdrawal

In many alcoholics, the severity of withdrawal symptoms increases after repeated withdrawal episodes. This exacerbation may be attributed to a kindling process. Kindling is a phenomenon in which a weak electrical or chemical stimulus, which initially causes no overt behavioral responses, results in the appearance of behavioral effects, such as seizures, when it is administered repeatedly. Both clinical and experimental evidence support the existence of a kindling mechanism during alcohol withdrawal (Becker, 1998). Withdrawal symptoms, such as seizures, result from neurochemical imbalances in the brains of alcoholics who suddenly reduce or cease alcohol consumption. These imbalances may be exacerbated after repeated withdrawal experiences. The existence of kindling during withdrawal suggests that even clients experiencing mild withdrawal should be treated aggressively to prevent the increase in severity of subsequent withdrawal episodes. Kindling also may contribute to a client's relapse risk as well as to alcohol-related brain damage and cognitive impairment (Becker, 1998).

Pharmacological Management of Detoxification

The APACN implements appropriate role behaviors in relation to pharmacologic interventions for detoxification. Most detoxification procedures are specific to particular drugs of dependence; others are based on general principles of treatment and are not drug-specific. The general principles for detoxification are presented in Table 7-12, followed by specific treatment regimens for each category of abused drug.

Alcohol Dependency

Alcohol Detoxification

Most alcohol-dependent individuals can be detoxified in a modified medical setting, as long as assessment is comprehensive, medical backup is available, and staff know when to obtain a medical consultation.

TABLE 7-12 Principles of Detoxification.

- Detoxification alone is rarely adequate treatment for alcohol and other drug (AOD) dependencies.
- When using medication regimens or other detoxification procedures, clinicians should use only protocols of established safety and efficacy.
- Providers must advise clients when procedures are used that have not been established as safe and effective.
- During detoxification, providers should control client's access to medication to the greatest extent possible.
- Initiation of withdrawal should be individualized.
- Whenever possible, clinicians should substitute a long-acting medication for short-acting drugs of addiction.
- The intensity of withdrawal cannot always be predicted accurately.
- Every means possible should be used to ameliorate clients' signs and symptoms of AOD withdrawal.
- When the level of severity indicates dependence, clients should begin participating in follow-up support therapy such as peer group therapy, family therapy, individual counseling or therapy, 12-step recovery meetings, and AOD recovery educational programs.

Detoxification episodes are often hospital-based and may begin with emergency treatment of an overdose. A large percentage of drug detoxification (an estimated 100,000 admissions annually) is now taking place in hospital beds (USDHHS, 1995). It is doubtful whether hospitalization (especially beyond a day or two) is necessary in most cases, except for the special problems of addicted neonates, severe sedative-hypnotic dependence, or concurrent medical or severe psychiatric problems. For clients with a documented history of complications or flight from detoxification, residential detoxification may be indicated. Detoxification may be undertaken successfully in most cases on a nonhospital residential, partial day care, or ambulatory basis (USDHHS, 1995).

Clients who score higher than 20 on the Clinical Institute Withdrawal Assessment (CIWA-Ar) instrument should be admitted to a hospital (see Table 7-13).

ASSESSMENT OF ALCOHOL WITHDRAWAL SYMPTOMS

Most clients can be detoxified from alcohol in 3 to 5 days. Providers should devise a withdrawal time frame in terms of when the client will need the most support; for alcoholics, this occurs the second day after the last ingestion. Other factors that influence the length of the detoxification period include the severity of the dependence and the client's overall health status. Clients who are elderly or medically debilitated may detoxify more slowly.

The signs and symptoms of acute alcohol abstinence syndrome generally begin 6 to 24 hours after the client takes his or her last drink. The acute phase of alcohol abstinence syndrome may begin when the client still has a significant blood alcohol concentration (BAC) level. Signs and symptoms of alcohol withdrawal may include:

- Restlessness, irritability, anxiety, agitation
- Anorexia, nausea, vomiting
- Tremor, elevated heart rate, increased blood pressure
- Insomnia, intense dreaming, nightmares
- Impaired concentration, memory, and judgment
- Increased sensitivity to sounds, alteration in tactile sensations
- Delirium (disorientation to time, place, and situation)
- Hallucinations (auditory, visual, or tactile)
- Delusions (usually paranoid)
- Grand mal seizures
- Elevated temperature

Symptoms do not always progress from mild to severe in a predictable fashion. In some clients, a grand mal seizure may be the first manifestation of acute alcohol abstinence syndrome.

Although many programs devise their own methods of monitoring clients' withdrawal signs and symptoms, there is considerable advantage to using a widely accepted validated instrument. The CIWA-Ar is commonly used in clinical and research settings for initial assessment and ongoing monitoring of alcohol withdrawal symptoms. It takes "2 to 5 minutes to administer, helps make the decision to hospitalize the client or to treat him or her as an outpatient, and is useful for monitoring and managing the client during withdrawal" (Fuller and Gordis, 1994, p. 558). It measures the severity of alcohol withdrawal by rating 10 signs and symptoms: nausea and vomiting; tremor; paroxysmal sweats; anxiety; agitation; tactile, auditory, and visual disturbances; headache; and orientation (see Table 7-13). The maximum score is 67.

TABLE 7-13 Clinical Institute Assessment (CIWA-Ar).

Patient: _____ Date: / _____ / _____ / _____ Time: _____

Y M D (24-hour clock, midnight = 00:00)

Pulse or heart rate, taken for one minute: Blood pressure:

NAUSEA AND VOMITING—Ask, "Do you feel sick to your stomach? Have you vomited?" Observation.	TACTILE DISTURBANCES—Ask, "Have you any itching, pins and needles sensations, any burning, or any numbness, or do you feel bugs crawling on or under your skin?" Observation.
0 no nausea and no vomiting	0 none
1 mild nausea with no vomiting	1 mild itching, pins and needles, burning, or numbness
2	2 mild itching, pins and needles, burning, or numbness
3	3 moderate itching, pins and needles, burning, or numbness
4 intermittent nausea with dry heaves	4 moderately severe hallucinations
5	5 severe hallucinations
6	6 extremely severe hallucinations
7 constant nausea, frequent dry heaves and vomiting	7 continuous hallucinations
TREMOR—Arms extended and fingers spread apart. Observation.	AUDITORY DISTURBANCES—Ask, "Are you more aware of sounds around you? Are they harsh? Do they frighten you? Are you hearing anything that is disturbing to you? Are you hearing things that you know are not there?" Observation.
0 no tremor	
1 not visible, but can be felt fingertip to fingertip	0 not present
2	1 very mild harshness or ability to frighten
4 moderate, with patient's arms extended	2 mild harshness or ability to frighten
5	3 moderate harshness or ability to frighten
6	4 moderately severe hallucinations
7 severe, even with arms not extended	5 severe hallucinations
	6 extremely severe hallucinations
	7 continuous hallucinations
PAROXYSMAL SWEATS—Observation.	VISUAL DISTURBANCES—Ask, "Does the light appear to be too bright? Is its color different? Does it hurt your eyes? Are you seeing anything that is disturbing to you? Are you seeing things that you know are not there?" Observation.
0 no sweat visible	
1 barely perceptible sweating, palms moist	
2	0 not present
3	1 very mild sensitivity
4 beads of sweat obvious on forehead	2 mild sensitivity
5	3 moderate sensitivity
6	4 moderately severe hallucinations
7 drenching sweats	5 severe hallucinations
	6 extremely severe hallucinations
	7 continuous hallucinations

(continued)

TABLE 7-13 (continued)

ANXIETY—Ask, "Do you feel nervous?" Observation.	**HEADACHE, FULLNESS IN HEAD**—Ask, "Does your head feel different? Does it feel like there is a band around your head?" Do not rate for dizziness or lightheadedness. Otherwise, rate severity.
0 no anxiety, at ease	
1 mildly anxious	0 not present
2	1 very mild
3	2 mild
4 moderately anxious or guarded so anxiety is inferred	3 moderate
	4 moderately severe
5	5 severe
6	6 very severe
7 equivalent to acute panic states as seen in severe delirium or acute schizophrenic reactions	7 extremely severe
AGITATION—Observation.	**ORIENTATION AND CLOUDING OF SENSORIUM**—Ask, "What day is this? Where are you? Who am I?" Observation.
0 normal activity	
1 somewhat more than normal activity	0 oriented and can do serial additions
2	1 cannot do serial additions or is uncertain about date
3	2 disoriented for date by no more than 2 calendar days
4 moderately fidgety and restless	3 disoriented for date by more than 2 calendar days
5	4 disoriented for place and/or person
6	
7 paces back and forth during most of the interview or constantly thrashes about	

Total CIWA-Ar Score:

Rater's Initials:

Maximum Possible Score: 67

Note: This scale is not copyrighted and may be used without permission.

Source: Addiction Research Foundation.

The CIWA-Ar should be repeated at regular intervals (initially every 1 or 2 hours) to monitor clients' progress. Increasing scores on the CIWA-Ar signify the need for additional medication or a higher level of treatment; decreasing scores suggest therapeutic response to medication or treatment milieu. Clients scoring less than 10 on CIWA-Ar do not usually need additional medication for withdrawal.

BENZODIAZEPINE TREATMENT OF ALCOHOL WITHDRAWAL

Benzodiazepines, such as chlordiazepoxide (Librium), clonazepam (Klonopin), clorazepate (Tranxene), and diazepam (Valium), are considered effective tools in ameliorating signs and symptoms of alcohol withdrawal because they decrease the likelihood and number of withdrawal seizures and episodes of delirium tremens. Chlordiazepoxide is "currently the most commonly administered medication for alcohol withdrawal in the United States" (Saitz et al., 1994). Oxazepam (Serax) and lorazepam (Ativan) are sometimes used with clients who have severe liver disease because neither is metabolized by the liver.

There are several acceptable pharmacologic regimens for treating alcohol withdrawal:

- **Gradual, tapering doses.** Oral benzodiazepines are administered on a predetermined dosing schedule for several days and gradually discontinued. This regimen is the one most commonly used. Dosing protocols vary widely among treatment facilities. As an example, clients may receive 50 mg of chlordiazepoxide (or 10 mg of diazepam) every 6 hours during the first day and 25 mg (or 5 mg of diazepam) every 6 hours on the second and third days. Doses of medication are usually omitted if the client is sleeping soundly or showing signs of oversedation.

- **Symptom-triggered therapy.** Using the CIWA-Ar, APACNs are trained to recognize signs and symptoms of alcohol withdrawal and to give benzodiazepine to their clients only when signs and symptoms of alcohol withdrawal appear. Studies have demonstrated that appropriate training of nurses in the application of the CIWA-Ar dramatically reduces the number of clients who receive symptom-triggered medication (from 75 percent to 13 percent).

- **Loading dose.** Staff administer a slowly metabolized benzodiazepine for only the first day of treatment. Clients in moderate to severe withdrawal receive 20 mg of diazepam (or 100 mg of chlordiazepoxide) every 1 to 2 hours until they show significant clinical improvement (such as a CIWA-Ar score of 10 or less) or become sedated. Oral diazepam loading alone may be sufficient to prevent withdrawal seizures in clients who have had them previously and who have no other reason for having seizures. Symptom-triggered therapy is an approach that can individualize and improve the management of alcohol withdrawal.

Some clients can be withdrawn from alcohol without medication treatment; however, guidelines for identifying clients who can safely be treated without medication have not been validated in controlled clinical trials. Clinically, it is safer to provide treatment for clients who may not need it than to withhold medication until clients develop severe withdrawal signs and symptoms.

Medication Management

Other medications that are used to address associated withdrawal symptoms are discussed here.

Carbamazepine (Tegretol)

Carbamazepine, a medication used for treatment of seizures, has been reported as effective in treatment of alcohol withdrawal. Anticonvulsants with antikindling properties may be superior to traditional benzodiazepines in preventing alcohol withdrawal seizures and in potentially reducing long-term neurologic, behavioral, and psychiatric complications of alcoholism. The usual dose is 80–1,200 mg/day in three to four divided doses.

Propranolol (Inderal) and Other Beta-Blockers

Some of the autonomic nervous system hyperactivity of alcohol withdrawal (such as rapid heartbeat, elevation of blood pressure, sweating, and tremors) is ameliorated by medications, such as propranolol (Inderal) and atenolol (Tenormin), that block beta-adrenergic receptors. Although effective in decreasing autonomic system symptoms, beta-blockers do not prevent hallucinations and confusion or withdrawal seizures. In addition, propranolol may increase the risk of delirium and hallucinations during alcohol withdrawal.

Treatment of Delirium and Seizures

DTs and seizures are two severe physiologic responses to withdrawal from sedative-hypnotics. Clients who develop DTs with auditory, visual, or tactile hallucinations may need antipsychotic medications to ameliorate their hallucinations and to decrease agitation. Haloperidol, known by the trade name Haldol, generally controls symptoms using doses of 0.5 to 2.0 mg every 4 hours by mouth or using intramuscular injections. Clients who are not vomiting may be given the medication by mouth; those who are severely agitated or vomiting may be administered Haldol intramuscularly. Clients should continue to receive benzodiazepines. Phenothiazines such as chlorpromazine (Thorazine) should not be used because of the increased risk of seizures.

MAGNESIUM SULFATE. Study findings suggest that magnesium sulfate does not reduce seizure frequency, even in clients with low serum magnesium levels. More recent studies have affirmed the use of benzodiazepines as most effective in treating DTs and seizures (Gorelick, 1993).

PHENYTOIN (DILANTIN). The therapeutic or prophylactic value of a routine prescription of phenytoin to prevent alcohol withdrawal seizures is not established. The current consensus is that phenytoin or other anticonvulsant therapy appropriate for the seizure type should be used for clients with an established history of seizure disorder (seizures not caused solely by alcohol withdrawal). Expert opinion is mixed as to whether phenytoin (or other anticonvulsants) should be used in addition to adequate sedative-hypnotic medication in clients who are at increased risk of alcohol withdrawal seizures because of a history of previous withdrawal seizures, head injury, meningitis, encephalitis, or family history of seizure disorder. Intravenous phenytoin is not beneficial for clients with isolated acute alcohol withdrawal seizures, but it may be indicated for clients who have multiple alcohol withdrawal seizures. It should be administered orally or intravenously because it is poorly absorbed when administered intramuscularly.

Phenobarbital

Phenobarbital is the drug of choice for alcohol detoxification when a client is physically dependent on both sedative-hypnotics and alcohol.

Naltrexone

Naltrexone has been approved by the Food and Drug Administration (FDA) as a treatment adjunct to reduce the likelihood of relapse to alcohol dependence among detoxified alcohol-dependent clients. Naltrexone, marketed under the trade name of Trexan, is now also marketed under the trade name ReVia.

Naltrexone is an opioid antagonist that has previously been used primarily to block the effects of heroin and thereby reduce the likelihood of relapse. Its mechanism of action in reducing alcohol consumption is not understood; however, clinical trials support its efficacy when it is used in conjunction with training in coping skills, cognitive therapy, and/or supportive therapy. It appears to reduce alcohol craving and thus is associated with less frequent and shorter relapses for individuals who abuse but are not physically dependent on alcohol.

The National Institute of Alcohol Abuse and Alcoholism cautions that naltrexone should be administered only by health care providers with knowledge of addiction treatment and as part of a structured treatment program. A central consideration is the severity of the addiction. ReVia is not a choice for an alcohol-dependent individual; rather, it appears to be most effective for alcohol abusers who have serious intent to reduce consumption.

VITAMIN SUPPLEMENTS

Alcohol-dependent clients often have vitamin deficiencies, particularly thiamine. Clients should receive thiamine in addition to high-potency multivitamins.

DECISIONS REGARDING OUTPATIENT TREATMENT

Increasingly, providers and clients are choosing the option of outpatient detoxification. These choices are being made because of cost and because hospitalization (for other than serious sedative dependence) is considered unnecessary when there are no concurrent medical or severe psychiatric problems. Nurse providers must take into account additional considerations when designing treatment plans for outpatients:

- Clients may have ready access to alcohol and other drugs (AODs) at home.
- Clients may continue to use alcohol in addition to the prescribed detoxification medications. If they develop withdrawal symptoms, they may self-medicate with AODs. The combination of detoxification medications and other drugs may result in overdose.
- Clients may have difficulty getting from their homes to their programs each day.
- Clients who are undergoing detoxification may experience side effects of withdrawal or breakthrough withdrawal.
- APACN and clinical social workers (CSWs) need collaborative protocols.

COMPLICATIONS OF ALCOHOL WITHDRAWAL

The APACN must observe complications during alcohol withdrawal and must monitor and treat these following problems.

Fluid and Electrolyte Imbalances

Maintaining the client's fluid and electrolyte balance is key during detoxification. Most clients can be given fluids orally, beginning with juices and progressing to other liquids, such as soups. Solid foods should be added to the client's diet only after he or she can tolerate liquids. Clients who are vomiting or having severe diarrhea should first be treated with sips of liquids that contain electrolytes. The amount can be increased to client tolerance. Clients who become dehydrated should receive intravenous fluids containing electrolytes, dextrose, and thiamine (100 mg/bottle).

Clients withdrawing from alcohol are not always dehydrated; in fact, many are overhydrated. Parenteral fluid therapy may be harmful in these cases and should be carefully monitored. During detoxification from alcohol, clients generally tolerate a mild degree of dehydration better than they do overhydration.

Hypoglycemia

Hypoglycemia is a significant danger during detoxification. Oral fluids should contain carbohydrates; orange juice may be one option. Parenteral fluids should contain 5 percent dextrose.

Fever

Observation for elevation of temperature in an individual who is undergoing withdrawal should be ongoing, and changes should be immediately investigated. If the elevated temperature is a result of withdrawal, there is a need for additional medication and reevaluation of the detoxification schedule. If a client has no other signs or symptoms of withdrawal, the elevated temperature may be indicative of an infection, and early aggressive antibiotic therapy may be necessary.

Psychiatric Comorbidity

Although medical concerns related to detoxification must be addressed first, any underlying psychiatric disorders must be dealt with as well. Failure to do so increases the risk of relapse. Evaluation of psychiatric conditions is determined by the drug of abuse and the clinical situation.

Suicidal clients can be detoxified, but they should be placed in an acute inpatient psychiatric setting rather than outpatient detoxification settings. These clients require close supervision by medical and nursing staff who understand both psychiatric and detoxification issues. The individual who takes the client's history should include questions about suicidal feelings, ideation, and plans, as well as previous suicide attempts.

Drug Interactions

Many drugs of abuse and certain medications used in detoxification may interact with others. Thus, it is important to obtain a history of any other medications that the client is taking and to consider potential drug interactions. Some examples of dangerous combinations include hypertensive medication and clonidine, phenytoin and methadone, and rifampin and methadone.

Opiate Dependency

WITHDRAWAL FROM OPIATES

All opiates—heroin, morphine, hydromorphone (Dilaudid), codeine, and methadone—produce similar withdrawal signs and symptoms; however, the time of onset and the duration of the abstinence syndromes vary. The severity of the withdrawal syndrome depends on many factors, including the drugs used, the total daily dose, intervals between doses, the duration of use, and the health and personality of the addict. The common signs and symptoms of opiate abstinence are summarized in Table 7-14.

Symptoms of withdrawal from opiates may be divided into four classes: 1) gastrointestinal distress, including diarrhea and (less frequently) nausea or vomiting; 2) pain, typically either arthralgias or myalgias or abdominal cramping; 3) anxiety; and 4) insomnia. The medications recommended for relief of these symptoms are presented in Table 7-15.

OPIATE ABSTINENCE SYNDROMES

Signs and symptoms of withdrawal from heroin or morphine begin 8 to 12 hours following the client's last dose. They subside over a period of 5 to 7 days.

Signs and symptoms of withdrawal from methadone begin 12 hours after the client's last dose. The peak intensity occurs on the third day of abstinence or later. Symptoms gradually subside but may continue for 3 weeks or longer. Methadone abstinence syndrome develops more slowly and is more prolonged, but it is usually less intense than other opiate abstinence syndromes.

TABLE 7-14 Signs and Symptoms of Opiate Abstinence.

Early	Advanced
Anxiety	Insomnia
Insomnia	Nausea and vomiting
Increased respiratory rate	Diarrhea
Sweating	Weakness
Lacrimation (tearing or crying)	Abdominal cramps
Yawning	Tachycardia
Rhinorrhea (runny nose)	Hypertension
Piloerection (goosebumps)	Muscle spasms
Restlessness	Muscle and bone pain
Anorexia	
Irritability	
Dilated pupils	

TABLE 7-15 Medications Recommended for Symptomatic Relief of Opiate Withdrawal.*

- Headache: Acetaminophen (Tylenol), 650 mg every 4 hours if needed
- Muscle, joint, or bone pain: Ibuprofen (Motrin, Advil), 600–800 mg every 8 hours
- Anxiety or insomnia: Hydroxyzine (Vistaril), 250 mg every 8 hours
- Abdominal cramps: Dicyclomine (Bentyl), 10 mg every 6 hours
- Constipation: Milk of Magnesia, 30 cc daily every other day
- Indigestion: Antacid (e.g., Mylanta), 30 cc between meals and at bedtime
- Loose stool: Bismuth subsalicylate (Pepto-Bismol), 30 cc after each loose stool, up to 8 doses total for no more than 2 days

*All doses are administered orally.

In July 1993, the FDA approved levo-alpha-acetylmethadol (LAAM) for use as a maintenance medication. It is a Schedule II controlled substance, which categorizes it as a medication with medical uses but also with a high potential for abuse. Withdrawal from LAAM produces symptoms similar to those produced by withdrawal from methadone.

MEDICATION TREATMENT FOR OPIATE WITHDRAWAL

Clonidine

Clonidine (Catapres), a medication marketed for the treatment of hypertension, has been used to treat the symptoms of opiate withdrawal since 1978. Although clonidine has not yet been approved by the FDA for treatment of opiate withdrawal, its use has become standard clinical practice.

Clonidine has some practical advantages over methadone for treating narcotic withdrawal, particularly in drug-free programs. These advantages include the following:

- It is not a scheduled medication.
- The use of opiates can be discontinued immediately in preparation for naltrexone induction or admission to a drug-free treatment program (e.g., a therapeutic community).
- It does not produce opiate euphoria, and the client's need for drugs is therefore reduced.

Although clonidine alleviates some symptoms of opiate withdrawal, it is not effective for muscle aches, insomnia, or drug craving. These symptoms require additional medication.

An appropriate protocol for clonidine is 0.1 mg administered orally as a test dose (0.22 mg for clients weighing more than 200 pounds). If the client's symptoms are acute, the sublingual route of administration may be used. The clinician should check the client's blood pressure 45 minutes after administration of clonidine. If diastolic blood pressure is normal for the client and the client has no signs of orthostatic hypotension (a drop in systolic blood pressure of 10 mm Hg upon standing), the client may continue clonidine, 0.1 to 0.2 mg orally every 4 to 6 hours. Clonidine is most effective when used for detoxification in an inpatient setting, as side effects can be monitored more closely.

In 1986, a transdermal patch containing clonidine (Catapres-TTS) was approved for use in the United States for the treatment of hypertension. Although the clonidine patch is commonly used for detoxification, there is concern that the safety of the patch for treatment of opiate withdrawal has not been sufficiently studied in controlled clinical trials. If clients receive too much clonidine from the patch and become hypotensive, the effects are not rapidly reversed even when the patch is removed. It is recommended that the use of clonidine be accompanied by regular blood pressure monitoring.

The clonidine patch is a 0.2-mm square that is applied in the same manner as a self-adhesive bandage. It is available in three sizes: 3.5, 7.0, and 10.5 cm^2. In a 24-hour period, these patches deliver an amount of clonidine equivalent to twice-daily dosing with 0.1, 0.2, or 0.3 mg of oral clonidine, respectively. Once the patch is in place on the epidermal surface, clonidine enters the circulatory system through the skin. A rate-limiting membrane within the patch governs the maximum amount absorbed. The patch supplies clonidine for up to 7 days. One application of the patch is sufficient.

In a recovery-oriented treatment program, the transdermal patch offers some advantages over oral clonidine:

- It minimizes drug cravings.
- The transdermal patch eliminates disruptions caused by administration of medication. Oral clonidine must be administered several times each day.
- The patch overcomes the problem of missed doses. Asymptomatic clients may forget to go to the nurses' station at scheduled times or may miss doses when they are attending outside activities.
- The patch prevents the buildup of withdrawal symptoms during the night. Clients who miss doses of oral clonidine during the night sometimes experience opiate withdrawal upon awaking.

For reasons such as these, staff and clients often prefer the patch over oral clonidine. Clients treated with oral clonidine appear to have more withdrawal symptoms than those treated with transdermal patches; however, controlled studies have not yet confirmed these findings.

Methadone

Methadone can be used for withdrawal from heroin, fentanyl, or other opiates. For certain client populations, including those with many treatment failures, methadone is the treatment of choice. Methadone generally is not used with adolescents because FDA regulations prohibit its use with this age group (there are rare exceptions). In this population, there are high risks of addiction and promotion of drug-seeking behavior.

Opiate-dependent inpatients who are being treated for an acute medical illness can be administered methadone for prevention of opiate withdrawal if opiate withdrawal would complicate treatment of their medical conditions. The withdrawal protocols using methadone vary, depending on the setting.

In an inpatient drug treatment program licensed for methadone detoxification, a starting dose of 30 mg to 40 mg per day of oral methadone is adequate to prevent severe withdrawal symptoms in most opiate-dependent clients. The methadone is administered four times daily, beginning with 10-mg doses, and the client is observed for 2 hours following each dose. If the client is sleepy, the next dose is decreased to 5 mg. If the client shows objective signs of opiate withdrawal, the dose is increased to 15 mg. After 24 hours, the methadone is withdrawn by 5 mg per day; thus, most clients are withdrawn over 8 days.

Methadone can be administered for detoxification only in a hospital or in an outpatient program that is licensed for methadone detoxification. Prescribing privileges are limited to nurse practitioners (NPs) and physicians who are part of the licensed treatment program.

OUTPATIENT METHADONE DETOXIFICATION CLINICS. In an outpatient clinic, treatment staff usually administer medication no more than twice a day. Thus, 20 mg of methadone, given orally twice daily, is a good starting point. To prevent an unacceptable level of withdrawal symptoms, some outpatients may need up to 60 mg of methadone per day administered in divided doses. After the second day, the methadone is tapered by 2.5 mg per day.

As of 1989, federal regulations allow short-term methadone detoxification of 30 days and long-term detoxification of 180 days. As the methadone state-licensing agencies develop regulations that parallel the federal regulations, state-licensed methadone programs will be able to implement long-term methadone detoxification.

Federal regulations allow physicians to administer (but not prescribe) narcotics for the purpose of relieving acute withdrawal symptoms while arrangements are being made for referral for treatment. Not more than 1 day's medication may be administered to the person or for the person's use at one time. Such emergency treatment may be carried out for not more than 3 days and may not be renewed or extended (USDHHS, 1995). Thus, under Drug Enforcement Administration (DEA) guidelines in states that allow the prescription of narcotics, a physician may administer methadone for 3 days without a special license if the client is experiencing acute withdrawal symptoms and cannot be immediately referred for treatment. This is considered an emergency situation.

In a short-term detoxification regimen, clients are not allowed to take methadone home. The initial treatment plan and periodic treatment plan evaluation required for maintenance clients are not necessary; however, the program must assign a primary counselor to monitor a client's progress toward the goal of short-term detoxification and to provide a drug treatment referral.

A client is required to wait at least 7 days between concluding a short-term detoxification treatment episode and beginning another. Before a short-term detoxification attempt is repeated, the program physician must document in the client's record that the client continues to be or is again physiologically dependent on narcotics. These requirements apply to both inpatient and outpatient short-term detoxification treatment programs.

For long-term detoxification, the opioid must be administered by the program physician or by an authorized agent who is supervised by and under the orders of the physician. The drug must be administered on a regimen designed to help the client reach a drug-free state and to make progress in rehabilitation in 180 days or fewer. The following six conditions apply (Banys et al., 1994):

1. During detoxification, the client must be under observation while ingesting the methadone for at least 6 days a week.
2. Before long-term detoxification can begin, the program physician must document in the client's record that short-term detoxification is not a sufficiently long treatment course to provide the client with the additional program services that will be necessary for the client's rehabilitation.
3. An initial drug screen is required for each client. At least one additional random urine test or analysis must be performed monthly.
4. An initial treatment plan and monthly treatment plan evaluation are required.
5. A client is required to wait at least 7 days after concluding a long-term treatment episode before beginning another. Before a long-term detoxification attempt is repeated, the program physician must document in the client's record that the client continues to be or is again physiologically dependent on narcotic drugs.
6. These requirements apply to both inpatient and ambulatory long-term detoxification treatment.

Levo-Alpha-Acetylmethadol

As mentioned previously, in July 1993 the FDA approved LAAM for use as a maintenance medication. The trade name of LAAM is Orlaam.

Until August 1993, LAAM was a Schedule I controlled substance, which is defined as a drug with a high abuse potential but with no recognized medical use. In August 1993, the DEA reclassified it as a Schedule II controlled substance, which defined it as a medication with medical uses as well as a drug with a high potential for abuse (USDHHS, 1995).

FDA methadone regulations have been revised (58 38706 Part, July 20, 1993) to allow use of LAAM (USDHHS, 1995). The regulations for LAAM are similar to those for methadone with two exceptions: Take-home doses of LAAM are not allowed, and LAAM cannot be administered to pregnant women. Clients who need take-home doses must be switched to methadone. Like methadone, LAAM may be dispensed only by licensed AOD treatment clinics (USDHHS, 1995).

LAAM is a prodrug with little opiate activity. This means that its opiate effects are produced by its long-acting metabolites, nor-LAAM and dinor-LAAM. Because LAAM itself is not a potent opiate, oral ingestion or intravenous injection of LAAM does not produce rapid onset of opiate effects as does the ingestion of methadone, heroin, morphine, and most other opiates.

DISCONTINUATION FROM LAAM MAINTENANCE. The metabolites of LAAM are long-acting, and gradual discontinuation of LAAM results in a slow decline in the plasma levels of nor-LAAM and dinor-LAAM and in the emergence of opiate withdrawal symptoms. Maintenance treatment with LAAM produces significant levels of dependence of the opiate type; therefore, discontinuation of LAAM requires management of opiate withdrawal. Few studies have addressed the medically supervised withdrawal of LAAM clients to a drug-free state; however, no evidence exists to suggest that withdrawal from LAAM is different from withdrawal from methadone or any other opioid. Because LAAM is longer acting than methadone, withdrawal will have a delayed onset and protracted course, although it may be less intense than withdrawal from methadone. Clients, however, tend to perceive a longer period as being worse, whether the actual intensity of symptoms is greater or not. Special counseling may be needed to address this aspect of withdrawal from LAAM.

The LAAM dose can be reduced gradually at a rate determined by the client's response. As an alternative, clients who want to withdraw from LAAM treatment can be converted to methadone (at 80 percent of their LAAM dose) with minimal difficulty. The key consideration may be the client's support system; take-home methadone entails fewer clinic visits. Although clients can visit the clinic on nondose days for support services only, they are less likely to do so without the incentive of receiving medication. Another option is the use of clonidine in the dosage regime, described previously for treatment of heroin withdrawal, to assist in discontinuing use of LAAM. When involuntary withdrawal from medication is unavoidable, clients should switch to methadone before withdrawal begins.

HEROIN DETOXIFICATION WITH LAAM. Although there is substantial medical literature reporting clinical trials with LAAM in treatment of heroin withdrawal, the FDA has not approved LAAM for use in heroin detoxification. It should, therefore, be used for heroin detoxification only under an Investigational New Drug (IND) exemption. Because LAAM takes from 8 to 12 hours to produce significant opiate effects, it is not a good choice for treatment of acute heroin withdrawal symptoms. Addicts may become impatient while waiting for LAAM to relieve their opiate withdrawal symptoms and may self-medicate their withdrawal symptoms with heroin. As the opiate effects of LAAM develop, the combined effects of heroin and LAAM may result in a life-threatening overdose. Treatment providers may prefer to begin heroin detoxification by stabilizing the client on methadone, then switch to LAAM for gradual discontinuation over 21 to 180 days. LAAM's long duration of effect makes it a logical option for this process. Additional research to determine how to optimally use LAAM for detoxification is necessary.

Buprenorphine

Buprenorphine is being investigated as a treatment for opiate dependence and detoxification. Buprenorphine is a potent analgesic that is available by prescription as a sublingual tablet in many parts of the world. Recently approved by the FDA in the United States, it is available by prescription as an analgesic in an injectable form (Buprenex). The doses of buprenorphine under investigation for maintenance treatment are considerably higher than those commonly prescribed for treatment of pain.

Buprenorphine's unusual pharmacological profile makes it attractive for the treatment of opiate dependence. The level of physical dependence produced by buprenorphine is not as great as that produced by methadone or heroin; therefore, most clients find buprenorphine easier to discontinue than methadone. Some clients can eventually be switched from buprenorphine maintenance to treatment with an opiate antagonist such as naltrexone. Buprenorphine is safer than methadone or LAAM if an overdose is ingested. Its opiate effects appear to be substantially less than those of methadone or heroin. Though it is currently an experimental drug with regard to its use in detoxification, buprenorphine may soon be approved by the FDA.

Buprenorphine produces physical dependence of the opiate type. The dosages of clients who have been maintained on buprenorphine for treatment of opiate dependence or chronic pain must be tapered. The onset of withdrawal symptoms is generally delayed for at least 24 hours, and peak intensity of withdrawal symptoms may not occur for 5 days or more. The intensity of withdrawal symptoms is generally less than that following methadone discontinuation. Buprenorphine can be discontinued by tapering the dosage to zero over 7 to 21 days. Symptoms also may be ameliorated with clonidine, particularly toward the end of the taper. Buprenorphine has been used successfully to detoxify heroin addicts to assist with methadone discontinuation. In 1985, buprenorphine was classified as a Schedule V narcotic (USDHHS, 1995). A narcotic is defined by the Controlled Substance Act of 1984 as a class of drugs containing opiates and cocaine (USDHHS, 1995). The narcotic classification is important because federal law permits prescription of a narcotic to narcotic addicts only in specially licensed treatment programs (USDHHS, 1995). The sole exception to this law is that when a client is admitted to a hospital for treatment of an acute medical condition (not solely addiction to drugs), he or she may be administered narcotics to prevent opiate withdrawal.

Buprenorphine has already been approved by the FDA for treatment of pain, so physicians can use it in clinical practice. Because it is classified as a narcotic, buprenorphine requires FDA approval for treatment of opiate dependence; therefore, it should be prescribed for opiate dependence only under an FDA-approved IND exemption. Others may be prosecuted for prescribing, dispensing, or administering buprenorphine for treatment of opiate dependence or withdrawal.

Propoxyphene

In the 1970s, propoxyphene (Darvon) was among the medications used for opiate withdrawal. Because of abuse of propoxyphene by addicts, the DEA reclassified it as a Schedule

IV narcotic (USDHHS, 1995). The narcotic classification prohibits its use for treatment of opiate dependency in routine clinical practice.

Termination of Opiate Maintenance Treatment

Clients on opiate maintenance are sometimes discontinued from medication for failing to comply with treatment program guidelines and requirements. This situation is awkward for both the program and the client, particularly if the client is abusive, threatening, and/or potentially violent. The program manager should develop and post prominently on the program premises at least one copy of a written policy covering criteria for involuntary termination of treatment. This policy should describe clients' rights and responsibilities as well as those of program staff. At the time a client enters treatment, a staff member designated by the program director should inform the client about the policy and where it is posted. The staff person should inform clients of the conditions under which they might be involuntarily terminated from treatment and of their rights under the termination procedure.

The medication discontinuation should not occur so rapidly that the client experiences severe opiate withdrawal symptoms. Treatment staff should taper the methadone dosage until the client is receiving 30 mg to 40 mg a day. At this point, treatment with clonidine and other medications may begin.

Voluntary Termination of Opiate Maintenance

Clients in methadone treatment, like others who are receiving daily medication on a long-term basis, should be evaluated periodically regarding the risks and benefits of their therapy. For some, eventual withdrawal from methadone maintenance is a realistic goal.

Research and clinical experience have not yet identified all the critical variables that determine when a client can be withdrawn from methadone and remain drug-free. A decision to withdraw voluntarily from methadone maintenance must therefore be left to the client and to the clinical judgment of the health care provider. Staff should encourage the client to remain in the program for as long as it is necessary and economically feasible.

NONPHARMACOLOGIC INTERVENTIONS

Acupuncture

Although some clinicians consider acupuncture an acceptable primary detoxification treatment for opiate abusers, there are few controlled studies to support this. Acupuncture can be a useful treatment adjunct to methadone or clonidine detoxification. According to Bullock and associates (1989): "Increased use of acupuncture therapy may be an effective adjunct to therapy in current programs for clients with persistent craving for alcohol but also may allow treatment to be extended to a large group of recidivist alcoholics for whom current therapies are not effective" (p. 28).

Auricular (ear) acupuncture has been used in treatment of opiate withdrawal since 1972, and it is done in clinics throughout the world. Brumbaugh (1993) stated: "The use of auricular acupuncture in treating acute drug withdrawal began in Hong Kong in 1972. It was used sporadically throughout the United States during the 1970s, and some experimentation with acupuncture was conducted at the Haight-Asbury Free Clinic in San Francisco. It began at Lincoln Hospital in New York where the protocol has been refined and expanded and has taken its firmer root" (p. 28).

Benzodiazepine and Sedative-Hypnotic Dependency

WITHDRAWAL FROM BENZODIAZEPINES AND OTHER SEDATIVE-HYPNOTICS

Barbiturates and the older sedative-hypnotics have been largely replaced by the benzodiazepines. Withdrawal syndromes from benzodiazepines and other sedative-hypnotics are similar, and the pharmacotherapy treatment strategies apply to both.

Dependence on benzodiazepines and other sedative-hypnotics usually develops as an unintended outcome of medical treatment. Benzodiazepines have many therapeutic uses. As therapy for some conditions, such as panic disorder, long-term treatment is appropriate medical practice. Physical dependency is sometimes unavoidable. Benzodiazepine dependency that develops during pharmacotherapy is not necessarily a substance use disorder. When the dependency results from clients taking the prescribed doses as directed by a physician, the term therapeutic discontinuation is preferable to the term detoxification. Abusers of heroin and stimulants often misuse benzodiazepines and other sedative-hypnotics, sometimes to the extent that they develop a physical dependence. In such cases, it is appropriate to think of withdrawal from the sedative-hypnotic as detoxification.

Use of either benzodiazepines or sedative-hypnotics at doses above the therapeutic range for a month or more produces physical dependence. Without appropriate medical treatment, withdrawal from benzodiazepines or other sedative-hypnotics can be severe and life-threatening. Withdrawal from benzodiazepines or other sedative-hypnotics produces a similar withdrawal syndrome, described in the section High-Dose Sedative-Hypnotic Withdrawal Syndrome. Some people will develop withdrawal symptoms after stopping therapeutic doses of benzodiazepines or other sedative-hypnotics after they have been used daily for 6 months or more. With low-dose withdrawal, the benzodiazepines and other sedative-hypnotics can produce qualitatively different withdrawal syndromes described in the section Low-Dose Benzodiazepine Withdrawal Syndrome.

High-Dose Sedative-Hypnotic Withdrawal Syndrome

Signs and symptoms of high-dose sedative-hypnotic withdrawal include anxiety, tremors, nightmares, insomnia, anorexia, nausea, vomiting, orthostatic hypotension, seizures, delirium, and hyperpyrexia. The syndrome is qualitatively similar for all sedative-hypnotics; however, the time course of symptoms depends on the particular drug. With short-acting sedative-hypnotics (e.g., pentobarbital [Nembutal], secobarbital [Seconal], meprobamate [Equanil, Miltown], and methaqualone) and short-acting benzodiazepines (e.g., oxazepam [Serax], alprazolam [Xanax], and triazolam [Halcion]), withdrawal symptoms typically begin 12 to 24 hours after the last dose and reach peak intensity between 24 and 72 hours after the last dose. Clients who have liver disease or who are elderly may develop symptoms more slowly because of decreased drug metabolism. With long-acting drugs (e.g., phenobarbital [Barbita], diazepam [Valium], and chlordiazepoxide [Librium]), withdrawal symptoms peak on the fifth to eighth day after the last dose.

Withdrawal delirium may include confusion as well as visual and auditory hallucinations. The delirium generally follows a period of insomnia. Some clients may have only delirium, and others only seizures; some may have both.

Low-Dose Benzodiazepine Withdrawal Syndrome

Low-dose benzodiazepine withdrawal syndrome may be referred to as therapeutic dose withdrawal, normal dose withdrawal, or benzodiazepine discontinuation syndrome. Knowledge about low-dose dependency is based on clinical observations and is still sketchy and controversial. As a practical matter, it is often impossible to know with certainty whether symptoms are caused by withdrawal or whether they mark a return of symptoms that were ameliorated by the benzodiazepine. Clients who are treated therapeutically with benzodiazepines often have symptoms such as anxiety, insomnia, or muscle tension before taking the benzodiazepine. When they stop taking the benzodiazepine, these symptoms may reappear. Some people who have taken benzodiazepines in therapeutic doses for months to years can abruptly discontinue the drug without developing symptoms. Others, taking similar amounts of a benzodiazepine, develop symptoms ranging from mild to severe when the benzodiazepine is stopped or the dosage is substantially reduced.

Although the risk factors associated with withdrawal are not completely understood, clients who develop the severe form of low-dose benzodiazepine withdrawal syndrome tend to be those who have a family or personal history of alcoholism, those who are daily alcohol users, or those who concomitantly use other sedatives. Many clinical studies and case reports published in the 1980s on withdrawal discussed therapeutic dose discontinuation. Most clients experienced only a transient increase in symptoms for 1 to 2 weeks after termination of a benzodiazepine. This transient increase in symptoms is known as symptom rebound and is defined as an intensified return of the symptoms (e.g., insomnia or anxiety) for which the benzodiazepine was prescribed. According to the American Psychiatric Association (APA) (1990): "The most immediate discontinuance symptoms tend to be a rebound worsening of the original symptoms. A more severe withdrawal syndrome consists of the appearance of new symptoms, including perceptual hyperacusis, psychosis, cerebellar dysfunction, and seizures" (p. 30). Original symptoms may reappear when the therapeutic medication is withdrawn, and it may be difficult to distinguish recurrence of original symptoms from rebound.

Physiological dependence on benzodiazepines, as indicated by the appearance of discontinuance symptoms, can develop with therapeutic doses. Duration of treatment determines the onset of dependence when typical therapeutic anxiolytic doses are used. Clinically significant dependence indicated by the appearance of discontinuance symptoms usually does not appear before four months of such daily dosing. Dependence may develop sooner when higher antipanic doses are taken daily.

Protracted Withdrawal, Severe Form

A few clients experience a severe, long-lasting withdrawal syndrome with symptoms such as paresthesia and psychoses that were never experienced before the benzodiazepines were taken. This condition may be quite disabling and may last many months; it has generated much of the concern about the long-term safety of the benzodiazepines. Many psychiatrists, however, believe that the symptoms that occur after discontinuation of therapeutic doses of benzodiazepines are not a withdrawal syndrome but a reemergence of the client's psychopathology.

Protracted Withdrawal, Mild Form

One additional form of withdrawal is sometimes attributed to the benzodiazepines and other sedative-hypnotics as well as to alcohol and opiates. This is a mild form of protracted withdrawal. Symptoms include irritability, anxiety, insomnia, and mood instability, and it may persist for months following the beginning of abstinence.

TREATMENT FOR BENZODIAZEPINE WITHDRAWAL WITH MEDICATION

The health care provider's response during benzodiazepine withdrawal is critical to a successful outcome. Some health care providers interpret clients' escalating symptoms as evidence of their need for additional benzodiazepine treatment. Consequently, they prescribe the benzodiazepine, often at higher doses, or switch the client to another benzodiazepine. Reinstitution of any benzodiazepine agonist may not achieve satisfactory symptom control and may, in fact, prolong the recovery process.

A common response, which is to declare clients addicted to benzodiazepines and refer them to primary chemical dependency treatment, is not appropriate unless the client has a substance use disorder.

Treatment of High-Dose Benzodiazepine Withdrawal

Discontinuation of the benzodiazepine of dependence should be done in medical settings. The client must be cooperative, be able to adhere to dosing regimens, and not be abusing AODs. Abrupt discontinuation of a sedative-hypnotic when a client is severely physically dependent on it can result in serious medical complications and even death. For this reason, medical management is always needed, and treatment is best provided in a hospital.

There are three general medication strategies for withdrawing clients from sedative-hypnotics, including benzodiazepines: (1) the use of decreasing doses of the agent of dependence; (2) the substitution of phenobarbital or another long-acting barbiturate for the addicting agent and the gradual withdrawal of the substitute medication (Smith and Wesson, 1970, 1971, 1983, 1985); and (3) the substitution of a long-acting benzodiazepine, such as chlordiazepoxide (Librium), tapered over 1 to 2 weeks. The method selected depends on the particular benzodiazepine, involvement of other drugs of dependence, and clinical setting in which detoxification takes place. Steps include gradual reduction of the agent of dependency and phenobarbital substitution.

GRADUAL REDUCTION OF THE AGENT OF DEPENDENCY. This is an appropriate strategy for managing clients who (1) are taking long-acting medications such as chlordiazepoxide (Librium) or diazepam (Valium), (2) can be expected to give accurate accounts of their use of medication, and (3) are not concurrently abusing alcohol or other drugs.

PHENOBARBITAL SUBSTITUTION. Phenobarbital is the best choice to substitute for clients who have lost control of their benzodiazepine use or who are polydrug-dependent. Phenobarbital substitution has the broadest use for all sedative-hypnotic drug dependencies and is widely used in drug treatment programs.

The phenobarbital method is the most generally applicable for high-dose benzodiazepine withdrawal. The pharmacologic rationale for phenobarbital substitution is that this agent is long-acting and produces little change in blood levels between doses. This allows the safe use of a progressively smaller daily dose. Phenobarbital is safer than the shorter-acting barbiturates; lethal doses of phenobarbital are many times higher than toxic doses, and the signs of **toxicity** (e.g., sustained nystagmus, slurred speech, and ataxia) are easily observable. Finally, phenobarbital intoxication usually does not produce disinhibition; consequently, most clients view it as a medication, not as a drug of abuse.

The client's history of drug use one month before treatment is used to compute the stabilization dose of phenobarbital. Although many clients exaggerate the number of pills they are taking, the client's history is the best guide to initiating pharmacotherapy for withdrawal. Clients who have overstated the amount of drug they have taken will become intoxicated during the first day or two of treatment. The treatment provider can easily manage intoxication by omitting one or more doses of phenobarbital and recalculating the daily dose.

The client's average daily sedative-hypnotic dose is converted to phenobarbital equivalents, and the daily amount is divided into three doses. (See Tables 7-16 and 7-17 for a list of benzodiazepines and other sedative-hypnotics, and their phenobarbital withdrawal equiv-

TABLE 7-16 Benzodiazepines and Their Phenobarbital Withdrawal Equivalents.

Generic Name	Trade Name	Therapeutic Dose Range (mg/day)	Dose Equal to 30 mg of Phenobarbital for Withdrawal (mg)[a]	Phenobarbital Conversion Constant
alprazolam	Xanax	0.75–6	1	30
chlordiazepoxide	Librium	15–100	25	1.2
clonazepam	Klonopin	0.5–4	2	15
clorazepate	Tranxene	15–60	7.5	4
diazepam	Valium	4–40	10	3
estazolam	ProSom	1–2	1	30
flumazenil	Mazicon	N/A	N/A	N/A
flurazepam	Dalmane	15–30[b]	15	2
halazepam	Paxipam	60–160	40	0.75
lorazepam	Ativan	1–16	2	15
midazolam	Versed	N/A	N/A	N/A
oxazepam	Serax	10–120	10	3
prazepam	Centrax	20–60	10	3
quazepam	Doral	15[b]	15	2
temazepam	Restoril	15–30[b]	15	2
triazolam	Halcion	0. 125–0.50[b]	0.25	120

[a]Phenobarbital withdrawal conversion equivalence is not the same as therapeutic dose equivalency. Withdrawal equivalence is the amount of the drug that 30 mg of phenobarbital will substitute for and prevent serious high-dose withdrawal signs and symptoms.

[b]usual hypnotic dose.

Sources: Reproduced with permission from U.S. Department of Health and Human Services (1995). Detoxification from alcohol and other drugs. *Treatment Protocol (TIP) Series, #19.* Rockville, MD: Author. Portions of the exhibit are reprinted with permission from the American Psychiatric Press. (1990). *Textbook of Substance Abuse Treatment,* Washington, DC.

TABLE 7-17 Sedative-Hypnotics and Their Phenobarbital Withdrawal Equivalents.

Generic Name	Trade Name(s)	Common Therapeutic Indication	Dose Equal to 30 mg of Phenobarbital Therapeutic Dose Range (mg/day)[a]	Phenobarbital for Withdrawal (mg)	Phenobarbital Conversion Constant
Barbiturates					
amobarbital	Amytal	Sedative	50–150	100	0.33
butabarbital	Butisol	Sedative	45–120	100	0.33
butalbital	Fiorinal, Sedapap	Sedative/ analgesic[b]	100–300	100	0.33
pentobarbital	Nembutal	Hypnotic	50–100	100	0.33
secobarbital	Seconal	Hypnotic	50–100	100	0.33
Others					
buspirone	BuSpar	Sedative	15–60	[c]	[c]
chloral hydrate	Noctec, Somnos	Hypnotic	250–1000	500	0.06
ethchlorvynol	Placidyl	Hypnotic	500–1000	500	0.06
glutethimide	Doriglute	Hypnotic	250–500	250	0.12
meprobamate	Equanil, Equagesic, Miltown	Sedative	1200–1600	1,200	0.025
methyprylon	Noludar	Hypnotic	200–400	200	0.15

[a]Phenobarbital withdrawal conversion equivalence is not the same as therapeutic dose equivalency. Withdrawal equivalence is the amount of the drug that 30 mg of phenobarbital will substitute for and prevent serious high-dose withdrawal signs and symptoms.

[b]Butalbital is usually available in combination with opiate or nonopiate analgesics.

[c]Not cross-tolerant with barbiturates.

Sources: Reproduced with permission from U.S. Department of Health and Human Services (1995). Detoxification from alcohol and other drugs. *Treatment Protocol (TIP) Series, #19.* Rockville, MD: Author. Portions of the exhibit are reprinted with permission from the American Psychiatric Press, *Textbook of Substance Abuse Treatment* (1990). Washington, DC.

alents.) The computed phenobarbital equivalence dosage is given in three or four doses daily. If the client is using significant amounts of other sedative-hypnotics, including alcohol, the amounts of all the drugs are converted to phenobarbital equivalents and added (e.g., 30 cc of 100-proof alcohol is equated to 30 mg of phenobarbital for withdrawal purposes). Before receiving each dose of phenobarbital, the client is checked for signs of phenobarbital toxicity (e.g., sustained nystagmus, slurred speech, or ataxia). Of these, sustained nystagmus is the most reliable. If nystagmus is present, the scheduled dose of phenobarbital is withheld. If all three signs are present, the next two doses of phenobarbital are withheld, and the daily dosage of phenobarbital for the following day is reduced by half.

If the client is in acute withdrawal and has had or is in danger of having withdrawal seizures, the initial dose of phenobarbital is administered by intramuscular injection. If nystagmus and other signs of intoxication develop 1 to 2 hours following the intramuscular dosage, the client is in no immediate danger from barbiturate withdrawal. Clients are maintained on the initial dosing schedule of phenobarbital for 2 days. If the client displays neither signs of withdrawal nor signs of phenobarbital toxicity (e.g., slurred speech, nystagmus, or unsteady gait), phenobarbital withdrawal is begun.

Unless the client develops signs and symptoms of phenobarbital toxicity or sedative-hypnotic withdrawal, phenobarbital is decreased by 30 mg per day. Should signs of phenobarbital toxicity develop during withdrawal, the daily phenobarbital dose is decreased by 50 percent and the 30-mg-per-day withdrawal is continued from the reduced phenobarbital dose. Should the client have objective signs of sedative-hypnotic withdrawal, the daily dose is increased by 50 percent and the client is restabilized before continuing the withdrawal.

Treatment of Low-Dose Benzodiazepine Withdrawal

Clinicians should make decisions regarding the treatment of low-dose benzodiazepine withdrawal based on the client's symptoms. Withdrawal seizures are not usually expected. Clients with an underlying seizure disorder must be maintained on full doses of anticonvulsant medications. Medications that lower seizure threshold should be avoided. Clients may need much reassurance that the symptoms are transient and that with continued abstinence they will eventually subside.

Clients who have the severe form of withdrawal may need psychiatric hospitalization if symptoms become intolerable. Phenobarbital in doses of 200 mg per day generally provides considerable reduction in symptoms. Phenobarbital is slowly tapered over several months.

Stimulant Dependency

WITHDRAWAL FROM STIMULANTS (COCAINE, CRACK COCAINE, AMPHETAMINES, AND METHAMPHETAMINE)

The two most commonly abused stimulants are cocaine and methamphetamine. Intermittent binge use of both agents is common. The withdrawal symptoms that occur after a 2- to 3-day binge are different than those that occur after chronic, high-dose use, although the withdrawal syndromes are similar.

Following a 2- to 3-day binge, stimulant abusers are dysphoric, exhausted, and somnolent for 24 to 48 hours. Because cocaine abusers commonly take alcohol, marijuana, or even heroin with cocaine to reduce the irritability caused by high-dose stimulant abuse, the withdrawal may be in response to the combination of drugs. The client may also have become dependent on more than one drug.

Following regular use, the withdrawal syndrome consists of dysphoria, irritability, difficulty sleeping, and intense dreaming. Often stimulant abusers experience signs and symptoms of the abuse of multiple drugs. The symptoms subside over 2 to 4 days of drug abstinence. There is no specific treatment for stimulant withdrawal. Mild sedation with phenobarbital or chloral hydrate for sleep may ameliorate clients' distress.

In the literature, descriptions of cocaine withdrawal can be confusing because some authors define cocaine craving as a prominent withdrawal symptom, although research findings do not support that. Cocaine craving usually rapidly diminishes when cocaine abusers are unable to get the drug and no longer come in contact with the environmental stimuli associated with cocaine use.

Although the mechanism of drug craving is not well understood, recent studies have demonstrated that environmental and other stimuli can trigger the physiological process of craving. Therefore, exposure to environmental and emotional stimuli (which include other drugs) must be limited by the client through behavioral change or inpatient hospitalization.

Dependency on Other Drugs

WITHDRAWAL FROM OTHER DRUGS

Marijuana

There is no acute abstinence syndrome associated with withdrawal from marijuana. Some clients are irritable and have difficulty sleeping for a few days when they discontinue chronic use of marijuana. Persons withdrawing from marijuana, like those withdrawing from cocaine, benefit from supportive environments during detoxification.

Nicotine

Two issues regarding tobacco smoking merit consideration by the APACN in all settings. The first is the program management's desire to establish a smoke-free treatment environment to comply with workplace ordinances and to safeguard the health and comfort of clients from exposure to second-hand smoke. The second issue is the client's dependence on nicotine as a drug of abuse. This is of particular concern in the acute care setting where the APACN routinely manages the care of individuals with chronic lung disorders as well as many cardiac disorders.

Many hospitals and rehabilitation programs have implemented smoke-free environments. Most programs provide education about nicotine and encourage clients to quit smoking. Some provide nicotine patches or other medication to manage physiological withdrawal symptoms. A more detailed treatment approach for nicotine dependency can be found in Chapter 6.

Hallucinogens

Lysergic acid diethylamide (LSD), dimethyltryptamine (DMT), psilocybin, mescaline, 3,4-methylenedioxymethamphetamine (MDA), and 3,4,-methylenedioxymethamphetamine (MDMA, also called XTC or ecstasy) do not produce physical dependence.

Treatment professionals have noted a recent resurgence in the use of hallucinogenic drugs such as LSD, phencyclidine (PCP), and MDMA. These drugs produce no acute withdrawal syndrome.

Phencyclidine

Chronic use of PCP can cause a toxic psychosis that takes days or weeks to clear; however, PCP does not produce a withdrawal syndrome.

Inhalants/Solvents

Individuals may become physically dependent on hydrocarbons, which include gasoline, glue, aerosol sprays (e.g., paint or waterproofing material), and paint thinner. There is clinical evidence that withdrawal from inhalant use is similar to that experienced by persons withdrawing from alcohol. Phenobarbital may be prescribed during detoxification.

Opiate-Barbiturates

Symptoms of withdrawal from opiates and barbiturates have some common features, making it difficult to assess the client's clinical condition when both drugs are withdrawn at the same time. Many clinicians prefer to gradually withdraw the sedative-hypnotic first, while administering methadone to prevent opiate withdrawal. When the client is barbiturate-free, the methadone is withdrawn at a level of 5 mg per day. If the sedative-hypnotic was a benzodiazepine (diazepam or chlordiazepoxide), some clinicians prefer to begin with a partial reduction of the sedative-hypnotic. While the client is still receiving a partial dosage of the sedative, methadone is withdrawn. Finally, the sedative-hypnotic is totally withdrawn.

Polydrug Use

Addicts rarely use just one drug. Typical combinations and the preferred modes of treatment are:

- Alcohol and stimulant: Treat alcohol abuse.
- Alcohol and benzodiazepine: Treat with phenobarbital.
- Cocaine and benzodiazepine: Treat benzodiazepine withdrawal.
- Cocaine and opiate: Treat opiate dependence.
- Cocaine and amphetamine: No detoxification protocol is known.

Special Situations

PAIN MANAGEMENT IN THE ADDICT AND THE RECOVERING INDIVIDUAL

Management of acute pain in the substance abuser is complex and an increasingly common clinical problem in acute care settings. As noted earlier, this population uses the health care system more than non–substance-abusing individuals for a wide variety of health problems.

An additional issue of concern is that a substantial proportion of nurses and other health professionals have beliefs and values about opioids and pain management that are not consistent with current knowledge in the field. This becomes even more complex when substance abuse is a factor in decision making about pain management. Health care professionals do not appear to be incorporating scientific knowledge of these two fields into the management plans for this client population. Guidelines for pain management for this population are provided in Table 7-18.

The client who is a recovering addict is concerned about relapse, and the health care team may also have concerns about reinducing addictive behaviors. These concerns may interfere with appropriate pain management. The recovering addict is usually managed in a manner like that used for the actively addicted client. The pain management plan for this client and all clients should be comprehensive and include all components needed and accepted by the client to control pain.

The complementary modalities in Table 7-19 should be considered and used as appropriate as part of the pain management plan.

TABLE 7-18 Guidelines for Pain Management in the Chemically Dependent Client.

• Emphasize philosophy of care and high-quality care for all clients. Assure clients they will receive medication as needed to relieve pain.
• Identify and plan promptly for chemically dependent clients experiencing pain.
• Identify resources for care.
• Specify team member responsible for client care. One physician should be assigned to write orders.
• Clarify inherent limitations.
• Schedule regular meeting times for all involved with care.

• Intervene as appropriate for the chemically dependent client by:
   • Defining pain as quickly as possible and treating primary problem
   • Preventing/treating withdrawal and considering polydrug use
   • Accepting the report of pain

• Provide pain relief by: Following current pharmacological principles for pain management and opioid use   Assessing pain regularly and as needed   Adjusting dosage as needed   Working with the client to relieve pain   Setting limits, avoiding excessive negotiation   Getting regular feedback, encouraging open communication   Considering around-the-clock (ATC) dosing   Recognizing the need for larger doses and more frequent doses related to drug tolerance   Using IV patient-controlled analgesia (PCA) with appropriate lockout doses and tamper-resistant equipment   Using nonsteroidal anti-inflammatory drugs (NSAIDs) as first line but not as replacement for opioids   Considering use of morphine   Using long-acting opioids as part of management plan   Combining NSAIDs and opiates   Avoiding Demerol and agonist/antagonist drugs (may precipitate withdrawal)   Using alternative modalities   Keeping client informed of changes, expectations, and progress
• Provide information and/or referral as needed for rehabilitation.
• Recognize drug abuse behavior and firmly deal with it.
• Respect client's refusal of narcotics.
• Establish a written treatment plan or contract.

Nursing Diagnoses Related to Substance Abuse

Nursing diagnoses appropriate for the substance-abusing client include the following (Lisanti, 1991):

- Alteration in nutrition (less than body requirements)
- Risk of infection
- Self-care deficit

TABLE 7-19 Complementary Modalities.

Cutaneous stimulation	• Massage of body, hands, or feet
	• Pain relief with heat, cold, or both
	• Ice application or massage for pain relief
Relaxation	• Deep breathe/tense, exhale/relax, yawn
	• Humor
	• Heartbeat breathing
	• Jaw relaxation
	• Slow rhythmic breathing
	• Peaceful past experiences
	• Meditative relaxation script
	• Progressive relaxation script
	• Simple touch, massage, or warmth
Distraction	• Visual concentration and rhythmic massage
	• Slow rhythmic breathing
	• Sing and tap rhythm
	• Active listening to music
	• Taking laughter seriously
	• Describing a series of pictures
Imagery	• Hypnosis and imagery
	• Emptying the sandbag
	• Breathing out pain
	• Ball of healing energy
	• Individualized imagery technique

Sources: Salerno, E., and Willens, J. (1996). *Pain Management Handbook.* St. Louis, MO: Mosby and U.S. Department of Health and Human Services. Public Health Service. Agency for Health Care Policy and Research. Clinical Practice Guideline. (1992). *Acute Pain Management: Operative or Medical Procedures and Trauma.* (AHCPR Publication No. 92-0032). Rockville, MD: Author.

- Risk of injury
- Sleep pattern disturbance
- Alteration in thought processes
- Ineffective individual coping
- Anxiety
- Fear
- Social isolation
- Risk of violence
- Spiritual distress
- Grief
- Powerlessness
- Hopelessness

Case Study

Mr. Lowell is a 35-year-old male admitted to the acute care setting with an uncared-for appearance, visible tremors, rapid heart rate, elevated temperature, nausea, and vomiting. As you begin taking his history, you also note that he is exhibiting irritability, agitation and restlessness.

1. What other data are needed to assess Mr. Lowell comprehensively?
2. What emergency situations should the APACN monitor for in Mr. Lowell?
3. What nursing interventions are appropriate for this client?
4. What considerations should precede pharmacologic interventions?
5. What long-term interventions should be considered?

CRITICAL THINKING QUESTIONS

1. Advanced Practice Nurses in acute care require skills in screening for substance-related problems. What key questions must be included in the health history and examination that indicate that substance use may be a problem for the patient? Briefly discuss some screening tools for substance use, and provide benefits and limitations.
2. Advanced Practice Nurses implement pharmacologic interventions for detoxification. Most detoxification procedures are specific to particular drugs of dependence; others are based on general principles of treatment and are not drug-specific. Briefly discuss the general principles of detoxification.
3. The Clinical Institute Withdrawal Assessment (CIWA-Ar) is commonly used for initial and ongoing assessment of alcohol withdrawal symptoms. Discuss how this tool is used in a clinical setting, how the scoring is monitored, and how the scoring is used to determine treatment.
4. A variety of pharmacotherapeutic treatments is available for the substance-abusing individual. There are risks and benefits to their use in treatment of substance abuse. Discuss the implications for the Advanced Practice Nurse and for client education.
5. Advanced Practice Nurses require knowledge and skills of patient management during intoxication, toxicity, and withdrawal in the acute care setting; however, they must also be knowledgeable about ongoing and long-term treatment. Discuss the various long-term health implications of substance abuse and the various resources available for ongoing support and treatment.

REFERENCES

American Psychiatric Association, Task Force on Benzodiazepine Dependency. (1990). *Benzodiazepine Dependence, Toxicity, and Abuse*. Washington, DC: Author.

Banys, P., Tusel, D.J., Sees, K.L., Reilly, P.M., and Delucchi, K.L. (1994). Low (40 mg) versus high (80 mg) dose methadone in a 180-day heroin detoxification program. *Journal of Substance Abuse Treatment 11*, 225–232.

Becker, H. (1998). Kindling in alcohol withdrawal. *Alcohol World Health and Research 22*(1), 25–33.

Bennett, G., and Thomas, S. (1998). Substance abuse interventions in general nursing practice. *Nursing Clinics of North America 33*(1), 1–104.

Brumbaugh, A.G. (1993). Acupuncture: New perspectives in chemical dependency treatment. *Journal of Substance Abuse Treatment 10,* 35–43.

Bullock, M.L., Culliton, P.D., and Olander, R.T. (1989). Controlled trial of acupuncture for severe recidivist alcoholism. *Lancet 1,* 1435–1439.

Compton, M. (1991a). Nursing care in acute intoxication. *Substance Abuse Education in Nursing 22,* 349–508.

Compton, M. (1991b). Nursing care in acute withdrawal. *Substance Abuse Education in Nursing 15-2463*(2), 412–419.

Fuller, R.K., and Gordis, E. (1994). Refining the treatment of alcohol withdrawal. Editorial. *Journal of the American Medical Association 272,* 557–558.

Geller, A. (1994). Neurological effects. In N.S. Miller (ed.), *Topics in Addiction Medicine 1*(1), 1–17.

Gorelick, D.A. (1993). Overview of pharmacologic treatment approaches for alcohol and other drug addiction: Intoxication, withdrawal, and relapse prevention. *Psychiatric Clinics of North America 10,* 171–179.

Kinney, J. (1996). *Clinical Manual of Substance Abuse* (2nd ed.). St. Louis, MO: Mosby.

Lisanti, P. (1991). Assessment of the adult client for drug and alcohol use. *Substance Abuse Education in Nursing 15-2407*(1), 151–167.

Muma, R., Lyons, B., Borucki, M., and Pollard, R. (1997). *HIV Manual for Health Care Professionals* (2nd ed.). Stamford, CT: Appleton & Lange.

Saitz, R., Mayo-Smith, M.F., Roberts, M.S., et al. (1994). Individualized treatment for alcohol withdrawal: A randomized double-blind controlled trial. *Journal of the American Medical Association 272,* 519–523.

Salerno, E., and Willens, J. (1996). *Pain Management Handbook.* St. Louis, MO: Mosby.

Smith, D.E., and Wesson, D.R. (1970). A new method for treatment of barbiturate dependence. *Journal of the American Medical Association 213,* 294–295.

Smith, D.E., and Wesson, D.R. (1971). A phenobarbital technique for withdrawal of barbiturate abuse. *Archives of General Psychiatry 24,* 56–60.

Smith, D.E., and Wesson, D.R. (1983). Benzodiazepine dependency syndromes. *Journal of Psychoactive Drugs 15,* 85–95.

Smith, D.E., and Wesson, D.R. (1985). Benzodiazepine dependency syndromes. In D.E. Smith and D.R. Wesson (eds.), *The Benzodiazepines: Current Standards for Medical Practice.* Hingham, MA: MTP Press.

U.S. Department of Health and Human Services. Public Health Service. Agency for Health Care Policy and Research. Clinical Practice Guideline. (1992). *Acute Pain Management: Operative or Medical Procedures and Trauma.* (AHCPR Publication No. 92-0032). Rockville, MD: Author.

U.S. Department of Health and Human Services. (1993). Screening for infectious diseases among substance abusers. *Treatment Protocol (TIP) Series #6.* Rockville, MD: Author.

U.S. Department of Health and Human Services. (1995). Detoxification from alcohol and other drugs. *Treatment Protocol (TIP) Series #19.* Rockville, MD: Author.

8

Substance Use in Community Health Nursing Practice

Carolyn E. D'Avanzo, RN, MSN, DNSc

LEARNER OUTCOMES

On completion of this chapter, the learner will be able to:

1. Identify *Healthy People 2000* goals that relate to legal and illegal substance use.
2. Apply primary, secondary, and tertiary levels of prevention to substance use in community settings.
3. Interpret epidemiologic information on legal and illegal substances to identify risks for substance abuse in various population groups.
4. Synthesize knowledge about adolescent behaviors basic to effective risk reduction programs for adolescents.
5. Compare and contrast theories that attempt to explain adolescent risk-taking behaviors to program planning.
6. Utilize knowledge of effective substance abuse prevention strategies to evaluate community programming.

KEY TERMS

community-based programming
substance abuse

substance abuse prevention
substance dependence

substance use

Since the trend of deinstitutionalization of the mentally ill in the 1960s, greater emphasis has been placed on outpatient versus in-patient treatment within managed care models. Services for substance-abusing clients are sometimes included within broader services for mental health but are more often based in separate agencies. Both are appropriate areas of practice for advanced practice nurses (APNs). The differences in levels of nursing involvement in community facilities that provide services to substance abusers, however, are quite striking. In facilities that specialize in mental health treatment, nurses are a large part of the staff. These nurses are often APNs: mental health clinicians who work with clients with mental health and substance abuse diagnoses. In facilities that provide **substance abuse** treatment primarily without other specific mental health services, the majority of the staff are counselors, few of whom are certified by national organizations to work with acutely ill and recovering substance abusers (Rouse, 1998). Counselors may be individuals who are themselves recovering and who have further education. Nursing roles in these facilities are often limited to monitoring the physical condition of individuals during detoxification, a potentially life-threatening process, and the administration of medications.

Unfortunately, like their colleagues in other settings, many of these nurses are unaware of the impact of substance abuse on the overall health of their communities. Research findings suggest that as many as 18 percent to 25 percent of the clients on general medicine, 25 percent of the surgical, 30 percent to 40 percent of the psychiatric, and 15 percent to 25 percent of those treated in outpatient settings may be alcoholics, other substance abusers, or dually diagnosed (Babor, 1990; Coleman, 1993; Coleman and Veach, 1990; Moore et al., 1989). Many are not recognized as having these conditions. It is estimated that only 1 in 20 clients with a substance abuse disorder will have it recorded on charts, and sequelae are often medically treated without identification and treatment of the underlying problem. As a result, substance abuse becomes chronic, medical costs increase, and successful outcomes of the initial treatment are compromised (Hyman, 1995).

Substance abuse is a widespread community problem. Addiction in individuals and families burdens service delivery and community infrastructures in a variety of ways, with local emergency department, firefighter, law enforcement, and judicial system personnel heavily impacted. Alcohol is involved in 53 percent of deaths from accidental falls, 50 percent of motor vehicle fatalities, 40 percent of industrial deaths, 64 percent of fatal fires, 50 percent of domestic violence arrests (Kinney, 1996), and 80 percent of suicides (American Psychiatric Association, 1995). Low-level drug dealing or prostitution in support of drug habits is common; drunk driving and boating accidents put further strain on law enforcement and judicial systems. Social services and welfare systems are also taxed as addicted individuals incur debt, and their families ultimately depend on public assistance for basic needs. As families struggle to cope, school systems are strained, and the resulting social and behavioral problems involve school nurses.

The prevalence of substance abuse in any given community will affect the provision of home care and program planning by community health nurses. As complex health care delivery systems expand in communities, the community health nurse is increasingly challenged by the need to prevent, recognize, and address substance-related problems.

Expansion of community health nursing in community health centers, occupational health and wellness centers, and church-based wellness programs should be guided by the professional practice standards for community health nursing as proposed by the American

Nurses' Association (ANA) and the Public Health Nursing Section of the American Public Health Association (APHA):

> Community health nursing is a synthesis of nursing and public health practice applied to promoting and preserving the health of populations. The practice is general and comprehensive. It is not limited to a particular population group or diagnosis, and is continuing, not episodic. The dominant responsibility is to the population as a whole; nursing directed to individuals, families or groups contributes to the health of the total population. Health promotion, health maintenance, health education, and management coordination, and continuity of care are utilized in a holistic approach to the management of the health care of individuals, families, and groups in the community (ANA, 1980, p. 2).

> Public health nursing synthesizes the body of knowledge from the public health sciences and professional nursing theories for the purpose of improving the health of the entire community. This goal lies at the heart of primary prevention and health promotion and is the foundation for public health nursing practice. To accomplish this goal, public health nurses work with groups, families, and individuals as well as in multidisciplinary teams and groups (APHA, 1981, p. 4).

The ANA and APHA recognize the aggregate, rather than the individual, as the primary unit of care. The focus of the specialty of community health nursing is on population aggregates (groups who share similar characteristics) and the promotion of well communities (ANA, 1980). When the community is the client, the nurse is concerned with the health of the community as a collective and seeks to improve the health of the community as a whole (Wallerstein and Bernstein, 1994).

While the focus for community health nurses is on the care, health education, and guidance of population aggregates, increased demand for individual care has resulted in the loss of a community focus and greater emphasis on individualized home care. This approach is short-sighted because individual and family data provide baseline information on the epidemiologic profile of the community, which should guide primary prevention efforts. The complexity of community problems and needs mandates that nurses adopt interdisciplinary approaches, collaborating with other health care providers who have expertise in related disciplines. As case manager for the client, the community health nurse coordinates planning and refers the client to other health providers such as nutritionists, social workers, and occupational and physical therapists. Substance-abusing clients in the community are often referred to advanced practice mental health nurses because alcohol abuse/dependence is the most prevalent diagnosis for all psychiatric disorders in the United States.

Contemporary roles of APNs in the community continue to be primarily as clinical specialists in traditional settings such as voluntary agencies (visiting nurses), proprietary, for-profit home health care agencies; home health care departments based in hospitals; city and state public health departments; and ambulatory settings such as occupational health centers, schools, or community centers. Nurse practitioners also practice in many of the same settings. Both practitioners are in prime positions to educate the public on substance abuse disorders and to assist in program planning for prevention.

Many objectives relate to the use of legal and illegal drugs in the U.S. government's prevention efforts for the year 2000 (*Healthy People 2000*, 1992); the use of community-based and public health services for drug treatment is strongly emphasized (see Table 8-1). In

TABLE 8-1 Selected *Healthy People 2000* Objectives That Relate to Tobacco and Drug Use.

Health Status Objectives

Tobacco
- Reduce coronary heart disease deaths to no more than 42 per 100,000 people.
- Slow the rise in lung cancer deaths to achieve a rate of no more than 42 per 100,000 people.
- Slow the rise in deaths from chronic obstructive pulmonary disease to achieve a rate of no more than 25 per 100,000 people.

Alcohol and Other Drugs
- Reduce deaths caused by alcohol-related motor vehicle crashes to no more than 8.5 per 100,000 people.
- Reduce cirrhosis deaths to no more than 6 per 100,000 people, and drug-related deaths to no more than 3 per 100,000.
- Reduce drug abuse–related hospital emergency department visits by at least 20 percent.

Risk Reduction Objectives

Tobacco
- Reduce the initiation of cigarette smoking by children and youth so that no more than 15 percent have become regular cigarette smokers by age 20.
- Increase smoking cessation during pregnancy so that at least 60 percent of women who are cigarette smokers at the time they become pregnant quit smoking early in pregnancy and maintain abstinence for the remainder of their pregnancy.
- Reduce to no more than 20 percent the proportion of children age 6 and younger who are regularly exposed to tobacco smoke at home.
- Reduce smokeless tobacco use by males ages 12 through 24 to a prevalence of no more than 4 percent.

Alcohol and Other Drugs
- Increase by at least 1 year the average age of first use of cigarettes, alcohol, and marijuana by adolescents ages 12 through 17.
- Reduce the proportion of high school seniors and college students engaging in recent occasions of heavy drinking of alcoholic beverages to no more than 28 percent of high school seniors and 32 percent of college students.
- Reduce alcohol consumption by people age 14 and older to an annual average of no more than 2 gallons of ethanol per person.
- Increase the proportion of high school seniors who perceive social disapproval associated with the heavy use of alcohol, occasional use of marijuana, and experimentation with cocaine.
- Increase the proportion of high school seniors who associate risk of physical or psychological harm with the heavy use of alcohol, regular use of marijuana, and experimentation with cocaine.
- Reduce to no more than 3 percent the proportion of male high school seniors who use anabolic steroids.

Service and Protection Objectives

Tobacco
- Establish tobacco-free environments and include tobacco use prevention in the curricula of all elementary, middle, and secondary schools, preferably as part of quality school health education.
- Increase to at least 75 percent the proportion of worksites with a formal smoking policy that prohibits or severely restricts smoking at the workplace.
- Enact in the 50 states comprehensive laws on clean indoor air that prohibit or strictly limit smoking in the workplace and enclosed public places (including health care facilities, schools, and public transportation).
- Enact and enforce in the 50 states laws prohibiting the sale, distribution, and associated advertising and promotion of tobacco products to youth younger than age 19.
- Establish and monitor in the 50 states comprehensive plans to ensure access to alcohol and drug treatment programs for traditionally underserved people.

TABLE 8-1 (continued)

Alcohol and Other Drugs

- Provide to children in all school districts and private schools primary and secondary school educational programs on alcohol and other drugs, preferably as part of quality school health education.
- Extend adoption of alcohol and drug policies for the work environment to at least 60 percent of worksites with 50 or more employees.
- Extend to the 50 states legal blood alcohol concentration levels of 0.04 percent over and 0.00 percent for persons under age 21 and administrative driver's license suspension or revocation laws or programs of equal effectiveness for people determined to have been driving under the influence of intoxicants.
- Increase to at least 75 percent the proportion of primary care providers who screen for alcohol and other drug use problems and provide counseling and referral as needed.

Source: U.S. Department of Health and Human Services. (1991). *Healthy People 2000.* Washington, DC: U.S. Government Printing Office.

addition, hospital downsizing has created a greater need for comprehensive and increasingly skilled home care services. Although they frequently encounter clients with substance use disorders, community health nurses have primarily focused on the physical illnesses caused indirectly or directly by drug use rather than the drug use itself.

Substance Use/Misuse and the Role of the Community Health Nurse

The principles of primary prevention define community health nursing practice, and the goal of primary prevention is to reduce the number of persons becoming first-time regular users of a drug in a given time period. It is essential, therefore, that adolescents be the major focus of community-based primary prevention of substance abuse. The onset of alcohol use by age 12 has been found to be associated with alcohol abuse later in adolescence and increased risks of other drug abuse. Behaviors that accompany early use include violence, drunk driving, and absenteeism from school or work. Primary prevention must begin in elementary school in order to help children develop an awareness as well as the skills to deal with introduction to drugs, because the preadolescent years from 10 to 12 seem to be a particularly vulnerable time for initiation into use (Gruber, DiClemente, Anderson, and Lodico, 1996).

The community health nurse begins the process of primary prevention by conducting a needs assessment in the community. This is followed by delineating at-risk groups, screening (secondary prevention), and getting answers to questions specific to that particular community. What factors may encourage initiation of substance use? How effectively do school or community programs educate adolescents about the use of gateway drugs such as nicotine, alcohol, and marijuana? What activities by employee assistance programs (EAPs) are directed toward preventing substance abuse in young adults? What are the political issues in the community that may influence resource allocation for prevention programming? In short, what do community health nurses need to know about their respective communities in order to address **substance abuse prevention** issues?

The Role of Social Reform in Prevention

Early efforts to control the use of illicit drugs can be perceived as prevention, and they occurred prior to the 1970s. Despite social concerns, the point was appropriately made in 1973 that a radical cultural transformation of the drug-using society must occur if attitudes about drug use are to be changed (Goshen, 1973). Efforts by government agencies to control the supply of drugs constitute one approach to prevention in law enforcement; efforts to change the demand for drugs are also addressed in prevention and treatment programs. Through the 1970s, the enforcement of legal sanctions against drug retailing was over-emphasized, and medical research focused on finding the causes and cure of addiction rather than on preventing or treating drug use. This trend continued into the 1980s. The call for reform of drug policies increased in tenor, however, based on the failure of the drug enforcement system to effectively curtail early initiation and ongoing use of drugs and alcohol in excess. The strengthening of treatment approaches for alcoholism had positive effects in public education and on education among health professionals. Federal funding supported the development of curricular models for physicians and nurses, and professional organizations began to acknowledge the lack of preparedness on the part of most health practitioners to treat illnesses of addiction.

Prevention at National and Private Levels

In the 1970s, government efforts directed at the demand side of the drug problem focused on coordination of local and state information programs, implementation of health information programs in schools, development of programs to provide information to adults, and provision of delinquent counseling services. Unfortunately, evaluation of formal educational programs was infrequent and lacked standardization. Currently, state agencies created in the early 1970s function as structures for the receipt, distribution, and utilization of federal grants in relation to alcohol and other drug projects. They continue under the 1981 Omnibus Reconciliation Act that consolidated all drug and alcohol funding into a block grant program handled by single state agencies. Noteworthy programs have also been developed by privately funded organizations.

Coombs and Ziedonis (1995) note that since 1986, with the development of the Center for Substance Abuse Prevention (CSAP), more recognition has been given to prevention as a tool in the War on Drugs at federal and state levels. They suggest the following eight areas in which prevention activities should take place:

1. *Law enforcement and regulatory agencies.* These agencies have the power to shape the environment by reducing the number of alcohol sales establishments and banning certain kinds of high-content alcohol products. Some measures already implemented by these agencies include revocation of drivers' licenses for driving while under the influence, mandated server training, and use of comprehensive health warnings, labels, and public service messages. Efforts are under way to stigmatize drunkenness, educate about safety, and criminalize abusive drinking or improper alcohol sales.

2. *Community-based programming.* **Community-based programming** shows promise and has the potential of developing population-specific programs. More research is needed, however, to demonstrate the efficacy of these programs.

3. *Schools.* Schools need to use a range of social influence approaches, including elementary school self-esteem-building programs, drug and alcohol education, and peer counseling in grades six to eight, with supplemental educational sessions through middle school and high school.

4. *Health professionals.* Health professionals should be educated to undertake prevention activities and should receive such training in professional schools through continuing education. They will then be in a position to shape educational and government policy in relation to program planning and funding.

5. *Religious organizations.* These can network with other groups and assist in the dissemination and evaluation of various types of drug use prevention programming.

6. *Volunteer consumer groups.* Groups with special interests and representatives from various regional age and ethnic groups can be encouraged to work individually or in groups to organize and/or sponsor prevention activities. Groups that have had considerable impact on increasing awareness of the consequences of driving while intoxicated are Mothers Against Drunk Driving (MADD) and Students Against Drunk Driving (SADD).

7. *Organized sports programs.* Sports organizations need to incorporate education about drug abuse and/or other prevention activities at every level of sports activities, with special attention to growth-enhancing drugs such as dehydroepiandrosterone (DHEA) and steroids.

8. *Systems interventions.* These interventions include media campaigns in a range of designs and techniques. Principles underlying campaigns already found to be successful should be utilized. Such principles should undergird the inclusion of culturally relevant, population-specific content and interventions.

During the late 1980s and 1990s, themes of user accountability, school-based education, the workplace, the media, and the community have been stressed. Design and implementation of future campaigns should target the needs of specific populations and delineate culturally relevant and realistic goals, both limited in scope and related to prevention activities.

Prevention: Early Approaches and Their Origin

The goal of health promotion and disease prevention is to decrease medical costs and loss of time from school or work and to increase the quality of life for individuals and their communities. A public health classification system of disease prevention was proposed in the 1950s (Commission on Chronic Illness, 1957) that described three levels of prevention: primary, secondary, and tertiary. Implicit in all three levels was that the causes of diseases could be linked with disease occurrence: a cause-and-effect model. Primary prevention has been slow to receive support by providers within the health care delivery system, even though its value has been touted by health educators and practitioners for decades. It consists of activities designed to prevent diseases or disorders, undertaken before manifestations of illness exist and when the individual is in a relative state of health (such as reduction of first-time regular drug use). Secondary prevention is directed toward the treatment of individuals identified as having a disorder. Also known as early intervention, the goal is to reduce the duration and severity of illness and to return the individual to a relative state of health. Tertiary prevention seeks to reduce the degree of impairment occurring as a result of illness and to maximize whatever level of health the individual can enjoy through rehabilitation.

Activities related to drug and alcohol problems have emphasized secondary and tertiary prevention. Within the health care delivery system, reimbursement for service continues to be limited to treatment and/or rehabilitation of substance abusers, with few financial resources for the development of programming in primary prevention. Debates continue among federal, state, and community governments about which branch should have the responsibility and financial burdens of prevention programming. Few policies delineate how these goals are best achieved at state and federal levels. Considerable frustration has resulted relative to the efficacy of primary prevention efforts within the three levels of the prevention model. For example, what specific interventions can be proven effective to prevent adolescent drinking? It is clear that knowledge about **substance use** may not affect actual behavior. If it did, the rates of adolescent drug use would be decreasing dramatically rather than increasing because most students attend health education classes in school. Historically, many of the primary prevention efforts that have been undertaken relative to this subject have been ineffective.

In the 1980s, an alternative classification was proposed that recognized the complex interaction of multiple risk factors and illness onset and stressed a risks versus benefits approach (Gordon, 1987). Costs, risks, and benefits of prevention efforts were considered in light of the individual's risk of developing a given disease. Within the public health classification of prevention, three categories were developed by Gordon that referred to the populations for which specific interventions could be targeted: universal preventive measures, selective preventive measures, and indicated preventive measures. Universal preventive measures, such as the use of seat belts, were those that could be directed at the entire population because the benefits clearly were greater than either costs or risks. Selective preventive measures would apply only to members of particular subgroups in the population at high risk for particular illnesses by reason of heredity, occupation, gender, or age, such as diabetes in certain Native American groups. Indicated preventive measures would be used only for those individuals known to be at high risk for development of certain disease, for example, individuals at high risk for heart disease who have been identified by blood lipid screening.

Factors Hindering the Success of Prevention Programs

A number of factors have negatively impacted the development, funding, and sustained support of prevention programs. One major factor relates to problems demonstrating the relationship between increased knowledge and decreased drug use. Follow-up studies of prevention programs frequently demonstrate increased knowledge about the risks of substance use, without subsequent behavioral change. The use of self-report results in both over- and underreporting, and is a methodological weakness that potentially compromises interpretation of data. Sustained support for prevention and prevention research is difficult in light of the fact that treatment still gets the major allocation of resources.

The present-day managed care model mandates targeted prevention activities that demonstrate that benefits clearly override costs or risks. Expanding on Gordon's classification, Mrazek and Haggerty (1994) proposed a slightly different prevention model they thought more appropriate for some conditions, such as substance abuse, that fall within mental disorder classifications. Therefore, universal preventive interventions for substance abuse would only be implemented if the entire population or a whole subset within the population would benefit. For example, all pregnant women could be targeted for substance abuse education. Selective preventive interventions could be targeted to subgroups of populations such as preadolescents, who are at high risk of initiating substance use. Lastly, indicated preventive interventions would target identified individuals at high risk who may already be using drugs or who have a hereditary predisposition to do so, such as the children of alcoholics. Such an approach may be more successful in producing cost-effective, measurable outcomes that will encourage further prevention efforts.

Epidemiology and Current Trends in Drug Use

Epidemiological trends delineate directions for community-based education and programming and are a major source of information available to support prevention strategies. The National Household Survey on Drug Abuse (NHSDA) is the broadest epidemiological profile of drug use in the United States; it reports the past-month (considered current use), past-year, and lifetime use of the total spectrum of both legal and illegal drugs for ages 12 to 17, 18 to 25, 26 to 34, and 35 and older. The 1997 survey reported on 216 million people (Substance Abuse and Mental Health Services Administration [SAMHSA], 1998). There are several other national surveys that are specific to the adolescent population. The Youth Risk Behavior Survey (YRBS) is a component of the Centers for Disease Control's (CDC) Youth Risk Behavior Surveillance System, which biennially measures the prevalence of priority health risk behaviors among youth. In general, this survey has found higher rates of alcohol, cigarette, marijuana, and cocaine use in youths than those found in the NHSDA. The National Longitudinal Study of Adolescent Health (Add Health) was conducted from 1994 to 1996 to measure the effects of family, peer group, school, neighborhood, religious institution, and community influences on health risks such as substance abuse. The Partnership Attitude Tracking Study (PATS) was conducted by the Partnership for a Drug-Free America in 1998. This is the only ongoing national research study that tracks drug use and drug-related attitudes among children as young as 8 and 9, as well as their parents. Another ongoing study that provides excellent information on adolescents specifically is the Monitoring the Future (MTF) study, which is funded by the National Institute on Drug Abuse of the National Institutes of Health. MTF has measured the extent of drug abuse among high school seniors annually since 1975. In 1991, the survey was expanded to include eighth- and tenth-grade students.

Nurses should be familiar with current trends in the use of legal and illegal drugs in their communities. Nurses must be knowledgeable about the entire population, but the following discussion serves as an example of one subgroup and places major emphasis on adolescents. Adolescents should be a major focus of primary prevention of drug abuse in all communities.

Adolescents: An Important Subgroup At Risk

LEGAL DRUGS

Alcohol

Alcohol has been the most commonly used psychoactive drug since the inception of the NHSDA. Of the 216 million persons surveyed in 1997, over 51 percent (more than 111 million people) reported past-month use. About 11 million current drinkers were 12 to 20 years old in 1997. Of these, almost 5 million were binge drinkers, including 2 million heavy drinkers. Among adolescents ages 12 to 17, the current rate of alcohol use was about 50 percent in 1979; it fell to 21 percent in 1992 and has remained at about that level. Young adults ages 18 to 25 were most likely to binge or drink heavily. About 46 percent of the drinkers in this age group were binge drinkers, and about 1 in 5 were heavy drinkers. The rate of initiation of alcohol use among the 12- to 17-year-old group increased from 113 to 165 new users per 1,000 potential new users. The age of first alcohol use decreased from age 19 in 1962 to age 16 in 1993.

The proportion of youth ages 12 to 17 reporting alcohol use is substantially higher in surveys of secondary school students such as the MTF study (Johnston, O'Malley, and Bachman, 1998). This is attributed to more underreporting in the household setting than in schools. Males are more likely to report lifetime or past-year use, except in the 12- to 17-year-old group, in which there are no gender or ethnic differences in use. Rates of heavy use were considerably higher among those who had not completed high school; this puts these individuals at risk for liver disease (cirrhosis, hepatitis), gastrointestinal bleeding, cancer, and Korsakoff's psychosis (Fontaine, 1999). In 1997, daily use of alcohol (four to five drinks) was associated with great risk of harm by 77 percent of the population; however, the perceived risk of having five or more drinks once or twice a week decreased from 70 percent to 60 percent over the same period for all groups, including youth ages 12 to 17.

ALCOHOL USE MAY PREDICT OTHER DRUG USE

For all age groups, the current use of alcohol is strongly associated with use of other legal/illegal drugs. For example, of the 11.2 million heavy drinkers (out of the total surveyed population of 216 million), 30 percent (3.3 million people) were current illicit drug users. Among binge (but not heavy) drinkers, 18 percent (3.7 million) were illicit drug users. Other drinkers (i.e., past-month but not binge) had a rate of 5.1 percent (3.7 million) for illicit drug use; only 2.3 percent (2.5 million) of nondrinkers were illicit drug users.

Nicotine

In the United States, rate of use of tobacco products is second only to that of alcohol. In 1997, an estimated 64 million people were current smokers, which represents a smoking rate of 30 percent for the population age 12 and older. About 4.5 million adolescents ages 12 to 17 were current smokers in 1997, with a rate of 20 percent, even though the percent reporting great risk in smoking one or more packs of cigarettes per day has steadily increased from 45 percent in 1985 to 54 percent in 1997. The mean age of first use has stayed fairly stable at 15 to 16 years old since the early 1960s. Use of cigarettes in the 12- to 13-year age group, however, increased from 7 percent in 1996 to almost 10 percent in 1997. Among adolescents ages 12 to 17, girls smoked more than boys: 21 percent versus 19 percent. The MTF survey also indicated that cigarette smoking is increasing in teens in general, and that girls are smoking at a younger age. This is of great concern to health professionals because active and passive smoking causes multiple health problems such as cardiovascular disease, cancer, emphysema, and chronic bronchitis. Caucasians continue to be more likely to smoke and are more likely to be heavy smokers than other ethnic groups. Level of education appears highly correlated with tobacco use; about 40 percent of adults who report they did not complete high school smoked cigarettes, as compared to 17 percent of college graduates. Over 2 million youths ages 12 to 17 reported using smokeless tobacco, with males having used it three times as much. Highest rates of use were in the South, and past-month use by whites was double the rate of use by Hispanics; use by blacks was extremely low.

TOBACCO USE MAY PREDICT OTHER DRUG USE

Adolescents ages 12 to 17 who currently smoke cigarettes were about 12 times as likely to use illicit drugs and 23 times as likely to drink heavily as nonsmoking youth.

ILLICIT/ILLEGAL DRUGS

Among youth ages 12 to 13, 4 percent were illicit drug users. The highest rates were in young people ages 16 to 17 (19 percent) and 18 to 20 (17 percent). The percentage of adolescents ages 12 to 17 using drugs increased from 9 percent in 1996 to 11.4 percent in 1997. The rate of past illicit drug use among youths was higher among those who were currently using cigarettes and alcohol, compared with nonusers. Furthermore, the increase in illicit drug use between 1996 and 1997 occurred only among youths who were using cigarettes and alcohol. In 1996 and 1997, 3.8 percent and 3.6 percent of youth nonsmokers used illicit drugs, respectively. Among youths who used cigarettes, the rates of past-month illicit drug use were 32.5 percent in 1996 and 42.8 percent in 1997. Similarly, the increase in illicit drug use occurred only among alcohol users. Illicit drug use remains highly correlated with educational level; those who had not completed high school have the highest rates of current use, and college graduates have the lowest.

Marijuana

The 1998 NHSDA survey determined that, in all age groups, marijuana was the most commonly used illicit drug in the United States. An estimated 2.5 million Americans used marijuana for the first time in 1996, and 11 million were current (past-month) marijuana/hashish users. This represents 5 percent of the population age 12 and older. The rising incidence during the 1990s seems to have been fueled primarily by the increasing rate of new use among youth ages 12 to 17 (from 37 new users per 1,000 potential new users in 1991 to 83 in 1996). In 1997, 58 percent of youth ages 12 to 17 reported that marijuana was easy to obtain. The rate of marijuana initiation for youth ages 12 to 17 is at its highest level ever, which is expected to impact the treatment system in future years, as many new drug users progress to addiction and require treatment. Approximately 80 percent of all current illicit drug users admitted to use of either marijuana or hashish. Nearly 1 in 10 of youth ages 12 to 17 (almost 10 percent) were current users in 1997, a trend that has been increasing steadily since 1992. Past-month use increased from 3.4 percent to 8.2 percent from 1992 to 1995, and it increased significantly between 1996 and 1997 (7.1 percent to 9.4 percent). These trends are evident across gender, race, and geographic areas.

When those surveyed were asked whether their use of marijuana was causing problems in their lives, about 43 percent admitted that it was. Among youth ages 12 to 17, the perceived risk of smoking marijuana once or twice a week decreased significantly between 1996 and 1997, which mirrors trends in use. As the perceived risk decreased, use increased, and vice versa. Other national surveys, including the MTF study, reflect a similar trend. The community health nurse should be aware that young people reporting current use of marijuana are more likely than nonusers to drink alcohol, smoke cigarettes, and use other illicit drugs.

Cocaine

After marijuana, cocaine (also crack ["rock" or "base"]) is used more than any other illicit drug. The annual number of new users of any form of cocaine increased from 1992 to 1996 but was at a lower level than during the 1980s. In 1996, there were an estimated 675,000 new cocaine users. In 1997, an estimated 1.5 million Americans were current cocaine users (0.7 percent of the population age 12 or over), and 682,000 were frequent users (defined as use on 51 or more days during the past year).

The initiation rate among youth ages 12 to 17 increased from 4.0 in 1991 to 11.3 in 1996, similar to the high rates of the early 1980s. Historically, most initiation of cocaine use takes place in the 18- to 25-year-old group; the rate in 1996 was 14.8 percent. The MTF and NHSDA reported that past-month use of cocaine rose significantly in the 12- to 17-year-old group (it doubled from 1993 to 1995). Monthly use in this age group has increased from 0.3 percent in 1994 to 0.8 percent in 1995, and to 1 percent in 1997. The highest rate of current cocaine use in 1997 was for young adults ages 18 to 25 years (1.2 percent). For the adolescent group only (12 to 17 years old), whites and Hispanics had similar rates of monthly use (1.1 percent versus 1.0 percent), with blacks at a considerably lower rate of 0.1 percent (over the age of 35, blacks have a considerably higher use rate than whites). College graduates had lower rates of use than high school graduates. Use of crack cocaine also is more prevalent in whites and Hispanics ages 12 to 17, although over 35 years of age, blacks report the most use. In 1985 and 1988, the perceived risk of monthly use of cocaine was 58 percent and 70 percent, respectively. Since 1990, the percentage of youth reporting great risk in using cocaine once a month had decreased once more to 54 percent. In 1997, there was a rate increase once again for those age 12 and older in the perceived risk of occasional (once-a-month) use of cocaine from 1996 to 1997 (76 percent to 77.9 percent, respectively), which theoretically should signal a future decrease in the use of cocaine. According to the Drug Abuse Warning Network (DAWN), which tracks emergency room episodes involving drugs, cocaine is the most frequently reported substance involved (47 percent of cases).

Hallucinogens

Lifetime use of hallucinogens was 9.6 percent overall in 1997, basically unchanged since the 1995 NHSDA (9.5 percent). There were an estimated 1.1 million new hallucinogen users in 1996, approximately twice the average annual number during the 1980s. The rate of initiation among youth ages 12 to 17 more than doubled between 1991 and 1996, from 12 to 26 new users per 1,000 potential new users. Over the same period, the rate for those ages 18 to 25 also increased from 14 to 21 new users per 1,000 potential new users. Both age groups had similar rates from 1995 to 1996.

Overall rates of current use of hallucinogens changed little between 1996 and 1997 (0.6 percent and 0.8 percent, respectively). Overall rates of use increased significantly from 1992 to 1995 (SAMHSA, 1996), but they remained steady from 1995 to 1997. Past-month use of hallucinogens is steadily rising in 12- to 17-year-olds, however (0.5 percent in 1994, 0.7 percent in 1995, 2.0 percent in 1996, and 1.9 percent in 1997).

In 1997, the majority of overall hallucinogen use in the 12- to 17-year-old group (6.5 percent) was accounted for by lysergic acid diethylamide (LSD) (5.2 percent). Psilocybin (mushrooms) also had high rates of use (2.6 percent, approximately half of LSD use). This was followed by ecstasy (3,4,-methylenedioxymethamphetamine [MDMA]) (1.3 percent), phencyclidine (PCP) (1.4 percent), mescaline (0.4 percent), and peyote (0.5 percent). In the 18- to 25-year-old group, hallucinogen use more than doubled overall (15 percent) and remained at 15 percent until age 34, when it decreased to levels similar to adolescent use (7.4 percent). In all age groups, LSD and psilocybin were the drugs of choice.

The western region of the United States had the highest rates of hallucinogen use for lifetime, past-year, and past-month use. Past-year use in this group almost doubled between 1994 and 1995, from 2.7 percent to 4.6 percent, and rose to 4.7 percent in 1997. In every age group, whites had the highest rates of use. Lower educational levels were associated with higher levels of use.

Inhalants

About 6 percent of those questioned in the 1997 NHSDA reported lifetime inhalant use, and 1 percent admitted to past-year use. Both current and past-year use were highest in 12- to 17-year-olds, especially in the north-central and western regions of the United States. Other age groups were basically unchanged; however, the 1997 survey showed an increase in inhalant use in the 12- to 17-year-old group from 5.9 percent to 7.2 percent, indicating more experimentation with these harmful substances. The use of inhalants by children and adolescents is of great concern because inhalants destroy organs and may cause death on the first use (Espeland, 1997). Between 1991 and 1996, the number of adolescents using inhalants almost doubled: 382,000 to 805,000 (from 10.3 to 21 new users per 1,000 potential new users). In addition to amyl nitrate (Poppers), nitrous oxide (Whippets), and anesthetics such as halothane or ether, common substances such as cooking spray, gasoline or lighter gases (butane, propane), glue, shoe polish or toluene, cleaning fluids and degreasers, spray paints, lacquer thinner and other paint solvents, aerosol sprays, and typewriter correction fluid may be used by youth to get a high. For ages 12 to 17, sniffing gasoline, lighter fluid, glue, shoe polish, or toluene is most common (2.7 percent). In 18- to 25-year-olds, rates of use increased to 10 percent, with dramatic increases in the lifetime use of nitrous oxide (6.6 percent). In the 18- to 25-year-old group, the rate of first use also increased from 1991 to 1996 (from 5 to 12 new users per 1,000 potential new users). Overall and across all age categories, whites report the most lifetime use.

Heroin

Reported estimates of heroin use probably fall below actual use because about 20 percent of users (the homeless and institutionalized) are not included in the NHSDA estimate. Estimates are subject to wide variability so they usually do not show clear trends, although there was a statistically significant upward trend in the number of new users from 1992 to

1996, a finding consistent with anecdotal reports and comparable to the increases seen in the epidemic of the late 1960s. In 1996, an estimated 171,000 people used heroin for the first time. The rate of heroin initiation for the 12- to 17-year-old group increased from below 1 new user per 1,000 potential new users in the 1980s to 4 in 1996. Rates of initiation also increased for young adults ages 18 to 25. The NHSDA data showed an increasing rate of past-month heroin use from 1993 to 1997, and an increasing rate of lifetime heroin smoking, snorting, or sniffing between 1994 and 1997 (SAMHSA, 1998). Most new heroin users in recent years had never injected heroin; rather, they were smoking, snorting, or sniffing.

Survey estimates of heroin use were higher in the 12- to 17-year-old group in 1997, as compared with previous years. Lifetime, past-year, and past-month use were 0.5 percent, 0.3 percent, and 0.2 percent, respectively. Of great concern is the MTF study finding that among twelfth-graders, lifetime, past-year, and past-month rates had risen significantly, with non-injectable forms of heroin accounting for the overall rise. Past-year use was more than double in whites, followed by blacks and Hispanics; percentages were highest in the western region of the United States. Overall rates were higher for those who had less than a high school education or who were unemployed.

DAWN reported that, between 1994 and 1995, there was a 19 percent increase in heroin-related emergency department episodes. Heroin was mentioned in 45 percent of the episodes involving male deaths, 41 percent of female deaths, and 11 percent of suicides; it was frequently used in combination with cocaine.

Psychotherapeutic Drugs

Nonmedical use of any prescription-type psychotherapeutic drug, such as stimulants, sedatives, tranquilizers, or analgesics, was lowest among those ages 12 to 17: Lifetime use was 7 percent, previous-year use was 5 percent, and previous-month use was 2.1 percent. Past-year and current use were highest in young adults ages 18 to 25, particularly in the western U.S. region. Individuals with college degrees had the lowest rates of use.

When the overall category of psychotherapeutic drugs is broken down, the lowest lifetime use of stimulants was in 12- to 17-year-olds (2.3 percent); only 0.6 percent of 12- to 17-year-olds were current stimulant users. Lifetime sedative use was lowest in 12- to 17-year-olds (0.8 percent), and only 0.1 percent were current users. Lifetime tranquilizer use also was lowest in those ages 12 to 17; only 0.5 percent were current users. Lifetime analgesic use was highest in the 18- to 25-year-old group (7.5 percent) and lowest in those ages 12 to 17 (5.2 percent); past-month use was 1.3 percent for both. Two new addictive sedative-hypnotic drugs to watch are Rohypnol (roofies, R2) and GHB (G-riffic, Liquid G), which have become popular in Europe and are increasing in use among adolescents in the United States. These drugs have been nicknamed the date rape drugs because they cause loss of consciousness and short-term memory loss. They are particularly dangerous when combined with alcohol because they may cause death.

Anabolic Steroids

Anabolic steroids are synthetic derivatives of the male hormone testosterone. They increase lean muscle mass and the growth of skeletal muscle, thereby improving physical appearance and enhancing the sports performance of athletes by maximizing both their strength and their ability to train longer and harder. Steroids are typically taken in cycles of weeks/months, a process called cycling, rather than continuously. Steroids are known to cause multiple health problems including liver tumors, jaundice, fluid retention, manic-like symptoms leading to violent episodes, impaired judgment stemming from feelings of invincibility, hypertension, severe acne, and trembling. In adolescents, growth may be halted through premature skeletal maturation and accelerated pubertal changes. The 1997 MTF study reported high school seniors' attitudes toward steroid use: Of those surveyed, 67.2 percent perceived great risk in taking steroids, and 91.4 percent said that they disapproved of people who use them.

According to the MTF study, between 1989 and 1997, lifetime prevalence of anabolic steroid use among high school seniors fluctuated between a 3 percent high in 1989 and a 1.9 percent low in 1996; annual prevalence rates remained relatively stable. In 1997, 1.8 percent of eighth-graders and 2.0 percent of tenth-graders had used anabolic steroids at least once in their lifetimes, and 1.0 percent of eighth-graders and 1.2 percent of tenth-graders had used them in the past year. In the class of 1997, 2.4 percent of high school seniors had used anabolic steroids at least once in their lifetimes—up from the class of 1996's 1.9 percent lifetime use. Past-year use among seniors has been stable at 1.4 percent from 1991 to 1997. Although the number of high school and college athletes who use steroids is relatively small, those who use them risk numerous threats to their health and dismissal from sports programs.

A natural testosterone booster, androstenedione (known as andro) received wide attention after Mark McGwire of the St. Louis Cardinals broke the home run record in baseball in the summer of 1998. Although banned in other sports, this substance, found naturally in meats, is considered legal in major league baseball. This metabolite of DHEA is converted directly into testosterone by liver enzymes, resulting in increased muscle mass, energy, and ability to sustain physical exercise. Widely available without prescription, its side effects are unknown.

SUMMARY

Trends in substance use continue to change, with increased cigarette smoking in girls; earlier and increased use of alcohol, marijuana, inhalants, cocaine, and hallucinogens by adolescents; and increased and earlier experimentation with illicit drugs, such as noninjected heroin. Other than the category of psychotherapeutics, the trends in overall drug use in 12- to 17-year-olds are alarming and point to the need for effective and early intervention strategies in this group. Polydrug use in adolescents is growing and is occurring at younger ages. Initiation of one drug frequently leads to use of others. For example, college students who use steroids report cigarette use, greater alcohol consumption overall, binge drinking, and use of a wide variety of illegal drugs as compared to nonsteroid users (Meilman, Crace, Presley, and Lyerla, 1995; Scott, Wagner, and Barlow, 1996).

Drug use is associated with high-risk sexual behaviors in adolescents. Estimates from the World Health Organization (WHO) indicate that about half of the individuals worldwide who become infected with the human immunodeficiency virus (HIV) do so between the ages of 15 to 24, although they may not become symptomatic for many years. Increases in HIV and acquired immunodeficiency syndrome (AIDS) among injecting adolescents and young adults in the United States are an important and underrecognized public health problem (Morse, Morse, Burchfiel, and Zeanah, 1998). Drinking and driving also continues to be problematic in adolescents, although the higher minimum drinking age of 21 resulted in declines in alcohol consumption and traffic accidents among people under 21 years old (SAMHSA, 1994). However, about 10 percent, or 18 million people, in the United States age 16 years and older who drove in 1991 through 1993 reported that they drove under the influence (DUI) of alcohol or other drugs.

Primary Prevention in Adolescents

Developmentally, adolescents are self-oriented and have a sense of invulnerability that is frequently inconsistent with reality. Adolescence is a time of momentous changes in cognitive, psychological, social, and physical functions, as well as a period of rapid growth. The adolescent's lack of concern for the future increases his or her potential for risk taking, even when exposed to information about alcohol and other drug use. Jessor (1992) states that the tendency for several risk behaviors to co-occur within the same adolescent may constitute a syndrome that requires broad interventions emphasizing health-promoting lifestyles incompatible with risk behavior syndromes. For example, significant increases in the number of adolescents carrying weapons and physically fighting have been associated with use of all types of substances (Dukarm, Byrd, Auinger, and Weitzman, 1996).

Theories Underlying Program Development

Two theories applied to developing prevention strategies for adolescents are social learning theory (Bandura, 1977) and problem behavior theory (Jessor and Jessor, 1977). These theories were developed 20 years ago, but their application continues to undergird prevention programming. Social learning theory states that children imitate the behavior of others and learn acceptable behavior by receiving positive or negative reinforcement. They also observe behaviors of others, and the consequences of such behaviors. If older siblings, peers, or high-status individuals appear to gain from the behavior (smoking, drinking, or taking drugs), these outcomes will be powerful motivators to try it. Affiliation with drug-using friends emerges repeatedly as a strong predictor of use (Jenkins, 1996). The adolescent who has low self-esteem/self-confidence, is impulsive, and has a greater need for social approval within his or her peer group will be at greatest risk (Fontaine, 1999; Jessor, Collins, and Jessor, 1972). Even well-adjusted adolescents, however, may experiment with drugs to be part of a peer group (Pipher, 1994). Peers, siblings, and parental attitudes strongly influence decisions to try or use drugs; strong family relationships and good social supports may lessen the need for drugs. There is also an increased likelihood of substance use (cigarettes, marijuana, alcohol) in teens who exhibit psychosocial behaviors such as bulimia, crime, or suicidal ideation (Wiederman and Pryor, 1996) or who were exposed to physical or sexual abuse during childhood.

Problem behavior theory integrates well with social learning theory and was developed in an attempt to explain why adolescents engage in risky behaviors. It includes physiological factors (e.g., heredity), personal factors (e.g., attitudes, beliefs), and environmental factors (e.g., school, home, community). Learned behavior observed in adolescence is purposeful and goal-directed, and it fulfills multiple goals central to adolescent life (Jessor, 1992). Problem behavior theory sees engaging in problem behavior as contributing to the adolescent's achievement of desired personal goals. It is important for the nurse to discern what purpose the problem behavior (e.g., smoking, drinking, or use of drugs) serves. It may provide entry to a peer group; it may be a way of coping with anxiety, frustration, or feelings of failure; or it may be a rejection of adult authority. This theory may also support healthy behaviors by emphasizing personal goals that are positive and future-oriented. Teens can be exposed to messages that communicate that the attainment of independence and control of one's life can be achieved in other ways, such as school or sports achievement or hobbies (e.g., community volunteerism, music, hiking, scouts). Present experiences may be seen as essential groundwork where choices made either enhance or inhibit future success. In this light, risk taking may be seen as too costly.

Given the contexts of both theories, it seems logical that enhancing characteristics that promote adolescent coping should be a part of prevention strategies. Many newer approaches to substance abuse prevention incorporate the concept of resistance to negative social influences into their programs. Prevention strategies, therefore, should focus on eliminating or minimizing the environmental influences that may either promote or facilitate legal and illegal drug use. This includes decreasing drug availability, decreasing visibility of drug-using role models while increasing visibility of non–drug-using high-status role models, altering social norms and attitudes about acceptability of drug use, and eliminating media promotion of drug use via advertising, movies, or television (Botvin, 1986, 1988; Botvin et al., 1995). The average adolescent views 21 hours of television weekly, which makes media influence a powerful force (National Campaign to Prevent Teen Pregnancy, 1996). Teaching specific skills designed to help adolescents resist advertising that glorifies smoking or drinking and peer pressure to use drugs has been shown to be effective. Teaching adolescents decision-making strategies, goal setting, social skills, and assertiveness can provide them with coping skills to reduce anxiety and promote problem solving, as alternatives to taking drugs to alleviate stress (Botvin, 1995). Botvin's more recent work indicates that these strategies are effective with Caucasian, inner-city African American, and Hispanic youths (Mathias, 1997). The "just say no" approach to the multifaceted problems of substance abuse represents an oversimplification of the many factors contributing to initiating and sustaining drug-using habits.

Current Approaches to Prevention in Adolescents

Most primary prevention efforts targeting adolescents have occurred in elementary and middle schools, usually through the incorporation of drug abuse curricula into health education classes. Evaluations of some popular curricula in use over the past decade have demonstrated that they are ineffective; others have never been evaluated.

A review of 47 drug abuse prevention curricula that met four specific criteria was recently done (Dusenbury, Falco, and Lake, 1997). In order to be included in the review, the curricula were required to focus on primary prevention of alcohol and/or drug use, be classroom-based and designed for any grade level, and be nationally and currently available; program distributors needed to be willing to provide samples of drug abuse content. Only 10 had been sufficiently evaluated, and 8 of the 10 showed varying degrees of success in drug use prevention. The authors reported that the Alcohol Misuse Prevention Project, Growing Healthy, Know Your Body, Life Skills Training Program, Project Northland, and Students Taught Awareness and Resistance (S.T.A.R.) had effects that lasted 2 or more years after the pretest. The Life Skills Training Program had positive effects into young adulthood. Both Project Alert and Drug Abuse Resistance Education (D.A.R.E.) (the most widely used program in the United States) had variable initial success (including no effects), and no sustained effects on use. Other reports also indicate that the seventh-grade D.A.R.E. program is one example of a program that seems to have comparatively poor outcomes (Clayton, Cattarello, and Johnstone, 1996; Hansen and McNeal, 1997). The All Stars program had significantly better outcomes when compared to D.A.R.E. (Hansen, 1996). Project Alert actually increased substance abuse in some high-risk adolescents (these results disappeared by the 10th grade).

It is important to discard program strategies that have not proven successful over time. There are newer and possibly more effective prevention strategies that should be evaluated for effectiveness. Prevention programs that include peer speakers who have become alcoholics or who are HIV-positive due to injectable drug use can be a powerful reality check. In one approach, live theater is used to stimulate thought and discussion with adolescents (Harding et al., 1996). Jump Start (Harrington and Donohew, 1997) and Black Pearls (Center for Substance Abuse Prevention, 1997a) are prevention programs geared to African American teens. Right Turns Only (Freimuth, Plotnick, Ryan, and Schiller, 1997), a video-based multicultural drug education series for seventh-graders, has been demonstrated effective. Electronic Zoot (Jackson, 1995), a computer bulletin board program that teaches users about risks associated with substance use and abuse, and the P.I.E.D. (People Involved in Education about Drugs) Pipers program are newer educational prevention efforts that should be reviewed by community health nurses involved in program planning (Gloss, 1995).

Community-Based Programming for Adolescents

Prevention programs should begin before adolescents become users; they are best given in early adolescence (between the ages of 10 and 14). Schools need to utilize a range of social influence approaches designed to fit the needs of their particular populations. Curricula that include social resistance skills (recognition of influences and the skills to resist them) and education positing that using drugs is not the norm have been successful (Dusenbury, Falco, and Lake, 1997). These curricula are further enhanced by including subjects such as decision making, coping skills, and anxiety reduction. Peer counseling has been found effective as early as grades 6 through 8, with supplemental sessions in high school (Coombs and Ziedonis, 1995).

Early adolescents are particularly concerned with identity formation and approval of peers, and their emotions can be extreme and highly changeable (Bragg, 1997). At this young age, program effects are difficult to assess unless samples are huge because base rates of drug use are low, causing statistical power to be too weak to identify program effects (Botvin, 1995). Efforts should be targeted at prevention of first use of tobacco, alcohol, and marijuana because use of these drugs occurs toward the beginning of the developmental progression of drug abuse. Also, these drugs are the most widely used; therefore, the base rates are higher than for other drugs, increasing statistical power and the probability that true program effects will be detected.

During the time of middle adolescence, young people endeavor to move away from their parents emotionally. In the process of becoming independent, they may reject the values of their parents and experiment with drugs to be cool, as well as because their peers are doing it. They may become narcissistic, self-reliant, defiant, and hard to tolerate (Bragg, 1997). During late adolescence (17- to 18-year-olds), some stabilization usually occurs; self-importance lessens, usually resulting in greater ability to consider the views of parents and others (Stevens-Simon and Reichert, 1994).

As is true for all educational programs, clear and logical objectives should provide a clear strategy for both the conduct and evaluation of the program. Advanced practice community health nurses will notice that the following objectives reflect standard, time-tested epidemiologic and public health principles stressed by graduate programs in community health nursing. Botvin (1988, 1995) proposes that these eight criteria should be met by all programs geared to school-age children and adolescents:

1. *Interventions should be acceptable.* The prevention model proposed should seem feasible to both the program providers and the target population. Most community health nurses have had an unfortunate experience with programs that failed because there was insufficient collaboration with the community in all phases of program planning, so that consensus about the goals of the program are never reached. Although the nurse may recognize a need for a particular program, its success will be limited unless the community has a stake in it. Goals need to be consistent with community norms and should not be overly complex, requiring skills the program providers do not possess. Program proponents being overly zealous or crusading, as well as being bored or disinterested, can be deadly to program success.

2. *Interventions can affect variables associated with drug abuse or drug abuse risk.* The program may focus on knowledge of the effects of drugs on health and drug-using behaviors or be concerned with variables associated with drug initiation, such as self-efficacy, self-esteem, or locus of control. The evaluation of such programs typically seeks to demonstrate that participants either leave knowing more than they did on arrival or have changed their attitudes about substance use in the desired direction. However, gains in either knowledge about drugs or attitude change have generally not affected actual drug use behaviors.

3. *Interventions can reduce the use or abuse of at least one drug.* Drug involvement is usually measured by assessing frequency and consequences of use. Does the approach used prevent or delay at least one form of drug-taking behavior? Because tobacco, alcohol, and marijuana are the most frequently used, an appropriate goal would be to prevent or at least delay use of at least one of these gateway drugs.

4. *Interventions can reduce the use or abuse of multiple drugs.* The goal of prevention is to prevent the onset of drug abuse; an appropriate goal for adolescents, however, is delaying experimentation or significantly reducing experimentation with new drug use. In older populations in which drug use rates are higher, a reasonable expectation is to demonstrate a decrease in more frequent use (weekly or daily) that leads to actual **substance dependence.**

5. *Interventions can produce lasting effects.* Even when a program finds that drug use has been statistically reduced at its end, this may be of little practical significance. Effects should last, an outcome that can only be demonstrated by longitudinal studies. Such studies are difficult due to problems in tracking of students, attrition, waning enthusiasm of the administrators and/or teachers responsible for overseeing data collection, and resistance on the part of students who may object to repeated testing. Short-term

interventions cannot be expected to have lasting effects on behavior. Ongoing interventions should occur throughout the school years and should be consistent with adolescent development and patterns of learning. Students unable to process complex information need other learning strategies.

6. *Interventions are adaptable to different conditions, providers, and delivery methods.* If specific interventions must be developed for different drugs or different classes of drugs, the sheer volume of interventions would negate their use. The etiology of drug use/abuse may be similar enough in variable populations that a generic intervention could be developed that would be reasonably effective with all or most forms of drug abuse. Interventions should have the ability to adapt to different scheduling formats, group sizes, and institutions. Interventions should be effective regardless of conditions (e.g., schools versus community agencies) or providers (e.g., nurses or teachers).

7. *Interventions are effective with several different populations.* Populations are defined by many characteristics such as race, ethnicity, socioeconomic status, age, or risk factors. If the causes of drug abuse are similar, perhaps the same intervention could be used with a variety of population groups with modifications (such as making them more culturally sensitive).

8. *Interventions are exportable and easy to disseminate.* Can the interventions be disseminated widely, or will they only work under a set of unique circumstances? Those that work in limited environments are of little value in national efforts.

Program planners must take into account the etiology of drug use, relevant theories, and the results of evaluation studies, as well as reasonable prevention objectives. The most effective prevention strategies are those that have multiple components and use program providers and delivery channels that effectively reach target populations and provide ongoing interventions throughout the critical period when drug use is usually initiated (Botvin, 1995). Media advocacy (strategic use of mass media) has been a potent tool for promoting social or public policy initiatives in some communities (Jernigan and Wright, 1996). Long-term follow-up evaluations of drug abuse prevention programs indicate that such programs, if conducted by middle school, can produce meaningful and lasting reductions in drug use by adolescents (Botvin et al., 1995).

Primary Prevention in Occupational Health

Occupational health nurses need to be strong advocates of primary prevention in the workplace. It makes good economic sense for companies to support employee assistance programs (EAPs), which are effective in reaching young adult populations. EAPs were designed to provide a source of health care for employees with emotional, family, or substance abuse problems. Approximately 33 percent of all private, nonagricultural worksites with 50 percent or more full-time employees offer such programs (Hartwell et al., 1996). Routine examinations may identify at-risk individuals who will benefit from primary prevention. The workplace is an excellent venue for the delivery of programs on legal and illegal drugs, and programs may be offered either during or after working hours. Support groups and promotion of smoking cessation programs, smoke-free environments, and alcohol-free parties are all ways the occupational health nurse can advocate for primary prevention and adoption of healthy lifestyles.

The cost of substance-related loss of productivity or illness is estimated at over $300 billion yearly (American Psychiatric Association, 1995). EAP figures indicate that 35 percent of individuals who abuse alcohol and 20 percent of those who abuse other drugs report frequent absenteeism or lateness to work. EAP clients who abuse alcohol also report more accidents both on and off the job (Blum and Roman, 1992). Marijuana and cocaine users also report frequent absenteeism. These observations supported the initiative of mandatory drug testing, primarily to maintain public safety (Hiner, 1996). Most drug users are employed part- or full-time; however, they use at lower rates than the unemployed. Of the 10.3 million persons 18 and older reporting past-month illicit drug use, 5.7 million were employed full-time, 1.7 million were employed part-time, 1.2 million were unemployed, and 1.7 million were in the "other" category (e.g., retired and disabled persons, homemakers, students) (SAMHSA, 1994). Although national data are an important guide, these figures suggest that all employers should consider the potential for employee drug use and implement an approach for detection and assistance.

Aggressive management by preferred provider organizations (PPOs) and other managed care approaches has resulted in decreased expenditures for alcohol, drug, and mental health treatment (National Survey of Employer-Sponsored Health Plans, 1994). At the same time, employer-based (not unlike managed care) health insurance coverage is generally less comprehensive for both mental health and substance abuse treatment than for other health problems. For example, 17 percent of full-time employees had hospital costs for other health problems paid in full, but only 2 percent received full coverage for in-patient mental health/substance abuse care (U.S. Department of Labor, Bureau of Labor Statistics, 1991). In the early 1990s, employers in medium and large companies expanded coverage for detoxification treatment to over 95 percent of their employees. This is a significant increase, but detoxification is only the first of many steps in treatment (Kronson, 1991; U.S. Department of Labor, Bureau of Labor Statistics, 1991).

Nurses in Primary Prevention in Community Health Centers

APNs are key linkages to health centers within their communities. Frequently, these are satellites of larger institutions such as teaching hospitals or health maintenance organizations (HMOs). Primary prevention services may be limited to immunizations or may cover a wide range of activities for health promotion and disease prevention, including substance abuse prevention and screening. Well-baby and family planning clinics provide broad secondary prevention. Women's health, mental health, walk-in clinics, emergency departments, and health departments may be community health centers for individuals with no other private or public health care resources.

In 1965, the U.S. Office of Economic Opportunity sponsored two grants to increase public access to community-based care. The Community Health Centers (CHC) grant (Section 330, Public Health Services [PHS] Act) and the Migrant Health Centers grant

(PHS Act, Section 329) were designed to fill gaps in the system. Over 500 centers operate more than 2,000 clinics (urban and rural) throughout the United States and provide a variety of primary health and prevention services. Community health nurses knowledgeable about such centers can help clients access comprehensive services, especially for the medically underserved and those abusing substances.

Another innovative approach that increases access to health care is the development of community nursing centers. The first, Loeb Center, was established in New York City in 1963; it was described as "public health nursing in an institutionalized setting" (Riesch, 1992, p. 16). Many nursing centers are staffed by nursing faculty and students, and they provide primary care and prevention primarily to individuals with limited access to health care. These centers are in schools of nursing, retirement communities, home care agencies, or hospital outreach satellites. Reimbursement comes from federal, state, or private sources. The Community Nursing Organizations Bill of 1987 mandated direct reimbursement to nurses at 10 demonstration sites in the United States. At the present time, clients contribute about 25 percent of the payment, 19 percent is paid by private insurance, Medicare or Medicaid pays about 24 percent, and 17 percent is provided by other sources; about 13 percent is not compensated (*American Journal of Nursing*, 1992). Because of nursing's commitment to primary prevention, nursing centers often do a better job than most agencies in organizing groups and resources for the primary prevention of substance abuse. These centers are usually located in regions where the negative effects of substance abuse are all too evident, and where nurses encounter frequent problems related to dependence and addiction. Community-based nursing centers are excellent settings for educational groups and counseling, as well as family-oriented, culturally sensitive care. The focus is on individuals and families rather than on the presenting illness (Pender, 1996).

Nurses have also developed an innovative practice model of clinical partnerships between nurse practitioners and community health nurses, integrating prevention with treatment. Jenkins and Sullivan-Marx (1994) have proposed a primary care delivery pyramid with principles of public health science as the foundation, community health nursing centers at the second level, and home and nursing home care at the third level; medical management and acute and critical care form the top of the pyramid

The Healthy Cities program, originating in Canada and endorsed by WHO in 1986, is another innovative approach to improving the health of communities. This program sought to develop healthier communities through grassroots analysis, consensus, and social action (Flynn, 1993). The unique needs of particular cities, such as inequities in health care, are addressed through the involvement of local citizens. The WHO Collaborating Center in Healthy Cities at the Indiana School of Nursing continues to promote these initiatives.

Most people with substance abuse disorders are treated in their own communities. When comparing types of facilities that individuals use for substance abuse treatment, one-day census figures may be more accurate than annual rates. This is because clients may be counted more than once in annual rates if they are admitted more than once a year, but one-day census clients are counted only once. There were more admissions to ambulatory treatment than to 24-hour care in facilities specializing in substance abuse treatment, whether measured by annual admissions or one-day census. According to 1995 one-day census figures, there were 1,009,000 total admissions to substance abuse treatment facilities. Of these, 864,000 were admitted to ambulatory facilities (which include outpatient and partial care), and 145,000 were admitted to 24-hour care facilities (which include in-patient and residential care). Of the total 1,009,000 admissions to specialty substance abuse facilities in 1995 (Rouse, 1998):

- 46 percent were to freestanding facilities that provide no medical or mental health services other than substance abuse treatment
- 25 percent were to mental health services, which include psychiatric and behavioral hospitals, community mental health centers, and psychiatric and mental health counselors, that directly provide a range of mental health services in addition to substance abuse treatment
- 17 percent were to physical health services, such as hospitals, medical centers, clinics, and HMOs, that directly provide medical services in addition to substance abuse treatment (these facilities may also provide mental health services)
- 9 percent were to the criminal justice system, which includes correctional facilities, juvenile residential facilities, community corrections facilities, probation, parole, DUI, and domestic violence programs
- 3 percent were to other community settings that provide social services in addition to substance abuse treatment, such as youth centers, schools, EAPs, and charitable organizations

Community health nursing is returning to social action. With proposed health care reform and cost cutting, nurses are helping communities create public health systems that emphasize health promotion and disease prevention. The encouragement of public participation in the coordination of community health services and policy is what Kang (1995) calls "building community capacity." Coalitions between consumers and health care providers are promoting solutions to alcohol, tobacco, and other drug abuse that are community-based, which have a greater likelihood of success (Butterfoss, Goodman, and Wandersman, 1996). The number of smaller community coalitions, such as Ohio Parents for Drug-Free Youth (Center for Substance Abuse Prevention, 1997b), are increasing. Many larger coalitions (such as the D.C. Community Prevention Partnership, a nonprofit organization addressing substance abuse and violence prevention) are also actively pursuing drug prevention in their communities. They have organized Black Pearls clubs and workshops through churches, schools, and youth summer programs in the District of Columbia (Center for Substance Abuse Prevention, 1991c).

The U.S. Department of Education formed the Partnership for Family Involvement in Education in 1994. This partnership has been promoting the conversion of schools into community learning centers and actively involving the community in educating children. The Partnership is a coalition of over 3,000 family, school, business, and community organizations. One of its programs—Extending Learning in a Safe, Drug-Free Environment Before and After School—advocates keeping schools open for extended hours. Consumer satisfaction and participation in coalitions are encouraged by shared decision making, linkages with other organizations, and positive climates. One community coalition, for example, impacted the sale of alcohol and tobacco products to minors in its community by issuing citations to clerks willing to sell to minors and commendations to those who did not. Alcohol sales to minors decreased from 83 percent to 33 percent (Lewis et al., 1996).

Secondary Prevention

Community health nurses aid in the assessment, screening, and early detection of substance misuse. Early interventions halt the progression of experimentation to dependence to abuse by appropriate and timely action. The nurse works with family members by explaining both the disease process and the relapsing nature of dependence and addiction, as well as by monitoring and coordinating resources and services during the initial stages of treatment. During the prolonged period of recovery, which is experienced by family members as well as the affected individual, the nurse interprets the process and provides support (Willenbring, Ridgely, Stinchfield, and Rose, 1991).

Community health nurses should attempt to form strong partnership roles with schoolteachers, helping them to recognize the early signs of drug use and providing consultation and referral to both treatment and support sources. Nurses and teachers should be aware of links between substance abuse and other presenting symptoms. For example, children of alcoholics are at risk for becoming alcoholics themselves; certain other adolescent groups, such as Native Americans, also are at greater risk. About 20 percent of Native American youth, especially school dropouts, are heavily involved with drugs, a pattern that has been true since 1980 (Beauvais, 1996). Suicide attempts occur three times more often in adolescent substance abusers than in the general adolescent population, with suicidal ideation usually occurring after the initiation of drug use. Depression and other self-destructive feelings, such as the post-high depression occurring with stimulant drugs, may be worsened by alcohol and drugs (Berman and Schwartz, 1990). In one study, 7 percent of cocaine-related deaths were suicides (Tardiff et al., 1989).

The nurse should be fully aware of community resources and self-help groups and should take an active role in empowering families to get the help they need. The *Diagnostic and Statistical Manual of Mental Disorders,* Fourth Edition (DSM-IV) (American Psychiatric Association, 1994) lists diagnostic criteria, including the range of symptoms, for problems of substance abuse. Substance abuse is defined as a "maladaptive pattern of . . . use indicated by one of the following: continued use despite knowledge of having a persistent or recurrent social, occupational, psychological, or physical problem that is caused or exacerbated by . . . use or recurrent use in situations in which . . . use is physically hazardous" (American Psychiatric Association, 1994, pp. 182–183). The DSM-IV also describes the range of symptoms that indicate dependence when an individual (American Psychiatric Association, 1994):

- Uses drug longer than intended, and amount of substance used escalates.
- Cannot control cravings for drug and has increased tolerance.
- Spends significant amounts of time using, obtaining, or recovering from drug use.
- Has withdrawal symptoms that interfere with activities of daily life.
- Continues to use drug regardless of physical or social consequences.

Substance abuse does not have to be at the level of dependence in order to be problematic. For example, nondependent alcohol abusers are estimated to be responsible for about half of drunk-driving incidents, drunkenness on the job, and alcohol-related violence (Hyman, 1995).

At the time of screening, the individual usually does not recognize the need for intervention. The community health nurse may assist in structuring a session during which the substance-using individual is confronted by family, peers, employer, schoolteachers, or the legal system. Information is shared about behaviors observed and their impact on the family, work, or school performance. A treatment program that has been preplanned is outlined for the individual by the participants. Following the intervention, the community health nurse continues to support the family and suggests programs that will assist their coping and self-help.

When an individual is already using drugs, the concept of harm reduction should be evaluated. It is estimated that only 5 to 10 percent of the drug-using population is ready to enter abstinence-based programs at any given time, so ways to work with the other 90 percent must be considered (O'Hare, 1992). Harm reduction or minimization (risk reduction) seeks to decrease the negative effects of drug use. This approach emphasizes strategies such as needle exchange programs to limit sharing injection equipment, encouraging a change from injectable to oral drugs, advocating reduction in the quantity of drugs taken, and eventually gaining the user's participation in an abstinence program (Newcombe, 1992). This approach decreases negative health effects for the user and consequences to the society as a result of drug use, such as crime and prostitution. Although abstinence is often a necessary goal, decreasing risks (e.g., by responsible drinking) has its merits.

Community Education

One of the best ways to gain community support is education. Nurses can be powerful forces for community change by encouraging primary prevention efforts. Through educating the public, nurses can advocate for primary prevention interventions that have been shown by research to be successful. The nurse is in an excellent position to determine what is acceptable in that community. Although the community health nurse is experienced in teaching individuals and their families, educating the aggregate requires different approaches and skills. Teaching is geared to small and large groups, necessitating knowledge of group process and adult learning strategies. A variety of community settings, such as schools, EAPs, clinics, and community centers, should be used. The nurse needs to be realistic about outcomes. If it is not possible to stop drug use in today's society, can the social and personal consequences of addiction be minimized? All or nothing interventions will inevitably fail. The Office of Substance Abuse Prevention (OSAP) is an excellent resource for community health nurses, providing information, strategies, and suggestions for community-based drug education. The National Clearinghouse for Alcohol and Drug Information is the source for OSAP materials, which are available free of charge. OSAP also provides information on the community empowerment system that is being encouraged for community prevention efforts.

Nurses need to determine the teaching needs and interests of the community by working collaboratively, planning strategies, and carefully evaluating programs. Coombs and Ziedonis (1995) state that health professionals need to be educated themselves to undertake prevention activities and should be active in shaping educational and government policy about drug abuse. They suggest, for example, that organized sports programs be encouraged to incorporate teaching about drug abuse at every level of sports activity. Innovative techniques such as motivational interviewing (Rollnick, Heather, and Bell, 1992) can be used by health professionals in group teaching. This technique, which takes from 5 to 15 minutes, was developed in the addictions field and is effective in helping clients articulate the need to change their substance use habits. The caregiver selects one strategy best suited to the client's perceived readiness to change from a menu of options.

General Community-Based Programming

SAMHSA has developed the following seven substance abuse prevention strategies for communities:

1. *Alternatives.* The use of alternative strategies provides for the participation of target populations in constructive activities that exclude alcohol, tobacco, and other drug use. They are intended to offset the attraction to substance use. Examples are drug-free dances and parties, youth/adult leadership activities, community drop-in centers, and community service activities.
2. *Community-based process.* This process aids communities in the provision of more effective prevention and treatment services for alcohol, tobacco, and drug abuse disorders. Activities may include organizing, planning, enhancing efficiency and effectiveness of implementation of services, and promoting interagency collaboration, coalition building, and networking. Examples include community and volunteer training (e.g., neighborhood action training), training of key people in the system, staff/officials training, systematic planning, multiagency coordination and collaboration, accessing services and funding, and community team building.
3. *Early intervention.* Early intervention uses activities designed to come between an early substance abuser and his or her actions in order to modify behavior. It may include a wide spectrum of activities from user education to formal intervention and referral to treatment from a substance abuse professional.
4. *Education.* Educational programs build critical life and social skills through structured learning processes. Critical life and social skills include decision making, peer resistance, coping with stress, problem solving, interpersonal communication, and systematic and judgmental abilities. Examples include classroom and/or small-group sessions, parenting and family management classes, peer leader/helper programs, and education programs for youth groups and children of substance abusers groups.
5. *Environment.* Environmental modification establishes activities to change written and unwritten community standards, codes, and attitudes that tend to tolerate, accept, or support the abuse of alcohol, tobacco, and other drugs used in the general population. This strategy is divided into two subcategories to permit distinction between activities that center on legal and regulatory initiatives and those that relate to the service and action-oriented initiatives. Examples include promoting the review of alcohol, tobacco, and drug use policies in schools; providing technical assistance to communities to maximize local enforcement procedures governing availability and distribution of alcohol, tobacco, and other drug use; and modifying alcohol and tobacco advertising practices and product pricing strategies.

6. *Information*. Information provides knowledge and increases awareness of the nature and extent of alcohol and other drug use, abuse, and addiction and their effects on individuals, families, and communities. This strategy also provides knowledge and increases awareness of available prevention and treatment programs and services. Examples include clearinghouse/information resource centers, resource directories, media campaigns, brochures, radio/television public service announcements, speaking engagements, health fairs/health promotion, and information lines.

7. *Problem identification and referral*. Problem identification and referral include activities to identify those who have engaged in illegal or age-inappropriate use of tobacco or alcohol and persons who have begun to use illicit drugs. This strategy assesses whether this early alcohol and drug use can be reversed through education. It does not include any activity designed to determine if a person is in need of treatment. Examples include EAPs, student assistance programs, and DUI and driving while intoxicated (DWI) education programs.

If community programming is to succeed, health professionals must establish a true partnership with citizens in their communities so that decision making is shared. Communities must have opportunities to identify and express their needs and contribute to their own well-being (Farley, 1993). Community health nurses and other health professionals can then take an active role in helping the community to achieve its goals.

Case Study

You receive a referral from the school nurse in your district to visit the Carraher family. Thirteen-year-old Michael has been expelled from school after admitting that he smoked marijuana on school grounds. When you visit Michael, he admits to smoking and inhaling several joints per day and sees no problem in doing so. His mother, a single parent, tells you that she isn't home very much because of her work schedule. She has noticed, however, that Michael seems to vacillate between euphoria and sleeplessness, but she attributed these behaviors to fluctuating hormones in adolescence. She also states that she has sometimes noted that the whites of his eyes appear red and that he lacks coordination on occasion, signs she also attributed to the adolescent period. She admitted to knowing that Michael sneaks smokes but thought he would never try drugs because he has always been well-behaved and responsible.

1. What are the biophysical, psychological, and social problems that may be caused by marijuana use?
2. What risk factors may be influencing Michael's use of marijuana and his adherence to continued use despite problems with school?
3. What secondary and tertiary interventions may be appropriate and effective in this situation?
4. How will you evaluate your interventions and provide follow-up care to this family?

CRITICAL THINKING QUESTIONS

1. What variables in your community increase or decrease the success of substance abuse prevention programs?
2. How may APNs use their skills to advocate for community-based treatment for substance abusers?
3. Should school nurses be mobilized to strategically plan for effective prevention programs for adolescents?
4. How can APNs in various clinical and academic settings appropriately apply primary, secondary, and tertiary levels of prevention to issues of substance abuse and dependence?

REFERENCES

American Journal of Nursing. (1992). News: Community nursing centers gaining ground as a solution to health issues. *American Journal of Nursing 92*(7), 70–71.

American Nurses' Association. (1980) *A Conceptual Model of Community Health Nursing Practice.* Kansas City, MO: Author.

American Psychiatric Association. (1994). *Diagnostic and Statistical Manual of Mental Disorders* (4th ed.). Washington, DC: Author.

American Psychiatric Association. (1995). Practice guidelines for the treatment of patients with substance use disorders. *American Journal of Psychiatry 152*(11), November Supplement, 5–59.

American Public Health Association. (1981). *The Definition and Role of Public Health Nursing in the Delivery of Health Care.* Washington, DC: Author.

Babor, T.F. (1990). Alcohol and substance abuse in primary care settings. In J. Mayfield and M. Grady (eds.), *Primary Care Research: An Agenda for the 90s.* Washington, DC: U.S. Department of Health and Human Services.

Bandura, A. (1977). *A Social Learning Theory.* Englewood Cliffs, NJ: Prentice-Hall.

Beauvais, P. (1996). Trends in drug use among American Indian students and dropouts, 1975 to 1994. *American Journal of Public Health 86*(11), 1594–1598.

Berman, A.N., and Schwartz, R. (1990). Suicide attempts among adolescent drug users. *American Journal of Diseases of Children 144,* 310–314.

Blum, T., and Roman, P. (1992). A description of clients using Employee Assistance Programs (EAP). *Alcohol Health and Research World 16*(2), 120–128.

Botvin, G.J. (1986). Substance abuse prevention research: Recent developments and future directions. *Journal of School Health 56*(9), 369–374.

Botvin, G.J. (1988). Defining "success" in drug abuse prevention. *NIDA Research Monograph 90,* 203–212.

Botvin, G.J. (1995). Principles of prevention. In R. Coombs and D. Ziedonis (eds.), *Handbook on Drug Abuse Prevention.* Boston: Allyn and Bacon.

Botvin, G.J., Baker, E., Dusenbury, L., Botvin, E.M., and Diaz, T. (1995). Long-term follow-up results of a randomized drug abuse prevention trial in a white middle-class population. *Journal of the American Medical Association 273*(14), 1106–1112.

Bragg, E.J. (1997). Pregnant adolescents and addictions. *Journal of Gynecologic & Neonatal Nursing,* September–October, 577–584.

Butterfoss, F.D., Goodman, R.M., and Wandersman, A. (1996). Community coalitions for prevention and health promotion: Factors predicting satisfaction, participation and planning. *Health Education Quarterly 23*(1), 65–79.

Center for Substance Abuse Prevention (CSAP). (1997a). Beautiful black pearls. *The Prevention Pipeline 10*(5), 8–9.

Center for Substance Abuse Prevention (CSAP). (1997b). Ohio is blazing a trail to curb drinking on college campuses. *The Prevention Pipeline 10*(5), 10–12.

Center for Substance Abuse Prevention (CSAP). (1997c). Schools and communities work together in new partnerships. *The Prevention Pipeline 10*(5), 2–4.

Clayton, R.R., Cattarello, A.M., and Johnstone, B.M. (1996). The effectiveness of drug abuse resistance education (Project DARE): 5-year follow-up results. *Preventive Medicine 25,* 307–318.

Coleman, P. (1993). Overview of substances. In R.D. Blondell (ed.), *Primary Care: Substance Abuse.* Philadelphia: Saunders.

Coleman, P.R., and Veach, T. (1990). Substance abuse and the family physician: A survey of attitudes. *Substance Abuse 11,* 84–93.

Commission on Chronic Illness. (1957). *Chronic Illness in the United States* (Vol. 1). Published for the Commonwealth Fund. Cambridge, MA: Harvard University Press.

Coombs, R.H., and Ziedonis, D. (1995). *Handbook on Drug Abuse Prevention.* Boston: Allyn and Bacon.

Dukarm, C.P., Byrd, R.S., Auinger, P., and Weitzman, M. (1996). Illicit substance abuse, gender, and risk of violent behavior among adolescents. *Archives in Pediatric Adolescent Medicine 150,* 797–801.

Dusenbury, L., Falco, M., and Lake, A. (1997). A review of the evaluation of 47 drug abuse prevention curricula available nationally. *Journal of School Health 67*(4), 127–132.

Espeland, K.E. (1997). Inhalants: The instant, but deadly high. *Pediatric Nursing 23*(1), 82–86.

Farley, S. (1993). The community as partner in primary health care. *Nursing and Health Care 14*(5), 244–249.

Flynn, B.C. (1993). Healthy cities: The future of public health. Restructuring how we live. *Healthcare Trends and Transition 4*(3), 12–18, 80.

Fontaine, K.L. (1999). Substance-related disorders. In K.L. Fontaine and J.S. Fletcher (eds.), *Mental Health Nursing.* Menlo Park, CA: Addison-Wesley.

Freimuth, V.S., Plotnick, C.A., Ryan, C.E., and Schiller, S. (1997). Right turns only: An evaluation of a video-based, multicultural drug education series for seventh graders. *Health Education and Behavior 24*(5), 555–567.

Gloss, E. (1995). Children and drug education: The P.I.E.D. Pipers. People Involved in Education about Drugs. *Nursing Outlook 43*(2), 66–70.

Gordon, R. (1987). An operational classification of disease prevention. In J.A. Steinberg and M.M. Silverman (eds.), *Preventing Mental Disorders.* Rockville, MD: Department of Health and Human Services.

Goshen, C.E. (1973). *Drinks, Drugs & DoGooders.* New York: Free Press.

Gruber, E., DiClemente, R.J., Anderson, M.M., and Lodico, M. (1996). Early drinking onset and its association with alcohol use and problem behavior in late adolescence. *Preventive Medicine 25*(3), 293–300.

Hansen, W.B. (1996). Pilot test results comparing the All Stars program with seventh grade D.A.R.E.: Program integrity and mediating variable analysis. *Substance Use and Misuse 31*(10), 1359–1377.

Hansen, W.B., and McNeal Jr., R.B. (1997). How D.A.R.E. works: An examination of program effects on mediating variables. *Health Education & Behavior 24*(2), 165–176.

Harding, C.G., Safer, L.A., Kavanagh, J., Bania, R., Carty, H., Lisnov, L., and Wysockey, K. (1996). Using live theater combined with role playing and discussion to examine what at-risk adolescents think about substance abuse, its consequences and prevention. *Adolescence 31*(124), 783–796.

Harrington, N.G., and Donohew, L. (1997). Jump Start: A targeted substance abuse prevention program. *Health Education and Behavior 24*(5), 568–586.

Hartwell, T.D., Steele, P., French, M.T., Potter, F.J., Rodman, N.F., and Zarkin, G.A. (1996). Aiding troubled employees: The prevalence, cost, and characteristics of employee assistance programs in the United States. *American Journal of Public Health 86*(6), 804–808.

Hiner, J. (1996). Mandatory drug testing in the workplace. *Kansas Nurse 71*(1), 2–3.

Hyman, S.E. (1995). Approach to the substance-abusing patient. In A.H. Goroll, L.A. May, and A.G. Mulley, Jr. (eds.), *Primary Care Medicine*. Philadelphia: J.B. Lippincott.

Jackson, J.E. (1995). A survey of a Canadian on-line substance abuse prevention initiative for adolescents and young adults. *Journal of Telemedicine and Telecare 1*(4), 217–223.

Jenkins, J.E. (1996). The influence of peer affiliation and student activities on adolescent drug involvement. *Adolescence 31*(122), 297–306.

Jenkins, M., and Sullivan-Marx, E. (1994). Nurse practitioners and community health nurses: Clinical partnerships and future visions. *Nursing Clinics of North America 29*(3), 459–470.

Jernigan, D.H., and Wright, P.A. (1996). Media advocacy: Lessons from community experiences. *Journal of Public Health Policy 17*(3), 306–330.

Jessor, R. (1992). Risk behavior in adolescence: A psychosocial framework for understanding and action. *Developmental Review 12*(4), 374–390.

Jessor, R., and Jessor, S.L. (1977). *Problem Behavior and Psychosocial Development: A Longitudinal Study of Youth*. New York: Academic Press.

Jessor, R., Collins, M.I., and Jessor, S.L. (1972). On becoming a drinker: Social-psychological aspects of an adolescent transition. *Annals of the New York Academy of Sciences 197*, 199–213.

Johnston, L.D., O'Malley, P.M., and Bachman, J.G. (1998). *National Survey Results on Drug Use from The Monitoring The Future Study, 1975–1997*. NIH Pub. No. 98-4345. Rockville, MD: U.S. Department of Health and Human Services, National Institute on Drug Abuse.

Kang, R. (1995). Building community capacity for health promotion: A challenge for public health nurses. *Public Health Nursing 12*(5), 312–318.

Kinney, J. (1996). *Clinical Manual of Substance Abuse* (2nd ed.). St. Louis, MO: Mosby.

Kronson, M.E. (1991). Substance abuse coverage provided by employer medical plans. *Monthly Labor Review 114*(4), 3–10.

Lewis, R.K., Paine-Andrews, A., Fawcett, S.B., Francisco, V.T., Richter, K.P., Copple, B., and Copple, J.E. (1996). Evaluating the effects of a community coalition's efforts to reduce illegal sales of alcohol and tobacco products to minors. *Journal of Community Health 21*(6), 429–436.

Mathias, R. (1997). This program reduces students' risk of drug use. *NIDA Notes*. NIH Pub. No. 97-3478, 1–6.

Meilman, P.W., Crace, R.K., Presley, C.A., and Lyerla, R. (1995). Beyond performance enhancement: Polypharmacy among collegiate users of steroids. *Journal of American College Health 44*(3), 98–104.

Moore, R.D., Bone, L.R., Geller, G., Mamon, J.A., Stokes, E.J., and Levine, D.M. (1989). Prevalence, detection, and treatment of alcoholism in hospitalized patients. *Journal of the American Medical Association 261*, 403–407.

Morse, E.V., Morse, P.M., Burchfiel, K.E., and Zeanah, P.O. (1998). Behavioral factors affecting HIV prevention for adolescent and young adult IDUs. *Journal of the Association of Nurses in AIDS Care 9*(3), 77–90.

Mrazek, P.J., and Haggerty, R.J. (1994). *Reducing Risks for Mental Disorders: Frontiers for Preventive Intervention Research*. Committee on Prevention of Mental Disorders, Division of Biobehavioral Sciences and Mental Disorders. Institute of Medicine. Washington, DC: National Academy Press.

National Campaign to Prevent Teen Pregnancy. (1996). *A Prospectus for the National Campaign to Prevent Teen Pregnancy: Mission, Leadership and Activities*. Washington, DC: Author.

National Survey of Employer-Sponsored Health Plans. (1994). New York: Foster Higgins.

Newcombe, R. (1992). The reduction of drug-related harm. A conceptual framework for theory, practice and research. In P.A. O'Hare, R. Newcombe, E.C. Buning, and E. Drucker (eds.), *The Reduction of Drug-Related Harm.* London, NY: Routledge.

O'Hare, P.A. (1992). Preface: A note on the concept of harm reduction. In P.A. O'Hare, R. Newcombe, E.C. Buning, and E. Drucker (eds.), *The Reduction of Drug-Related Harm.* London, NY: Routledge.

Pender, N. (1996). Settings for health promotion. In N.J. Pender (ed.), *Health Promotion in Nursing Practice* (3rd ed.). Stamford, CT: Appleton and Lange.

Pipher, M. (1994). *Reviving Ophelia: Savings the Selves of Adolescent Girls.* New York: Ballantine Books.

Riesch, S.K. (1992). Nursing centers: An analysis of the anecdotal literature. *Journal of Professional Nursing 8*(1), 16–25.

Rollnick, S., Heather, N., and Bell, A. (1992). Negotiating behavioral changes in medical settings: The development of brief motivational interviewing. *Journal of Mental Health I,* 25–37.

Rouse, B.A. (ed.) (1998). *Substance Abuse and Mental Health Statistics Sourcebook.* DHHS Pub. No. (SMA) 98-3170. Rockville, MD: Substance Abuse and Mental Health Services Administration.

Scott, D.M., Wagner, J.C., and Barlow, T.W. (1996). Anabolic steroid use among adolescents in Nebraska schools. *American Journal of Health-System Pharmacy 53*(17), 2068–2072.

Stevens-Simon, C., and Reichert, S. (1994). Sexual abuse, adolescent pregnancy and child abuse: A developmental approach to an intergenerational cycle. *Archives of Pediatric and Adolescent Medicine 148,* 23–27.

Substance Abuse and Mental Health Services Administration (SAMHSA), Office of Applied Statistics. (1994). *Preliminary Estimates from the 1993 Household Survey on Drug Abuse (NHSDA), Advance Report No. 7.* Rockville, MD: Author.

Substance Abuse and Mental Health Services Administration (SAMHSA), Office of Applied Studies. (1996). *National Household Survey on Drug Abuse (NHSDA): Main Findings 1995.* Rockville, MD: Author.

Substance Abuse and Mental Health Services Administration (SAMHSA), Office of Applied Studies. (1998). *Preliminary Results from the 1997 National Household Survey on Drug Abuse (NHSDA).* Rockville, MD: Author.

Tardiff, K., Gross, E., Wu, J., Stajic, M., and Millman, R. (1989). Analysis of cocaine positive fatalities. *Journal of Forensic Science 43,* 53–63.

U.S. Department of Health and Human Services. (1991). *Healthy People 2000.* Washington, DC: U.S. Government Printing Office.

U.S. Department of Labor, Bureau of Labor Statistics. (1991). Employee benefits in medium and large private establishments. *Bulletin 2422* (Table 39). Washington, DC: Author.

Wallerstein, N., and Bernstein, E. (1994). Introduction to community empowerment, participatory education, and health. *Health Education Quarterly 21*(2), 141–148.

Wiederman, M.W., and Pryor, T. (1996). Substance use and impulsive behaviors among adolescents with eating disorders. *Addictive Behaviors 21*(2), 269–272.

Willenbring, M.L., Ridgely, M.S., Stinchfield, R., and Rose, M. (1991). *Application of Case Management in Alcohol and Drug Dependence: Matching Techniques and Populations.* DHHS Pub. No. (ADM) 91-1766. Washington, DC: Alcohol Abuse and Mental Health Administration.

9

Substance-Related Problems and Childbearing

Deborah Mahony, ScD, RN, CSPNP
Sophronia Larig, CNM, MSN, CNP

LEARNER OUTCOMES

On completion of this chapter, the learner will be able to:

1. Describe the prevalence of licit and illicit drugs most frequently used during pregnancy.
2. Discuss the risk factors and their potential relationships to outcomes associated with neonatal drug exposure.
3. Analyze findings from the history, physical examination, laboratory data, and screening instruments to identify pregnant women who abuse licit and illicit drugs.
4. Describe the mode of action of common alcohol, tobacco, illicit drugs, and over-the-counter medications on pregnancy.
5. Discuss obstacles to drug treatment and rehabilitation for pregnant and parenting women.
6. Describe key characteristics of fetal alcohol syndrome (FAS) and alcohol-related birth defects (ARBDs).
7. Discuss ethical considerations associated with mandatory drug testing of pregnant women and/or their infants and the reporting of positive drug screens to criminal justice authorities.
8. Develop and implement management plans based on research evidence for pregnant and postpartum women who are identified as high-risk drug users and their infants.
9. Evaluate and modify management plans for pregnant and postpartum women identified as high-risk drug users and their infants.

KEY TERMS

child protective services
criminal justice system
drug rehabilitation

drug toxicology screens
fetal alcohol syndrome (FAS)
neonatal abstinence syndrome (NAS)

prevalence
risk factors

The use of tobacco, alcohol, and illicit drugs during pregnancy is a major concern for certified nurse-midwives (CNMs), nurse practitioners (NPs), and other advanced practice nurses (APNs) who care for women and their children. Although researchers have identified specific consequences of tobacco and alcohol use, as many as 40 percent of women of childbearing age use these drugs, and many women continue this use into pregnancy. The **prevalence** of heroin, cocaine, and marijuana remains low, but there is mounting evidence that the use of these drugs is associated with maternal complications and poor infant outcomes.

Identification before pregnancy, and treatment directed at abstinence or decreased use, is ideal. If pregnancy has occurred, early interview and screening followed by comprehensive management are essential. Some women may be identified but are lost to follow-up due to transient lifestyles or failure to comply with prenatal care. Infants born to these women may be affected by prenatal drug exposure and require intensive interventions. Methods of identification raise ethical questions as many women may not be informed of screening or the consequences of a positive screen. In some settings, providers may be mandated by law to report a positive toxicology screen to the **criminal justice system,** potentially interfering with opportunities to obtain necessary health care for the mother and her infant.

APNs have a unique opportunity to work with women who use substances. A plan of treatment and rehabilitation needs to address medical, social, psychological, and environmental factors. APNs need to have a working knowledge of methods of assessment, treatment protocols, and services available for the substance-using woman in order for prenatal care and treatment to be effective.

This chapter discusses the prevalence, **risk factors,** and outcomes associated with drug use during pregnancy; details screening and assessment processes; and describes the prenatal, postpartum, and newborn components of the management plan.

Scope of the Problem

Prevalence

Even though there has been a steady decline in the use of cigarettes, alcohol, and illicit drugs among women of childbearing age since 1985, a significant number of women continue to use these substances during their pregnancies. Data from the 1996 and 1997 National Household Survey of Drug Abuse (NHSDA) on pregnant women reported that 19.9 percent of those surveyed smoked cigarettes, 14 percent drank some alcohol, 1.3 percent engaged in binge drinking, and 2.5 percent used some kind of illicit drug in the past month

(SAMHSA, 1998). In the illicit drug category, only 1.5 percent of pregnant women surveyed reported that they used marijuana, 0.2 percent used cocaine or crack, 0.1 percent used hallucinogenic drugs such as lysergic acid diethylamide (LSD) or methylenedioxymethamphetamine (MDMA [ecstasy]), and 0.2 percent used heroin.

Women who were pregnant at the time of interview reported a significantly lower prevalence of past-month use than nonpregnant women. The 1996–1997 NHSDA further reports that the rate of tobacco, alcohol, and illicit drug use was higher for nonpregnant women with children than for pregnant women. This difference in prevalence suggests that women may have reduced or stopped use of cigarettes, alcohol, and illicit drugs during pregnancy but increased use of these substances after they gave birth.

When the 1996–1997 survey data were compared with the 1994–1995 NHSDA, the rate of drug usage in pregnant women is approximately the same (SAMHSA, 1997). Pregnant women's cigarette and alcohol use decreased slightly; illicit drug use increased from 2.2 percent to 2.5 percent. Table 9-1 summarizes past-month use from the 1996 and 1997 combined survey data.

In 1992–1993, the National Institute of Drug Abuse (NIDA) conducted a national survey of hospitals to determine the extent of drug abuse among women in the United States (NIDA, 1996). The National Pregnancy and Health Survey (NPHS) gathered self-report data from a national sample of 2,613 women who delivered babies at 52 urban and rural

TABLE 9-1 Demographic Characteristics of Women Reporting Last-Month Use of Licit and Illicit Drugs, NHSDA Combined Data, 1996 and 1997

Characteristic	Pregnant			Nonpregnant		
	Illicit Drugs %	Alcohol %	Cigarettes %	Illicit Drugs %	Alcohol %	Cigarettes %
Total prevalence	2.5	14.1	19.9	7.0	52.5	33.5
Age						
15–25	4.4	12.9	23.3	11.9	47.1	32.7
26–44	1.2	15.0	17.7	4.7	55.2	33.2
Race/ethnicity						
White	2.4	15.5	22.1	7.3	58.5	36.8
Black	5.4	16.7	28.8	8.0	41.7	28.9
Hispanic	1.2	7.1	10.0	4.7	38.2	22.3
Marital status						
Married	0.7	3.2	14.6	3.2	53.2	28.6
Not married	7.2	11.2	33.5	11.2	51.9	37.8
Adult education						
< High school	7.8	21.2	40.1	9.0	39.6	46.7
High school graduate	0.4	8.9	20.2	6.4	52.6	41.0
Some college	No estimate	No estimate	15.9	5.6	56.8	32.0
College graduate	No estimate	No estimate	7.8	4.4	66.1	16.7

Source: Substance Abuse and Mental Health Administration [SAMHSA]. (1998). *Preliminary Results for the 1997 National Household Survey on Drug Abuse.* Rockville, MD: National Clearing House for Alcohol and Drug Information.

hospitals. Based on these data, 5.5 percent of these women used illicit drugs, 18.8 percent used alcohol, and 20.4 percent smoked cigarettes at some time during their pregnancies. In addition, researchers found a strong link among cigarette, alcohol, and illicit drug use.

Smaller regional studies that use either toxicology screen, self-report, or both, have estimated the prevalence of illicit substance use among pregnant women to range between 3.0 percent and 27.0 percent for marijuana, 3.3 percent and 17.0 percent for cocaine, 0.3 percent and 1.7 percent for heroin, and 4.8 percent and 24.0 percent for use of any illicit drug during pregnancy. When meconium was analyzed, the prevalence for cocaine was even higher, between 11.8 percent and 30.7 percent. A summary of these studies is found in Table 9-2. The dramatic difference in the prevalence between the small studies and the NHSDA is related to the study site (small, inner-city, high-risk population versus large national random sample) and the method of identification (toxicology screens versus self-report).

Risk Factors

Women from any social, economic, or racial background can be at risk for substance abuse during pregnancy. Substance abuse in pregnancy is defined differently from substance abuse in a nonparturient state as the effects of alcohol and drugs are known to be damaging to the fetus in proportion to the amount and frequency of the drug used. In general populations, abuse is defined by regular use of amounts of the drug in patterns that result in negative interpersonal, legal, and health outcomes. Demographic attributes of women who use illicit drugs during pregnancy vary across studies. The NHSDA data indicate that pregnant women reporting cigarette smoking or alcohol use in the past month were more likely to be white, be of childbearing age (18–34), have 12 years of education or less, be employed, and be married (SAMHSA, 1998). In the NPHS, the estimated rate of cigarette and alcohol use was also highest among white women. The same survey found a higher percentage of illicit drug use for African American women. In a study using anonymous urine testing, alcohol use during pregnancy was most common in older, low-income women; marijuana use was most common in older white mothers; and cocaine use was most common in African American women in their mid-30s (Vega, Kolody, Porter, and Noble, 1997).

Certain factors have been linked to an increased risk for substance abuse in pregnancy; an awareness of these factors can be helpful in identifying women in need of special treatment (Bragg, 1997; Chasnoff, Griffith, Greier, and Murray, 1992; Daley and Argeriou, 1997; DeVille and Kopelman, 1998). These are:

- Lack of education
- Low self-esteem
- Depression
- Family problems and/or family history of substance abuse
- Financial problems and poverty
- Abusive relationships
- Poor housing
- Feelings of hopelessness
- Drug-abusing partner

Domestic violence, low self-esteem, and lack of a good social support system may lead to substance use as a coping mechanism. Violence in the form of sexual and physical abuse has

TABLE 9-2 Prevalence of Drug Use in Selected Studies

Study Location/Author	N	Method of Screening	Prevalence (%)		
Boston, MA (Frank et al., 1988)	679	Self-report/urine	Maternal	Marijuana Cocaine	27.0 8.0
Chicago, IL (Neerhoff et al., 1989)	1,776	Self-report/urine	Maternal	Cocaine toxicology only Self-report	 8.0 3.3
San Francisco, CA (Osterloh and Lee, 1989)	601[a] 339[b]	Urine	Maternal Infant	Any drug Cocaine Any drug Cocaine	68.0 46.0 63.0 42.0
New York State (Matera et al., 1990)	509	Self-report/urine	Maternal	Any drug Cocaine Marijuana Heroin	24.0 10.0 2.6 0.9
Rhode Island (Hollinshead et al., 1990)	495	Urine	Maternal	Any drug Cocaine Marijuana Heroin	7.5 2.6 3.0 1.7
Pennsylvania (Shutzman et al., 1991)	316[a] 500[b]	Self-report/meconium	Maternal Infant	Cocaine Cocaine	0.016 11.8
Detroit, MI (Ostrea et al., 1992)	3,010	Self-report/meconium	Maternal Infant	Any drug Any drug Cocaine	11.1 44.4 30.7
Jacksonville, FL (Vaughn et al, 1993)	1,062	Urine	Maternal	Any drug Cocaine	7.1 2.1
California (Vega et al., 1994)	29,494	Urine	Maternal	Any drug Cocaine	5.16 1. 11
Alabama (Pegues et al., 1994)	3,554	Urine	Maternal	Any drug Cocaine	8.4 1.3
New York State (Ryan et al., 1994)	903[a] 1,030[b]	Urine/meconium	Maternal Infant	Cocaine Cocaine	4.3 5.0
Minneapolis, MN (Yawn, 1994)	1,333	Meconium	Infant	Cocaine	2.0

Louisville, KY (Bibb et al., 1995)	554[a]
	532[b]
		Urine (all mothers)
		Urine (all infants)
		
		Meconium (386 infants)
			Maternal
			Infant
				Cocaine
				Cocaine:
				    Urine
				    Meconium
					4.8
					
					2.7
					4.5

[a]Mother
[b]Infant

also been linked to substance use. Barnet and colleagues (1995) studied the alcohol and illicit drug-using patterns of 125 parenting adolescents attending a pregnancy and parenting program. Of the adolescents screened, 42 percent tested positive for illicit drugs or reported use of alcohol at either a 2- or 4-month postpartum visit. When compared to nonusers, pregnant adolescents who used illicit drugs were found to be more depressed, to experience more stress, and to report a higher need for social support. They were also more likely than nonusers to have friends who used illicit drugs and alcohol. In a large nursing research study, alcohol and illicit drug use was reported by 42 percent of abused women and 21 percent of those not abused (McFarlane, Parker, and Soeken, 1996). In another nursing research study, Curry (1998) found that abused women used more tobacco and had lower self-esteem, higher stress, and less support from their significant other than did nonabused women.

A number of studies have linked depression to substance use before and after pregnancy (Hanna, Faden, and Dufour, 1994; Hutchins and DiPietro, 1997). Kelley (1998) found that a higher number of substance users (48 percent) than nonusers (3 percent) scored high enough on a stress index to warrant a mental health evaluation. In addition to depression, women who use substances are more likely to be involved in sexual risk taking. Women who use illicit drugs during pregnancy have been described as having past histories of sexually transmitted diseases (STDs) and therapeutic abortions (Amaro, Zuckerman, and Cabral, 1989; Marcenko, Spence, and Rohweder, 1994). They risk human immunodeficiency virus (HIV) when they exchange sex for drugs, engage in prostitution to earn money for drugs, or share intravenous drug-using paraphernalia (Jessup, 1997). Characteristics of pregnant women with positive drug tests were compiled from a review of 24 studies by Abercrombie and Booth (1997). There were positive associations among minority race, multiple pregnancies, single marital status, inadequate prenatal care, and substance abuse in several cases reviewed.

The research literature on adolescent health provides findings that have identified predictors of drug use. Susceptibility to peer pressure has been one of the most frequent correlates of adolescent drug use (Bush and Iannotti, 1993; Hansen et al., 1986; Hays and Revetto, 1990; Kandel, 1973; Kandel and Andreus, 1987). Initiation of use has been highly correlated with parental use (Gfroerer, 1987; Kandel, Kessler, and Marguiles, 1978), and pattern of early cigarette and alcohol use has been predictive of future use of illicit drugs (Kandel and Andreus, 1987; Yamaguchi and Kandel, 1984). A study of adolescent girls in a chemical dependency program revealed a high prevalence of sexual abuse prior to entering the program (Edwall, Hoffman, and Harrison, 1989). Many studies have concluded that multiple risk factor models are necessary to understand the correlates of drug use.

Maternal and Infant Outcomes

Tobacco use, the most common form of substance use by pregnant women, has long been associated with adverse maternal and infant outcomes. Smoking is a risk factor for preeclampsia, abruptio placentae, placenta previa, spontaneous abortion, ectopic pregnancy, and premature rupture of membranes (Fried, 1995). The more cigarettes smoked, the greater is the risk. The cost of these complications has been estimated to be as high as $135 million to $167 million (Adams and Melvin, 1998). Effects on the infant include intrauterine growth retardation (IUGR), premature delivery, and small-for-gestational-age (SGA) size (Zhang and Ratcliffe, 1993). In addition, nonsmoking women who are exposed to smoke in their homes have been found to have infants whose birth weight is 30 grams to 60 grams less than those of women who are not exposed to smoke in their homes (Das et al., 1998; Nafstad, Fugelseth, Qvistad, and Ershoff, 1997; Peacock et al., 1998; Perkins, Belcher, and Livesay, 1997). In one study, women who smoked fewer than nine cigarettes per day appear to have the same risk for low-birth-weight infants as nonsmokers (Nafstad, Fugelseth, Qvistad, and Ershoff, 1997). Smoke in the environment can lead to many problems for the infant, including predisposition to sudden infant death syndrome (SIDS), an increase in respiratory illness and otitis media, and the potential for an increased risk for cancer later in life (Committee on Environmental Health, 1997; Soyseth, Kongerud, and Boe, 1995). Infants and children exposed to maternal smoking have experienced some developmental delay, decreased mental function, and reduced growth in the first year (Boshuizen et al., 1998; Mascola, et al., 1998; Obel et al., 1998; Richardson, Day, and Goldschmidt, 1995). Quitting smoking either during pregnancy or within the first year of life has been found to reduce many of these long-term complications.

Alcohol consumption has been associated with a number of health-related problems in childbearing women. One study found that drinking more than three drinks per week increased the risk of spontaneous abortion in the first trimester (Windham et al., 1997). Prenatal alcohol exposure can cause subtle morphological and neurological problems that may not be discovered until the child attends school. The cost of caring for children exposed prenatally to alcohol can potentially reach $756 million to $9.7 billion annually (MMWR, 1997; Stratton, Howe, and Battaglia, 1996).

In 1973, two physicians who studied birth defects observed a pattern of complex physical and behavioral manifestations that they labeled **fetal alcohol syndrome** (FAS) (Jones and Smith, 1973). They identified a group of characteristics, including intrauterine growth retardation, craniofacial abnormalities, slow physical growth, and delayed development, that caused dysmorphic development of the fetus (Waterson and Murray-Lyons, 1990). The term *fetal alcohol effects* (FAE) applies to an infant who was exposed in utero to alcohol but who manifested some but not all of the effects of FAS. A related term, *alcohol-related birth defects* (ARBDs), is now used to describe less severe forms of FAS. Abel (1998) suggests that although alcohol is a teratogen, only heavy alcohol consumption is responsible for the effects that have been associated with FAS over the past two decades. In contrast, a longitudinal study followed children whose mothers were social drinkers (0–1 ounce of alcohol per day, including occasional binges of five or more drinks per day) as well as heavier drinkers and nondrinkers. Many of these children did not meet the criteria for FAS at birth, but subtle, neurobehavioral effects persisted even in the social drinkers. These effects included poor academic performance, antisocial behavior, and lower IQ scores (Olson et al., 1997). Given the conflicting data, there is no safe amount of alcohol that can be ingested during pregnancy described in the literature.

The effects of illicit drugs are less well-known than those for tobacco and alcohol because research is relatively recent and the number of women who use illicit drugs is relatively small. There has not been enough time to follow a large number of exposed children into adolescence; therefore, long-term implications are limited. Many of the studies come from small, nonrepresentative samples with significant bias. Often research studies take place in inner-city environments with a variety of social problems that confound associations between pregnancy drug use and maternal and infant outcomes. In addition, polydrug use (the use of more than one licit or illicit drug) can further confuse the outcome. Treatment decisions should be based on the physical and psychological assessments rather than on the preliminary findings regarding the harmful effects of these drugs.

Given these limitations, several studies have reported an association between the use of heroin (and methadone) during pregnancy and the obstetrical complications of eclampsia, placental abruption, IUGR, intrauterine death, postpartum hemorrhage, preterm labor, and premature rupture of membranes (deCubas and Field, 1993; Finnegan, 1981; Kaltenbach and Finnegan, 1992; Ostrea, Ostrea, and Simpson, 1997; Zebaleta, Jhaveri, and Rosenfield, 1995). Infants exposed to opiates may experience a variety of symptoms at birth, such as jitteriness, hyperreflexia, restlessness, sleeplessness, poor feeding pattern, vomiting, diarrhea, and a shrill cry, that are associated with **neonatal abstinence syndrome** (NAS) (Finnegan, 1981; Levy and Spino, 1993).

More recently, effects of neonatal exposure to cocaine have been found to be associated with increases in precipitous labor, placental abruption, premature rupture of membranes, and vaginal bleeding (Burkett, Yasin, and Palow, 1990; Delaney, Larrabee, and Monga, 1997; Dogra et al., 1994; Eyler et al., 1998; Macones et al., 1997; Mirochnick et al., 1995; Oro and Dixon, 1987; Spence et al., 1991; Sprauve, Lindsay, Herbert, and Graves, 1997; Zebaleta, Jhaveri, and Rosenfield, 1995). Infants exposed to cocaine are more likely than others to have gestational age less than 35 weeks, decreased birth weight, decreased length and head circumference, and IUGR (Bateman, Ng, Hansen, and Haegarty, 1993; Coles et al., 1992; Hite and Shannon, 1992; Kliegman et al., 1994; Ostrea, Ostrea, and Simpson, 1997; Pettiti and Coleman, 1990; Racine, Joyce, and Anderson, 1993; Zuckerman et al., 1989). Data suggest that infants exposed to cocaine may have abnormal cardiorespiratory patterns, may be neurologically compromised, and may have an increased risk for SIDS (Bender et al., 1995, Dogra et al., 1994; Eyler et al., 1998; Fares, McCulloch, and Raju, 1997; Jacobson et al., 1996; Lester et al., 1991a; Lipshultz, Frassica, and Orav, 1991; Singer et al., 1994).

In contrast, findings of studies on marijuana use are contradictory. Some researchers have found that marijuana use during pregnancy is associated with prematurity, IUGR, symptoms similar to FAS, and subsequent developmental delay (Cornelius, Taylor, Geva, and Day, 1995; Ostrea, Ostrea, and Simpson, 1997; Richardson, Day, and Goldsmidt, 1995). Other researchers have found no increased risk of maternal or infant complications (Dreher, Nugent, and Hudgins, 1994; Oro and Dixon, 1987).

Recent reports evaluate the long-term effects of neonatal drug exposure. The effects have contradictory outcomes related to methodological concerns and consideration of several confounding social factors that may lead to less preventive health maintenance (Forsyth et al., 1998; Neuspiel, 1994). Two studies have reported an association both between opiate use and poor attention span and between methadone use and greater anxiety, aggression, rejection, and behavior problems (deCubas and Field, 1993; Hickey et al., 1995). Most studies did not find any association between opium exposure and cognitive ability (Schneider and Hans, 1996). Cocaine exposure evaluated using the Bayley Scale of Infant Development has been associated with mental and motor development delays, poor recognition memory and information processing, and some visual impairment (Bender et al., 1995; Jacobson et al., 1996; Richardson, Conroy, and Day, 1996). Other studies have reported no relationship between language acquisition or cognitive ability, intelligence, or gross motor tests and cocaine use (Bender et al., 1995; Hurt et al., 1997; Richardson, Conroy, and Day, 1996).

The effects of marijuana exposure prenatally consistently have been shown to have no long-term consequences, until recently. Some reports suggest that there is an association between marijuana exposure in the second and third trimesters of pregnancy and intelligence and disrupted sleep patterns (Dahl et al., 1995; Day et al., 1994; Fried, 1995).

Polydrug use appears to be associated with cognitive impairment and behavioral problems as well as language delay in older children (Hurt et al., 1997; Johnson et al., 1997). Although there has been speculation that children exposed to multiple drugs may be at risk for SIDS, there appears to be no association with an increased mortality at two years of age (Fares, McCulloch, and Raju, 1997; Ostrea, Ostrea, and Simpson, 1997).

In summary, the short- and long-term effects of tobacco and alcohol have been widely studied for several decades and need to be considered when developing any treatment plan. Illicit drug use during pregnancy has been identified as a public health problem only in the past 15 years. Because the research has many methodological concerns, data from these research studies must be used cautiously.

Identification of Substance Abuse

Screening

Health care providers should attempt to identify mothers who use substances during pregnancy by toxicology screens, self-report, or a combination of both. These methods have advantages and limitations but are preferred over no pattern of inquiries, which frequently occurs.

TOXICOLOGY SCREENS

Drug toxicology screens can be performed on the mother and her infant. The accuracy of the screen depends on the laboratory chosen, the test used, the minimum drug in the sample considered positive, the reliability of the testing procedure, and the drug use pattern of the person being tested (one-time dose, moderate use, or daily use) (Christmas et al., 1992; Coombs and West, 1991). The most common type of drug screen is the urine toxicology, in which a sample of urine is assayed for the presence of drugs. More recently, meconium, infant hair samples, and amniotic fluid and umbilical cord tissue have also been used to detect both marijuana and cocaine metabolites (Bibb et al., 1995; Kline et al., 1997; Mirochnick et al., 1995; Ostrea, Romero, and Yee, 1993; Winecker et al., 1997).

The limitation of any urine test is that it measures only recent use. For example, drug metabolites are found in the urine up to 5 days after moderate marijuana use, 3 days after cocaine use, 2 days after heroin use, but only 12 hours after alcohol use. Moreover, urine tests cannot measure the quantity or frequency of drug use (Libscomb et al., 1992).

Unlike urine, meconium accumulates throughout pregnancy. This screen, therefore, appears to be highly sensitive and includes early exposure, detecting up to three times as many drug users during pregnancy as urine screens (Ostrea, Romero, and Yee, 1993). Unfortunately, this method is not available at many hospital laboratories.

Infant hair analysis also detects long-term maternal drug use (Callahan et al., 1992; Graham et al., 1989; Kline et al., 1997). A sample of the infant's hair can be collected and analyzed after preparation with a variety of chemicals by radioimmunoassay. The estimated sensitivity of hair analysis in a recent study was 92 percent, 3.1 times higher than that of a urine test.

A study in Florida examined the effectiveness of screening using amniotic fluid and umbilical cord tissue (Winecker et al., 1997). Specimens were subjected to solid-phase extraction and analyzed for cocaine and its metabolites. Cocaine was detected in 28.1 percent of the amniotic fluid and 18.5 percent of the umbilical cord specimens.

SELF-REPORT

Self-report combines one-on-one interview techniques with specific questions to elicit drug-using patterns (Lindsay et al., 1997). The advantage of this technique is that duration and frequency of any drug use, as well as alcohol and tobacco use, can be assessed conveniently and inexpensively. The disadvantage is that it relies on the accuracy of the respondent.

There are several self-report screening tools that have been used successfully in prenatal care settings. These screening tools are designed to be brief and simple to administer. The CAGE questionnaire (see Table 6-2) is a four-item, yes-no alcohol screen that assesses the extent of alcohol abuse (Ewing, 1984). The T-ACE (see Table 6-5), a revision of the CAGE, is designed to detect alcohol abuse specifically in women (Russell, 1994; Sokol, Martier, and Ager, 1989).

Nursing Care of Substance-Abusing Pregnant Women

Role of the Certified Nurse-Midwife and Nurse Practitioner

The American Academy of Nurse Practitioners, in a role position statement, includes CNMs and NPs in their description of APNs (American Academy of Nurse Practitioners, 1993).

Both the CNM and the women's health NP are responsible for independent care and management of healthy women throughout the prenatal, intrapartum, and postpartum periods, as well as newborn care (American College of Nurse Midwives, 1993). In addition, the CNM is responsible for active management of the labor and delivery of the client. These expert clinicians work within their specialty area in a variety of settings. However, if medical, obstetrical, or gynecological complications arise, a physician will comanage or collaborate with the APN (American College of Nurse Midwives, 1997).

The neonatal nurse practitioner (NNP) is responsible for management of the high-risk newborn in the intensive care unit. The pediatric nurse practitioner (PNP) provides an advanced level of care to children and their families that includes counseling on normal development and behavioral problems, the prevention of illness and preventable injuries, and the care of children with acute or chronic conditions (NAPNAP, 1990). PNPs may also work in specialty clinics where children with long-term problems related to maternal substance use are managed.

Women with known substance use during pregnancy are considered high risk and are followed closely by the collaborating physician prenatally, during labor and delivery, and in the immediate postpartum/newborn period.

Prenatal Care Assessment and Management

The APN should assess the specific needs of each prenatal client. Identifying substance use or abuse is only the first step. Establishing a strong nurse-client relationship is essential for any successful intervention and should be initiated during the early assessment process.

Fostering an atmosphere of trust and credibility with the client facilitates honest disclosure and client compliance throughout the prenatal course, and during **drug rehabilitation** if necessary. If the client believes her care provider is nonjudgmental and concerned for her and her baby's well-being, a more successful relationship will evolve.

Prenatal care and appropriate intervention for the substance-using client are dependent on the type of drug, the amount of use or abuse, and the client's current use pattern or withdrawal phase. A comprehensive nursing assessment helps identify the amount, frequency, and type of substance and provides the foundation for establishing individualized prenatal care and intervention. Observing the client during the interview and physical assessment phase can uncover a wealth of information, even in the absence of self-report or disclosure. It is important to recognize specific deviations in the client's affect, evident in slurred speech or abnormal speech patterns, and signs of disorientation, decreased alertness, or fatigue. Even when a client voluntarily admits to substance use or abuse, the disclosure may not be complete because clients minimize the frequency of use, quantity, or number of drugs used.

If prenatal care and drug treatment can be initiated within the first trimester of pregnancy, the chances for a positive outcome for the newborn are greatly improved. Close monitoring of maternal nutritional status, rehabilitation progress, and fetal well-being can be maintained and has been shown to reduce the incidence of IUGR. In addition, early maternal involvement and validation of the pregnancy promote maternal role identification, which is necessary for developing parenting skills. Table 9-3 lists the essential components to assess when drug use is suspected in the pregnant woman.

Prenatal Care

The initial prenatal screening starts with routine prenatal tests and cultures, with drug toxicology testing included (Delaney, Larrabee, and Monga, 1997; Glanz and Woods, 1991; Medoff-Cooper and Verklan, 1992; Wheeler, 1993). With baseline values in place, a treatment plan can be established to focus intervention where it is most needed. Initial prenatal laboratory tests and screening should include:

- Complete blood count (CBC)
- Serology
- Hepatitis B screen
- Liver function tests
- Fasting blood glucose
- Type and rhesus
- Toxoplasmosis, other infections, rubella, cytomegalovirus, and herpes (TORCH screen)
- Urine for culture and sensitivity
- Rubella screen
- Papanicolaou (PAP) smear
- Chlamydia and gonorrhea cultures
- Tuberculosis (TB) skin test
- Chest x-ray, if needed

Genetic screening may be offered on an individual basis. Referrals to a nutritionist should be made as needed, utilizing the Women's, Infants', and Children's (WIC) program

TABLE 9-3 Essential Components to Assess When Drug Abuse During Pregnancy Is Suspected

Physical appearance and demeanor

- Appearance of pregnancy not coinciding with stated gestational age
- Client physically exhausted
- Pupils extremely dilated or constricted
- Track marks, abscesses, or edema visible in lower or upper extremities
- Nasal mucosa inflamed or indurated
- Client slightly confused and not well oriented

Medical history

- Cellulitis
- Cirrhosis
- Acquired immunodeficiency syndrome
- Endocarditis
- Hepatitis
- Pneumonia
- Pancreatitis

Obstetric history in prior pregnancies

- Sexually transmitted disease
- Spontaneous abortion
- Premature labor
- Premature rupture of membranes
- Meconium staining
- Abruptio placentae
- Fetal demise
- Low-birth-weight infant

Current pregnancy

- History or evidence of early contractions
- Inactive or hyperactive fetus
- Poor maternal weight gain
- Sexually transmitted disease
- Spotting or vaginal bleeding

Sources: Chasnoff, I.J., Burns, W.J., Schroll, S.H., and Burns, K.A. (1985). Cocaine use in pregnancy. *The New England Journal of Medicine 313*(11), 666–669; and Lynch, M., and McKeon, V.A. (1990). Cocaine use during pregnancy: Research findings and clinical implications. *Journal of Obstetric, Gynecologic, and Neonatal Nursing 19*(4), 285–292.

to supplement the client's nutritional intake. Referrals to support groups are helpful in establishing resources for the client within her community and has been shown to facilitate success in abstinence and rehabilitation. HIV testing and urine toxicology testing should also be offered at intervals throughout the pregnancy. At 15 to 18 weeks' gestation, an alpha-fetoprotein (AFP) test is useful to evaluate for Down syndrome and possible neural tube defects, specifically spina bifida.

An early baseline ultrasound evaluation of the fetus and placenta is important. A glucose tolerance test should be done at 28 weeks' gestation to rule out gestational diabetes. As the pregnancy progresses, periodic ultrasound monitoring and use of a biophysical profile evaluation are helpful in identifying decreases in fetal growth and other physiological changes that may suggest that alcohol/drug use has resumed. A nonstress test (NST) can be used during the last trimester for continued evaluation of fetal status. Because the fetus could be at risk for IUGR, low birth weight, premature rupture of membranes, and abruptio placentae, these tools help monitor fetal well-being and can alert care providers to early changes in fetal status before there is a crisis (Feldman, Minkoff, McCalla, and Salwen, 1992; Glanz and Woods, 1991; Hanna, Faden, and Dufour, 1997; Lundsberg, Bracken, and Saftless, 1997; Medoff-Cooper and Verklan, 1992; Miller, Boudreaux, and Regan, 1995; Wheeler, 1993). Table 9-4 lists the sequence of testing by week of gestation.

Labor Management

Management of the labor and delivery of a substance-using client who has received prenatal care, is in drug rehabilitation, and is known to clinic personnel is like that of any other laboring woman. She should be screened for the presence of any illicit drugs and/or alcohol before labor. If all parameters are assessed and she is found to be stable, routine labor management protocols are followed. For pain management in labor, the client can be administered narcotic drugs but may need a higher dose of these medications due to cross-tolerance, which she may have developed while using alcohol and/or other drugs (Finnegan, 1991; Kaltenbach, Berghalla, and Finnegan, 1998; Wheeler, 1993). Fetal monitoring and assessment should be maintained continuously, and delivery should be accomplished with maternal involvement to facilitate maternal-infant bonding. Pediatric or neonatal specialists should be present at the time of delivery to assess for potential crises and to provide emergency care.

Many women who use drugs go to the clinic or hospital for the first time when they are in labor, having received no previous prenatal care. Timely diagnosis and treatment are necessary to achieve a satisfactory outcome and to minimize further complications. Co-management protocols between medicine and nursing should be implemented to optimize treatment for these high-risk obstetric clients. Assessment of maternal and fetal status is the first priority. If possible, a medical history should also be obtained that includes questions about the mother's most recent use of substances. Observing the client for signs of drug or alcohol intoxication or withdrawal is critical.

TABLE 9-4 Sequence of Testing for Suspected Substance Abuse During Pregnancy

Gestational Age in Weeks	Tests and Procedures
8–12 (or first visit)	CBC, blood type and antibody screen, sickle cell, tuberculin test, hepatitis B surface antigen, syphilis serology (STS) urine culture, cultures for gonorrhea and chlamydia, smear for cervical cytology, rubella titer, liver function tests, offer HIV test, consider the drug screen at all visits, consider high-risk obstetric consult.
16–18	Maternal serum AFP testing, HIV test counseling, ultrasound, and gestational age confirmation.
18–24	Consider ultrasound for congenital anomalies.
28	CBC, STS, O'Sullivan test, urine culture, cervical cultures, liver function tests (if woman abuses opiates).
28–32	Rho(D)immune globulin administration if Rh-negative and sensitized.
32–34	Repeat ultrasound for fetal growth, begin weekly NST (further tests as indicated).
36–38	Repeat STS, cervical cultures, and liver function tests (if woman abuses opiates), consider repeat ultrasound, consider possible need for neonatologist and special care nursery after delivery.

Source: Adapted with permission from Glanz J.C., and Woods H.R. (1991). Obstetrical issues in substance abuse. *Pediatric Annals 20,* 531–539.

Determining the stage of labor and fetal gestational development is important for prioritizing client management and intervention. Many heavy substance users experience amenorrhea long before the onset of pregnancy, which makes historical dating of the pregnancy very difficult. The fundal height measurements of the pregnant uterus may not coincide with the stated gestational age for a variety of reasons. Fetal growth is often compromised with substance abuse due to the mother's poor eating habits and the altered blood flow through the placenta as a result of drug-induced vasoconstriction (Bateman, Ng, Hansen, and Hagerty, 1993; Feldman, Minkoff, McCalla, and Swalen, 1992; Lynch and McKeon, 1990; Pettiti and Coleman, 1990; Racine, Joyce, and Anderson, 1993). If possible, an ultrasound should be performed on admission to identify the level of fetal maturity, IUGR, obvious fetal anomalies, or placental disorders.

The more information obtained about the fetus before delivery, the more prepared the care provider will be to address problems and optimize positive outcomes. Routine baseline laboratory tests and drug toxicology tests should be performed on the mother upon admission. A blood type and cross-match should also be done in case a blood transfusion becomes necessary during labor and delivery. An IV line should be started and a large-bore needle used to provide maximum access. Women who use substances such as alcohol or illicit drugs often have rapid labors (most often if crack cocaine is used). They also have a higher risk for intrapartum hemorrhage due to the increased incidence of placenta previa and abruptio placentae (Macones et al., 1997; Mishra, Landzberg, and Parente, 1995; Parente, Gaines, and Lockridge, 1990). Continuous fetal monitoring should be maintained through labor to provide assessment of fetal status. Once the newborn is stable, he or she is transferred to the neonatal intensive care unit (NICU) for further evaluation and observation.

Assessment and Management of the Newborn

Neonatal drug withdrawal varies with the type of drug used by the mother, variations in maternal and infant metabolism, and the amount of drug(s) ingested by the mother immediately before the onset of labor. Symptoms of withdrawal in the newborn are relatively minor if more than one week has elapsed between the last ingestion and delivery. Onset of withdrawal is determined by the half-life of the drug: The longer the half-life of the drug, the longer it takes for withdrawal to set in. Table 9-5 is a timetable for the onset of drug withdrawal for four selected drugs. Drug withdrawal is treated with supportive nursing care. Pharmacologic support of the newborn should also be considered for heroin, barbiturate, benzodiazepine, and methadone withdrawal.

TABLE 9-5 Onset of Drug Withdrawal Symptoms

Drug	Onset of Withdrawal Symptoms After Delivery
Alcohol	3–12 hours after delivery
Narcotics (heroin, methadone)	48–72 hours; may be as late as 4 weeks
Barbiturates	4–7 days on average (1–14 days possible)
Cocaine	48–72 hours

Source: American Academy of Pediatrics, Committee on Drugs. (1998). Neonatal drug withdrawal. *Pediatrics 101*(6), 1079–1088.

Management of the Drug-Exposed Infant

Infants born to substance-using mothers are at risk for developmental and behavioral problems. These problems are due both to the biophysical response of the infant to drug exposure and to the unstable environment and dysfunctional parenting that may occur as an outcome of continued substance use. These children may need to be involved with **child protective services,** early intervention, and home nursing care. A collaborative effort is necessary to help parents care for an infant who may be hard to console or feed because of drug-induced behavioral effects. Close monitoring and teaching of parenting skills as well as monitoring of parent drug addiction is essential.

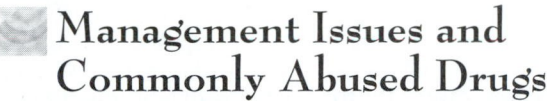

Management Issues and Commonly Abused Drugs

Tobacco Smoking and Nicotine

Tobacco use is of serious concern for maternal and fetal health. Federal law mandates that a warning label for pregnant women appear on all cigarette packages, stating the dangers of smoking and its effects on the developing fetus. Despite these warnings, approximately 25 percent of all American women continue to smoke throughout their pregnancy (Garland, 1998; Lee, 1998; McFarlane, Parker, and Soeken, 1996; Weimann, Berenson, and San Miguel, 1994; Wheeler, 1993). Nicotine use, along with alcohol use, is the most preventable cause of low-birth-weight infants. In addition, it is now realized that exposure to secondhand smoke may be as detrimental to mother and fetus as firsthand cigarette smoking. Approximately 4,000 different compounds have been identified in cigarette smoke. Of known compounds, carbon monoxide, nicotine, and cyanide are the elements believed to pose the greatest risk to mother and fetus.

Respiratory disease, lung cancer, cardiovascular disease, and gastrointestinal disorders are known to occur at a higher rate in smokers than in the general population (Parente, Gaines, and Lockridge, 1990; Wheeler, 1993). An increased incidence of respiratory infection, chronic bronchitis, emphysema, pneumonia, and influenza occurs as a result of direct toxic effects on the epithelium of the respiratory tract and decreased ciliary movement. Cigarette smoking has been shown to increase the incidence of squamous cell and oat cell carcinoma in lung tissue. Approximately 80 percent of all lung cancer deaths can be linked to cigarette smoking. Carbon monoxide is a gaseous component of cigarette smoke that combines to form carboxyhemoglobin. Levels of this toxic compound have been measured at 3 to 10 times higher in smokers than nonsmokers. The effects of smoking on the cardiovascular system include an increase in platelet aggregation, vasospasm and constriction of the coronary blood vessels, and episodes of angina induced in coronary clients due to an imbalance between the oxygen supply to cardiac muscle and demand. Smokers also report a higher incidence of gastric and duodenal ulcers.

Effects of smoking on the developing fetus are widely documented. Cigarette smoking is associated with an average birth-weight reduction in neonates whose mothers smoked during pregnancy (Garland, 1998; Lee, 1998; McFarlane, Parker, and Soeken, 1996;

Wheeler, 1993). As few as five cigarettes per day can cause fetal growth retardation. The primary physiological basis for the growth retardation is fetal hypoxia and/or ischemia that results from the increased levels of carbon monoxide and nicotine transported to the fetus through maternal circulation (Garland, 1998; Lee, 1998; Wheeler, 1993). Vasoconstriction of placental and fetal blood vessels is caused by the presence of nicotine, and it decreases vital blood circulation to the fetus. Carbon monoxide binds to fetal hemoglobin, decreasing the amount of oxygen available to the fetus for tissue growth and development.

APNs have a key role in educating adolescent and adult females on the potential dangers and long-term health consequences of smoking. Such education should precede pregnancy to influence preexisting behaviors with regard to health. Some women are motivated to modify or terminate unhealthy smoking practices in support of better health for their unborn child. Realistic goals include reduction in the number of cigarettes smoked per day. Positive reinforcement for this behavioral modification should be provided, and women should be praised for the effort involved and their commitment to improving positive birth outcomes.

During the initial history-taking process, it is important for the nurse practitioner or certified nurse-midwife, to identify:

- The client who smokes
- The number of years she has smoked (quantity)
- The number of cigarettes she smokes per day (frequency)
- The level of tar and nicotine of cigarettes she smokes (intensity of dose)
- The number of other smokers who are in the household (other drug sources)

Most women do not volunteer accurate smoking histories. Feelings of mistrust or guilt may interfere with frank self-disclosure. Indirect or nonthreatening questions (e.g., Have you ever smoked? How long did you smoke? How much did you smoke?) can obtain information about actual smoking behaviors. Any preexisting health conditions should be noted and followed up. When assessing and evaluating the prenatal client, the practitioner identifies any physiological changes that impact on maternal and/or fetal well-being and develops an appropriate plan of management. Encouraging a reduction in amount, if cessation is not possible, is an important component of management.

Prenatal Management

Prenatal care should incorporate education on health-related behaviors to decrease dangerous effects of smoking on maternal and fetal well-being. Written materials such as pamphlets and handouts may be useful to reinforce teaching. At each prenatal visit, the APN should reiterate the need to reduce cigarette consumption. Referral to a Quit Smoking group is indicated when the client expresses the desire to stop smoking. Use of the nicotine transdermal patch is appropriate for those wishing to terminate very heavy smoking during pregnancy. Although the transdermal patch has been associated with adverse outcomes in pregnant animals (but not in humans), the benefits of quitting may outweigh the risk in heavy smokers (Wright et al., 1997).

Nutritional counseling and vitamin supplements should be prescribed for the client. Evaluation of the fetus at each prenatal visit includes observation for signs of growth retardation, premature rupture of membranes, threatened preterm labor, and/or abruptio placentae.

Vaginal secretions should be checked for pH values; cervical cultures may identify premature rupture of membranes. Serial ultrasounds are used to identify decreased fetal growth and fluid volume as well as early signs of abruptio placentae. Education of the mother about the danger and warning signs that should be reported to the health care provider can improve the chance for early diagnosis and treatment of life-threatening obstetric emergencies.

MANAGEMENT OF THE NEWBORN

It is important for the mother to continue smoking cessation or reduction after delivery. Mothers who want to breastfeed should be advised that nicotine is passed on to the infant in breast milk. Secondhand smoke also causes respiratory problems in the newborn. Many of the infants whose mothers smoked are preterm or small-for-gestational-age and may experience previously described related problems. They will be at high risk for respiratory problems such as asthma that is aggravated by smoke. If the mother and other family members are unable to quit, agreements should be made with them to not smoke near the infant. Mothers should also be taught or referred to group teaching modalities to handle the feelings which support smoking. These include relaxation therapies, acupuncture, and meditation.

Alcohol Use and Abuse

Alcohol is frequently used and abused during pregnancy; an estimated 15 percent to 26 percent of pregnant women continue to drink. The significant risks to the mother and infant increase with the length of time and the amount of alcohol regularly ingested. The APN must observe the client for indications of the severity of the problem. Assessment should include identification of any alcohol-related problems in the client's psychosocial, physical, or family history or work environment as well as physical or nutritional deficits. Because alcoholism is frequently transgenerational, histories of the parents' families of origin are helpful.

Nutritional status of both mother and fetus is compromised with alcohol use. Wernicke-Korsakoff syndrome is an encephalopathy that results from decreased thiamine levels secondary to alcohol abuse in pregnancy (Bragg, 1997; Cross and Hennessey, 1993; Flandemeyer, Kenner, Bragg, and Campinha-Bacote, 1992; Lundsberg, Bracken, and Saftless, 1997; Medoff-Cooper and Verklan, 1992). As a result of poor nutritional intake, a depletion of the B vitamins occurs, leading to life-threatening complications. Marchiafava-Bignami disease, another nutritional problem of alcohol abuse, is the degeneration of the corpus callosum with cerebral atrophy (Bragg, 1997; Chavkin and Breitbart, 1997; Cross and Hennessey, 1993; Lundsberg, Bracken, and Saftless, 1997). Additional effects on the central nervous system (CNS) are seen in central positive myelinosis; however, this is only manifested in severely malnourished women with alcoholism.

Alcohol affects the maternal desire for food intake, and malnutrition can quickly impact the nutritional status of mother and fetus. The liver is the primary organ impaired by alcohol abuse, but general absorption of nutrients is also decreased. Common complications of liver impairment include hypoglycemia, fatty liver, hypertriglyceridemia, and impaired gluconeogenesis (Bragg, 1997; Flandemeyer, Kenner, Bragg, and Campinha-Bacote, 1992; Lundsberg, Bracken, and Saftless, 1997; Pettiti and Coleman, 1990). Gastritis and pancreatitis are common in alcoholics (Cross and Hennessey, 1993; Flandemeyer, Kenner, Bragg, and Campinha-Bacote, 1992).

Toxic ingestion of alcohol can increase the client's risk for coma. When treating these clients during a crisis situation, maintaining an open airway and providing supportive care are the most immediate needs to address (see Chapter 7 for detailed treatment protocols). A client suffering from alcohol withdrawal is at risk for experiencing tremors and seizures.

Minor alcohol withdrawal usually peaks at 24 hours to 36 hours after last alcohol intake (Cross and Hennessey, 1993; Flandemeyer, Kenner, Bragg, and Campinha-Bacote, 1992; Wheeler, 1993). The client also may show signs of coarse tremor, tachycardia, anxiety, mild autonomic hyperactivity, and anorexia. These symptoms are usually short term.

Major alcohol withdrawal occurs after 24 hours and usually peaks at 50 hours after the last alcohol intake. Characteristics include a more pronounced degree of autonomic hyperactivity, fever, disorientation, diaphoresis, and hallucinations.

In more extreme cases of alcohol withdrawal, the client may experience true seizure activity. These seizures are typically of the grand mal type and may occur singularly or in clusters. Delirium tremors is a rare complication and is not seen before the third day postabstinence (Cross and Hennessey, 1993; Wheeler, 1993). Characteristics of this period are profound confusion, incontinence, frightening visual hallucinations, gross tremor, and fever.

Seizures can be experienced at any point in the withdrawal process, are usually of the grand mal type, and may occur singularly or in clusters. Because it is important to maintain client observation and contact during the alcohol withdrawal period, hospitalization is recommended to maintain maternal and fetal assessment at this critical time.

PRENATAL MANAGEMENT

A comprehensive health history includes a social history that contains specific questions on past and present alcohol and drug use. Additional information as to the amount used, number of years of use or addiction, social and family stressors, and any underlying health problems must also be addressed in an individualized plan of prenatal care. Because there are strong correlations between heavy alcohol use and adverse fetal outcome, all heavy consumers should be seen in a high-risk clinic setting. Additional toxicology screens should be performed during assessment as alcohol use during pregnancy is highly correlated with the use of other illicit drugs.

In-patient detoxification to monitor maternal and fetal status in a safe environment is the best treatment option. The use of therapeutic medications in the maternal detoxification process should be evaluated carefully. A short-acting barbiturate (e.g., pentobarbital) can be used, if necessary, to manage the withdrawal process. Disulfiram and benzodiazepines are to be avoided in pregnancy due to their possible teratogenic and sedative effects (Cross and Hennessey, 1993; Grant, Ernst, and Streissquth, 1996).

Nutritional support and vitamin supplements are important parts of the initial maternal treatment plan. WIC programs also provide supplemental intake and nutritional counseling and can be continued after delivery. Referrals to support groups such as Alcoholics Anonymous are important for continued abstinence.

In addition to the special testing discussed above, all routine prenatal screening tests are performed. A glucose tolerance test should be done at 28 weeks' gestation to rule out gestational diabetes. Alcoholic clients can have alcoholic ketoacidosis and dehydration with normal blood glucose levels. As the pregnancy progresses, periodic ultrasound monitoring and use of biophysical profile evaluation are helpful in identifying decreases in fetal growth and other physiological changes. NST can be used during the last trimester for continued evaluation of fetal status.

Impact of Alcohol Exposure on the Newborn

Exposure of the fetus to alcohol in any amount introduces risk because the mechanism and timing of drug effect are not clearly understood as yet. FAS includes a wide range of physiological and behavioral characteristics. Current recommendations for diagnosis of FAS take into account the alcohol consumption pattern as well as the characteristics. The following are five categories currently being considered (Hess and Kenner, 1998; Stratton, Howe, and Battaglia, 1996):

1. FAS with confirmed maternal history of excessive alcohol intake
2. FAS with phenotypic features but unconfirmed history of maternal alcohol intake
3. Partial FAS, when there is confirmed maternal alcohol intake and some evidence of facial anomalies and any other evidence of prenatal alcohol exposure, such as growth retardation, CNS neurodevelopmental abnormalities, or some of the cognitive disabilities associated with FAS
4. ARBDs to indicate adverse birth outcomes related to alcohol consumption during pregnancy
5. Alcohol-related neurodevelopmental disorders when there is evidence of CNS abnormalities that have been associated with prenatal alcohol exposure

The estimated incidence of FAS in the United States ranges from 1 to 3 per 1,000 live births. Among heavy drinkers (two drinks per day, or five to six drinks per occasion), 43.1 cases were reported per 1,000 live births in a compilation of 39 studies from 15 countries (Abel, 1998). Risk factors include:

Binge drinking
Poor maternal health status
Increased maternal age
Increased parity
Increased production of acetaldehyde from alcohol
Low socioeconomic status
Genetic susceptibilities
Smoking
Undernutrition

Psychological and Physical Stressors

APNs can intervene with mothers who are at potential risk of having an infant with FAS by educating them about the risks associated with alcohol abuse during pregnancy. Early identification of infants with FAS/ARBDs is important to make sure multidisciplinary services are accessed to reduce the long-term effects on the mother and infant. Early intervention is essential to help with developmental needs. The mother may also want assistance with alcohol treatment services. The family may benefit from appropriate support services such as those provided by visiting nurse services and respite care for caregivers. The APN can help manage these complex cases with prevention, early recognition, and treatment of FAS, FAE, and ARBDs.

Opiates

Heroin and methadone are the two most commonly used narcotics in the childbearing population. Heroin (diacetylmorphine) is the most commonly used illegal narcotic (Finnegan, 1991; Haegerman and Schnoll, 1991, Kaltenbach, Berghalla, and Finnegan, 1998; Macones et al., 1997; Mishra, Landzberg, and Parente, 1995; Parente, Gaines, and Lockridge, 1990). It is highly soluble, enters the CNS faster than morphine, and can be inhaled, smoked, or injected intravenously, intramuscularly, or subcutaneously. Heroin is much stronger than morphine and readily crosses the placental barrier. Methadone, heroin's legal substitute, is a synthetic opiate used as a medical treatment for heroin addiction; it also crosses the placental barrier.

Opiate addiction is a serious and life-threatening problem. It exists in members of all socioeconomic levels and poses significant risks in pregnancy to mother and fetus. Each year, over 300,000 infants are exposed prenatally to either heroin or methadone (Cross and Hennessey, 1993; Flandemeyer, Kenner, Bragg, and Campinha-Bacote, 1992; Macones et al., 1997; Wheeler, 1993). Women who are addicted to heroin are likely to be polydrug users. They often add nicotine, barbiturates, alcohol, or marijuana to their daily intake of heroin. They suffer from malnutrition and may have numerous medical problems. Due to transient lifestyles, they may face unstable housing and living conditions, with few family or social supports.

An acute overdose of an opiate can be life-threatening. Signs of an overdose in the adult include unresponsiveness, bradycardia, respiratory depression, cyanosis, pupil dilation, and (in severe cases) circulatory failure (Botelho and Novak, 1997; Chang, 1992; Finnegan, 1991; Kaplan, 1993; Wang, 1998). Withdrawal symptoms vary according to the duration of the addiction and the dose taken, but they are rarely fatal. Early signs of withdrawal usually manifest 8 hours to 16 hours after the last dose and include restlessness, anxiety, nausea, diarrhea, yawning, tearing, and abdominal cramping (Chang, 1992; Dyer, 1998; Seoane, 1997; Stinus, 1998). For 1 to 3 days, these symptoms worsen. As withdrawal continues, the addict develops vomiting, diarrhea, severe anxiety, tremors and muscle spasms, fever and chills, and hypertension. By the end of the seventh day, all symptoms are resolved. The fetus goes through the stages of withdrawal with the addicted mother. If withdrawal is sudden and severe, it can be fatal to the fetus.

Treatment for heroin addiction often involves admission to a methadone maintenance program (Chang, 1992; Dyer, 1998; Finnegan, 1991; Haegerman and Schnoll, 1991; Hanna, Faden, and Dufour, 1997; Kearney, 1996). Methadone has effects similar to those of heroin and is also addictive. It is taken orally and is longer-acting than heroin. If detoxification is to be initiated during pregnancy, methadone treatment is less threatening to the fetus, but it should only be used in the second trimester. Treatment can be implemented in a clinic, but in-patient settings may provide a better opportunity for determining methadone dosage. The dosage of methadone should be decreased at a rate of 2 mg to 5 mg per week (Chang, 1992; Cross and Hennessey, 1993; Hanna, Faden, and Dufour, 1997). Fetal movement is an indicator of successful withdrawal and must be monitored carefully. Increased fetal movement is a sign of withdrawal, whereas excessive movement is a sign of fetal distress.

Once the client is stabilized on the treatment program, a target methadone maintenance dose of 20 mg per day can be administered in a clinic setting. The client benefits from this daily treatment and also can utilize social services, prenatal care, and medical treatment at the clinic site. Stable methadone maintenance also reduces the stress on the infant that may occur from sudden withdrawal secondary to periodic heroin use.

Obstetrical risks for opiate addicts include increased chance of placenta previa and abruptio placentae, either of which can lead to antepartal hemorrhage and/or preterm delivery of the fetus (Bragg, 1997; Chang, 1992; Daley and Argeriou, 1997; Feldman, Minkoff, McCalla, and Salwen, 1992; Finnegan, 1991; Hanna, Faden, and Dufour, 1997; Kaltenbach, Berghalla, and Finnegan, 1998). Intrauterine deaths may result from repeated episodes of withdrawal secondary to erratic maternal drug use. Intrauterine hypoxia occurs with these episodes and, if severe enough, can result in fetal death. Opiate-exposed fetuses tend to have small-for-gestational-age head circumferences and low birth weight (Coles and Smith, 1993; Hanna, Faden, and Dufour, 1997; Kaltenbach, Berghalla, and Finnegan, 1998). This decreased size is a result of an insult that occurs at an early stage of pregnancy and that causes a reduction of organ cells.

PRENATAL MANAGEMENT

Like other substance abusers, women using opiates need to be identified early and enrolled in intervention programs as soon as possible. Drug treatment and rehabilitation, social services, and nutritional counseling are essential components of prenatal care. Prenatal assessment and evaluation are the same as with other clients, with special attention to signs of IV drug use, including cellulitis, track marks, skin abscesses and necrosis, signs of septicemia, and drug withdrawal. Women who use injectable drugs are at a higher risk for pulmonary infections, so TB skin testing and chest x-ray may be necessary (Glanz and Woods, 1991; Haegerman and Schnoll, 1991; Kaltenbach, Berghalla, and Finnegan, 1998; Wheeler, 1993). Routine prenatal tests as previously described should be followed. It is especially important that HIV testing and urine toxicology testing be repeated at intervals throughout the pregnancy.

Methadone maintenance continues throughout the pregnancy, with adjustments in dosage if necessary. The mother will be given her daily dose on the day of delivery. During the labor process, she must be monitored for signs of withdrawal and treated promptly if they occur. Labor management is standard in most cases, with continuous fetal monitoring maintained and consideration of the possible need to increase narcotic dosing for pain management, as previously described.

The infant will be transferred to the NICU for observation and treatment of withdrawal symptoms. Maternal and infant bonding should be encouraged as soon as possible after delivery. If the mother continues her drug addiction or methadone maintenance, breastfeeding is discouraged as the infant may become opiate-dependent.

MANAGEMENT OF THE NEWBORN

Neonates chronically exposed to heroin, methadone, or other opiates are at high risk for NAS. A urine toxicology screen may be necessary to determine if other drugs, such as cocaine, were used in conjunction with the opiate. The use of additional drugs will increase the severity of NAS. Among infants exposed to opiates, withdrawal signs will develop in 55 percent to 94 percent. The signs and symptoms usually occur 72 hours after birth, but they can appear from shortly after birth up to 2 weeks of age. Severity of clinical symptoms often varies according to the drug used, the timing, and the amount last ingested. If longer than 1 week has elapsed between the last maternal use and delivery, withdrawal symptoms are relatively low. Large methadone dosages in later pregnancy have been accompanied by greater neonatal concentrations and increased risk for withdrawal.

Infants experiencing withdrawal from opiates will experience CNS irritability that may be accompanied by seizures and abnormal electroencephalograms, as well as gastrointestinal irritability. Signs of NAS are described using the mnemonic WITHDRAWAL (see Table 9-6). Identification of infants at risk for withdrawal is essential. If an infant is exhibiting some of the symptoms of neonatal withdrawal, urine or meconium should be screened for the presence of drugs. Because urine screens have a high incidence of false-negative results, it is important to assess the potential for withdrawal by obtaining a thorough maternal history, including prescription and nonprescription drugs received and social habits. It is important to differentiate the symptoms of withdrawal from other potential problems such as hypoglycemia and hypocalcemia.

Treatment should initially be supportive and includes swaddling to decrease sensory stimulation and observing sleeping habits, temperature instability, and weight gain or loss. A high-calorie diet may be necessary because of the increased energy expenditure related to activity, crying, or decreased sleep. Calories may also be lost through vomiting, drooling, and diarrhea. Intake should provide 150 kcal/kg to 250 kcal/kg per day for growth in neonates in withdrawal.

The decision to use pharmacologic therapy is based on the assessment of the individual infant and the severity of withdrawal; it is made in collaboration with the neonatologist or pediatrician. The purpose of pharmacologic therapy is to reduce life-threatening symptoms of drug withdrawal. Infants who have been exposed to opiates but who do not have the signs of withdrawal do not need therapy. Indications for therapy are weight loss, inability to sleep, fever as a direct result of seizures, poor feeding, diarrhea, and vomiting. An abstinence scoring method to measure the severity of withdrawal can be used to make the decision to treat

TABLE 9-6 Assessing for Neonatal Abstinence Syndrome

The following signs may exist in minimal, moderate, or marked degree.

Tremors (muscle activity of the limbs)	Range from disturbed to seizure-like movements
Irritability (excessive crying)	Varies from slightly, moderately when disturbed, to marked even when undisturbed.
Reflexes	Normal, increased, or markedly increased
Stools	Normal or explosive
Muscle tone	Normal to rigidity
Skin abrasions	None to redness to skin breakdown
Respiratory (rate/min)	<55 to 76–95
Repetitive sneezing	No . . . . Yes
Vomiting	No . . . . Yes
Fever	No . . . . Yes

TABLE 9-7 Neonatal Abstinence Syndrome Scoring System

Signs	Score			
	0	1	2	3
Tremors (muscle activity of limbs)	Normal	Minimally ↑ when hungry or disturbed	Moderate or marked ↑ when undisturbed, subside when fed or held snugly	Marked even when undisturbed, going on to seizure-like movements
Irritability (excessive crying)	None	Slightly ↑	Moderate to severe when disturbed or hungry	Marked even when undisturbed
Reflexes	Normal	Increased	Markedly increased	
Stools	Normal	Explosive, but normal frequency	Explosive, more than 8/day	
Muscle tone	Normal	Increased	Rigidity	
Skin abrasions	No	Redness of knees and elbows	Breaking of skin	
Respiratory rate/min	<55	55–75	76–95	
Repetitive sneezing	No	Yes		
Repetitive yawning	No	Yes		
Vomiting	No	Yes		
Fever	No	Yes		

Scoring: Identification of newborn with narcotic withdrawal when Score >17 (78% probability).

Source: Lipsitz, P.J. (1975). A proposed narcotic withdrawal score for use with newborn infants: A pragmatic evaluation of its efficacy. *Clinical Pediatrics 14,* 592.

the infant with pharmacologic therapy (see Table 9-7). If this method is chosen, a very specific therapy regime is developed, preferably using a drug from the same class as that causing withdrawal. Table 9-8 lists the drugs used to reduce opioid withdrawal in neonates.

When stable, infants will be discharged either to parents or family or to some form of foster care. Parents need to develop various strategies to cope with the many behaviors unique to the infant who has experienced drug withdrawal. Feeding problems, including vomiting and uncoordinated sucking and swallowing, are a major concern in the infant exposed to drugs. Strategies include giving small quantities of formula and learning proper positioning during and after feeding. Long-term neurological problems include weak development, irritability and difficulty sleeping, tremors, stiffness, and rigidity. Some helpful strategies include decreasing stimulation, swaddling, giving a pacifier, and holding the baby firmly. Table 9-9 lists infant behaviors and strategies that parents can employ.

The PNP will evaluate these infants in the primary care setting. Monitoring growth and development and nutritional status and performing a thorough neurological and behavioral screen are important parts of the well-child assessment. Assessing family coping strategies and subsequent drug use and treatment should be part of each scheduled outpatient visit.

TABLE 9-8 Drugs Used to Reduce Opioid Withdrawal in Neonates

Name	Dosing	Recommendations
Tincture of opium	0.1 ml/kg or 2 drops/kg with feedings every 4 hours. After 3–5 days stabilization, taper by decreasing dose without altering frequency.	Preferred over paregoric; 25-fold dilution contains same concentration of morphine found in paregoric.
Paregoric	0.1 ml/kg or 2 drops/kg with feedings every 4 hours; may be increased by 2 drops/kg every 3–4 hours until stabilized. After 3–5 days stabilization, taper by decreasing dose without altering frequency.	Infants have greater physiologic sucking and weight gain. Use of paregoric declined because of potential toxic effects of ingredients.
Morphine	Parenteral: 0.1 mg/kg. Oral: 4 mg/ml.	Oral route provides less analgesic than parenteral. Respiratory depressant; can be life-threatening.
Methadone	0.05 to 0.1 mg/kg every 6 hours with increases of 0.05 mg/kg until stable. After controlled, dose every 12 to 24 hours. Discontinue after weaning to 0.05 mg/kg per day.	Treat NAS from opioid withdrawal.
Clonidine	Oral: 0.5–1.0 mg/kg single dose. Maintenance: 3–5 mg/kg/day in divided doses every 4–6 hours.	May have immediate reversal of symptoms. Treatment shorter than phenobarbital. Oral liquid not available.
Chlorpromazine	IM/PO: 0.55 mg/kg every 6 hours.	CNS and GI signs produced by withdrawal are controlled. Multiple side effects.
Phenobarbital	Loading dose: 16 mg/kg per 24 hours. Maintenance: 2–8 mg/kg per 24 hours. When stabilized, decrease by 10–25% per day. Blood levels 24 to 48 hours after loading dose: 20–30 mg/ml .	Good choice for nonnarcotic-related withdrawal signs. Does not relieve GI symptoms.
Diazepam	1.0–2.0 mg every 8 hours.	Multiple side effects.

NAS, neonatal abstinence syndrome; CNS, central nervous system; GI, gastrointestinal.

Source: Adapted from American Academy of Pediatrics, Committee on Drugs. (1998). Neonatal drug withdrawal. *Pediatrics 101*(6), 1079.

Cocaine and Crack

Cocaine was reported by 0.2 percent of pregnant women according to a 1998 national survey. Other smaller studies using toxicology screens as well as self-report found the rate of cocaine use to be between 6 percent and 11 percent in metropolitan and suburban settings (Chasnoff, Landress, and Barrett, 1990; Matera et al., 1990; Shutzman, Frankenfiled-Chernicoff, Clatterbaugh, and Singer, 1991). Although studies have been small and results

TABLE 9-9 Strategies for Caring for Infants Prenatally Exposed to Drugs

Infant Behavior	Behavior Description	Strategies
Vomiting or poor feeding	Infants frequently display gastrointestinal difficulties throughout their first year of life. Vomiting is frequent during the first 6 to 9 months, as are intermittent constipation and diarrhea. These difficulties tend to increase irritability and discomfort. If allowed to, some infants sleep up to 20 hours per day during the first 6 months of life and miss feedings. They are therefore at risk for inadequate nutrition and failure to thrive.	• If necessary, wake infant for feeding. • Give small quantities of food. • Allow infant to rest frequently during feeding. • Have infant upright for feeding. After feeding, place infant in side-lying or prone position to prevent aspiration of milk. • If infant vomits, clean skin immediately to prevent irritation from stomach acid.
Uncoordinated sucking and swallowing	A variety of abnormal oral-motor behaviors have been observed, including a preemie-like suck pattern, poorly coordinated suck/swallow patterns, inability to stabilize tongue in midline, and (occasionally) tongue thrusting and tongue tremors. These abnormal patterns increase feeding time. Consequently, a great deal of infant energy is required, and stress and frustration may occur in mother and infant.	• Hold infant in sitting position with arms forward in slight trunk flexion (curve) during feeding. • Keep infant's chin tucked downward. Infants prenatally exposed to drugs often push head back, which causes an abnormal swallow pattern. • If sucking is difficult for infant, support infant's chin or chin and cheeks with your hand. • Play soft, rhythmic music to help infant relax and to facilitate rhythmic sucking.
Weak pull-to-sit development	Infants often are slow learning pull-to-sit movement; frequently, it is accomplished with head lag or excessive effort after 6 months of age. (Infants normally pull-to-sit with no head lag by 4 months.) Some prenatally exposed to drugs who are able to pull-to-sit with no head lag may compensate by pulling their arms back into a strong "W" position. Usually pull-to-sit is accomplished with arms forward and some trunk flexion. The skill is a developmental milestone that indicates abdominal and neck muscle strength; it later affects the quality and endurance of balance, sitting, walking, and protective reflexes.	• Move infant from supine to sitting position, supporting the head so that it does not lag. • While moving infant into sitting position, support shoulders close to infant's body with head forward (neck flexion). With infant semireclined (45° angle), encourage infant to assist with pull-to-sit. Give additional head support if needed to prevent head lag and bring infant's arms forward into midline position. • Place infant in supported sitting position, and move infant slowly backward within the range of head control. Then slowly rock or move infant back and forth to strengthen neck and abdominal muscles.

(continued)

TABLE 9-9 (continued)

Infant Behavior	Behavior Description	Strategies
Irritability and difficulty sleeping	Exposure to drugs in utero can cause infant's state to vary from highly irritable to very passive. Most of these infants, however, are highly irritable and often have difficulty sleeping. Irritable infants can reach a frantic-cry state, which needs to be avoided. If infant is passive, interaction needs to take place during quiet alert, not hyperalert, states. Caregivers need to monitor their interactions by being alert to infant behavioral and psychological cues that indicate stress and adjust interactions appropriately. Caregivers will be affected by infant irritability, resulting in frustration and feelings of inadequacy in the mothering role and in infant/caregiver attachment. The caregiver needs to be made aware of behavior typical in infants prenatally exposed to drugs. Subsequently, the quality of their relationship will improve, negative judgments about infant will be reduced, and the likelihood of child abuse will be decreased.	• Reduce noise in environment. • Turn down lights. • Swaddle infant in a cotton blanket in flexed position with arms close to body. • Hold swaddled infant close. • Put infant in bunting-type wrapper and carry close to body. • Rock infant slowly and rhythmically, either horizontally or with head supported vertically, whichever soothes. • Place in a front-pack carrier. • Walk with infant. • Give child pacifier. • Provide hydrotherapy (warm bath). • Respond to stress cues by stopping activity with infant. This response will give infant a timeout. • Provide firm, calm touch to the midchest, back, or soles of infant's feet. • Play soft music or sing or hum quietly. • Provide background noise (for example, a hair dryer or vacuum cleaner), often called white noise, which may calm infant. • If all else fails, place infant in a quiet, darkened room with no outside stimulation. (Caregivers report this works with both premature and full-term infants exposed prenatally to drugs.)
Tremors, trembling, and extraneous movement	Tremors of the hands, arms, legs, chin, and tongue are commonly observed in infants prenatally exposed to drugs, although usually more pronounced and intense in younger infant. Tremors and tremulousness of movements have been observed in infants older than 1 year, but the intensity is diminished. In younger infants, tremors are primarily observed when infants are at rest. As they get older, fewer and less intense at-rest tremors occur, and intention	• Swaddling and holding infant close may be helpful for early at-rest tremors and extraneous movement. • Hold infant semireclined (almost sitting) with arms and shoulders forward to reduce the effort exerted by infant to maintain arm at midline while reaching for, holding, or manipulating toys. • Touch tremulous area firmly and calmly. Touch chest firmly and calmly.

(continued)

TABLE 9-9 (continued)

Infant Behavior	Behavior Description	Strategies
Tremors, trembling, and extraneous movement (continued)	tremors emerge. They tend to increase as the infant tires. Intention tremors occur when the infant is actively attempting a specific motor movement, for example, reaching for a toy. Intervention is often successful with intention tremors of arms and hands. Signs of stress often occur after persisting with an activity that elicits intention tremors because physical movements are difficult, and more energy and time are required to accomplish a task. Fine-motor development is at risk. Some infants prenatally exposed to drugs exhibit constant extraneous movements that make it difficult for them to soothe themselves. These extraneous movements slow acquisition of organized intentional motor control and visual-motor skills.	
Stiffness and rigidity	Stiffness and rigidity, or increased extensor tone, are often seen in infants prenatally exposed to drugs. The increased muscle tone, which causes these infants to frequently roll over at a few weeks of age, interferes with normal motor development, ability to cuddle, and pull-to-sit, and it delays control of arms at midline. Increased extensor tone in infants tends to diminish slowly. By 1 year of age, some degree of increased tone usually remains and diminishes the quality and smoothness of gross-motor patterns, as well as balance and protective reactions. These infants often arch their backs when held in a variety of positions, or when being fed. Arching occurs up to 12 months of age. More energy is used to accomplish fine- and gross-motor tasks; thus, some level of frustration is created.	• Bathe infant in warm water. • Try gentle, calming massage. • Swaddle in flexion with shoulders and arms close to body. • Place infant in baby hammock to help ease rigidity, to maintain infant in slight spinal flexion, and to inhibit abnormal extension pattern. • Do not leave infant supine if the position maintains or increases stiffness, for example, head pushing back with scapular retraction (shoulder blades pinching together), or arms pushing into "W" position. Instead put infant in cloth, sling-type seat, as this position inhibits abnormal extension pattern. • Discourage the use of baby walkers, as they are known to further increase extensor tone.

(continued)

TABLE 9-9 (continued)

Infant Behavior	Behavior Description	Strategies
Arms in "W" position	A large majority of infants prenatally exposed to drugs exhibit scapular retraction and/or resistance or weakness when attempting to bring arms to midline. When supine, arms are typically widespread and in a "W" position or one arm is in a unilateral "W" position. As these infants develop, difficulty continues in bringing arms to midline or sustaining a midline position. Younger infants compensate by locking their hands together, but when they release them, their arms snap backward into a "W" position, much like a rubberband effect. When infants are older, they can use their arms against increased extensor tone and, thus, use large amounts of active energy to maintain control. Fine-motor performance is compromised, and development of bimanual skills is difficult. Maintaining hands at midline is an important developmental step in acquiring fine-motor skills.	• Swaddle infant with arms in midline position. • Carry or hold infant in a semireclining position with shoulders forward so that infant will experience arms at midline without excessive effort. • Place infant in cloth, sling-style infant seat. • Use reverse figure-eight strap to sustain arms in forward position while infant is in cloth, sling-style seat or in prone or sitting position. Infant can have successful experience without struggling for control. • Use a Form™ infant feeder chair to position child and assist in keeping arms at midline. This strategy can be used for infants who cannot tolerate the reverse figure-eight strap.

Source: Lewis, K.D., Bennett, B., and Schmeder, N.H. (1989). The care of infants menaced by cocaine abuse. *American Journal of Maternal Child Nursing 14,* 324–329.

inconsistent, it appears that prenatal exposure is potentially dangerous for the mother and fetus (Hulse et al., 1997; Sprauve, Lindsay, Herbert, and Graves, 1997).

Cocaine acts as a CNS stimulant (Haegerman and Schnoll, 1991; Kwong and Shearer, 1998; Lynch and McKeon, 1990; Wheeler, 1993). Crack, a freebase form of cocaine, can be smoked. Cocaine acts to block the reuptake of neurotransmitters, specifically norepinephrine and dopamine. The effect of decreased reuptake of dopamine acts on the CNS to stimulate the cerebral cortex, creating a feeling of euphoria.

The physiological effect of cocaine use in pregnancy involves several of the major body systems, and cocaine crosses the placental barrier easily (Garland, 1998; Haegerman and Schnoll, 1991; Lynch and McKeon, 1990). Decreased reuptake of norepinephrine acts through the hypothalamus to decrease appetite; poor nutritional intake can lead to IUGR. Stimulation of the peripheral nervous system leads to increases in maternal body temperature, blood pressure, heart rate, and respiration. Any prolonged increase in maternal blood pressure can lead to abruptio placentae. Vasoconstriction is also manifested and can lead to uterine contractions and fetal hypoxia. These factors, over the course of a pregnancy, increase the risk for IUGR, spontaneous abortion, and fetal death. Fetal anomalies include deformities of the upper limbs, microcephaly, myelomeningocele, growth retardation, increased blood velocity in the cerebral artery, ambiguous genitalia, prune belly syndrome, congenital heart defects, necrotizing enterocolitis, and ileal atresia (Bateman, Ng, Hansen, and Hagerty, 1993; Prank et al., 1990;

Haegerman and Schnoll, 1991; Hanna, Faden, and Dufour, 1997; Kenner and D'Apolito, 1997; Lopez, Taeusch, Findlay, and Walther, 1995; Richardson and Day, 1994).

PRENATAL MANAGEMENT

Ideally, drug-using women should be identified and treated before pregnancy. Most are identified when they are pregnant and enter the health care system after the first trimester. These clients are high-risk cases and should be managed under joint protocols by the APN and obstetrician. A plan of treatment should be initiated with documentation of treatments and interventions, followed by periodic reevaluation of the plan. Because cocaine abuse is a multidimensional problem, drug treatment and rehabilitation, social services, and nutrition counseling are all essential components in prenatal care.

Basic prenatal assessment and evaluation are the same as for all other clients. Cocaine can be snorted or injected; however, observation of the status of nasal mucous membranes and any signs of IV drug use as previously described are important. Routine prenatal blood work is performed.

As with opiate addiction, narcotics may be used for pain relief during labor and delivery, but the client may require higher doses for effect. After evaluation by neonatal specialists in the delivery room, the infant is transferred to the NICU for observation and treatment of withdrawal symptoms.

Appropriateness of breastfeeding should be determined based on the mother's desire to breastfeed and time of last maternal intake of cocaine or crack. Cocaine easily passes through the membranous barrier into the milk supply and remains in the breast milk for up to 60 hours after last maternal use (Howard and Lawrence, 1993; Matera et al., 1990). If there is any significant doubt as to the mother's continued abstinence from cocaine use, breastfeeding should not be advised.

COCAINE INTOXICATION

An acute overdose of cocaine or crack can be a life-threatening event for mother and fetus and may require hospitalization. Signs of an overdose include paranoia, frank psychosis, agitation, or sleeplessness (Bateman, Ng, Hansen, and Hagerty, 1993; Botelho and Novak, 1997; Cross and Hennessey, 1993; Matera et al., 1990; Medoff-Cooper and Verklan, 1992). The client should be maintained with supportive care in a quiet environment; the fetus should be maintained on continuous fetal monitoring throughout the acute withdrawal phase. Seizures, hypertension, hyperthermia, and tachycardia may also occur. Each of these problems is serious and must be addressed separately when implementing care. Many of the deaths that occur with cocaine overdose are results of uncontrolled seizures, hyperthermia, and rhabdomyolysis.

Seizures in the mother may be short-lived or persistent in nature. Care must be taken to maintain an open airway. If medication intervention becomes necessary, phenobarbital can be utilized at 15 mg/kg to 20 mg/kg intravenously over 15 to 20 minutes; it is relatively safe for the fetus (Cross and Hennessey, 1993; Medoff-Cooper and Verklan, 1992; Wheeler, 1993). Seizures due to cocaine intoxication can be refractory and must be controlled as quickly as possible.

Hypertension may be resolved with the use of sedatives. If longer treatment is necessary, any antihypertensive medication must be short-acting and titratable. Stroke, subarachnoid hemorrhage, and ruptured aneurysm can occur due to the extraordinary blood pressure changes attributed to cocaine abuse (Cross and Hennessey, 1993; Medoff-Cooper and Verklan, 1992; Wheeler, 1993). When implementing therapy, any sudden decrease in maternal blood pressure will decrease uteroplacental profusion and can lead to fetal distress.

Hyperthermia is treated with cold water baths and air fans. Cardiac arrhythmias and myocardial infarctions can also occur with cocaine abuse (Medoff-Cooper and Verklan, 1992; Wheeler, 1993). An increase in the presence of catecholamines can result in increased heart rate, sinus tachycardia, ventricular premature beats, and ventricular tachycardia. Cardiac arrest has been documented in healthy individuals who have abused cocaine. Anyone with underlying cardiac disease or congenital weakness is at a significantly increased risk for cardiovascular complications.

Preterm labor, abruptio placentae, and fetal distress occur as a result of the dramatic changes triggered by vasoconstriction, altered uteroplacental circulation, and fetal hypoxia (Garland, 1998; Lynch and McKeon, 1990; Mishra, Landzberg, and Parente, 1995). Preterm labor can be stopped with the use of magnesium sulfate tocolysis. The use of ß mimetics (e.g., ritodrine or terbutaline) should be avoided with suspected cocaine overdose (Garland, 1998; Lynch and McKeon, 1990; Mishra, Landzberg, and Parente, 1995). Abruptio placentae and fetal distress can cause intrauterine death, and immediate delivery of the fetus is required for any chance of survival.

COCAINE WITHDRAWAL

Withdrawal occurs with the loss of the cocaine effect on the midbrain. Depression, sleep dysfunction, loss of appetite, and generalized irritability are signs of cocaine withdrawal. Addicts experience strong cravings for cocaine, and the drive to obtain it results in extreme behavior. Withdrawal is not life-threatening, but stained abstinence is long and difficult to achieve without rehabilitation and support services. The severe depression that frequently results from discontinuation of use often triggers a return to use.

MANAGEMENT OF THE NEWBORN

Treatment of the newborn exposed to cocaine in utero is based on symptom management and usually does not require pharmacotherapeutics. Many exposed infants suffer from the consequences of preterm delivery because cocaine stimulates early and precipitous labor. These infants may be on respirators and may receive IV fluids and parenteral nutrition. They may suffer intracranial hemorrhages, hydrocephaly, seizures, and possibly cerebral palsy (Bateman, Ng, Hansen, and Hagerty, 1993; Chavkin and Breitbart, 1997; Feldman, Minkoff, McCalla, and Salwen, 1992; King et al., 1995; Pettiti and Coleman, 1990; Racine, Joyce, and Anderson, 1993). All these problems are consistent with preterm delivery. All infants, whether preterm or full-term, may experience the symptoms of NAS and need to be evaluated. For infants who are easily aroused, environmental stimuli should be at a minimum, with swaddling and frequent feeding recommended.

These mothers and babies need supportive services, including those of the visiting nurse and child protective and early intervention services. Although research findings on the long-term effects of cocaine exposure in utero are inconsistent, the high-risk environments of some of these children put them at risk for cognitive and behavioral deficits; they may require intensive multidisciplinary management (Bender et al., 1995; Eyler et al., 1998;

Jacobson et al., 1996; Lester et al., 1991b). Referral sources are available by calling 1-800-COCAINE for treatment directories in all states.

Marijuana

Marijuana, smoked in cigarettes, produces relaxation, euphoria, and an increased appetite. Although it is the most frequently used reported illicit drug in national surveys, only 1.5 percent of pregnant women used this drug (SAMHSA, 1998). Smaller studies that used toxicology screens in the early 1980s reported prevalence rates of marijuana use during pregnancy as high as 20 percent to 30 percent (Day and Richardson, 1991; Hansen et al., 1986; Zuckerman et al., 1989).

The active chemical ingredient in marijuana is delta-9-tetrahydrocannabinol (THC). This psychoactive chemical is present in marijuana smoke; it is estimated that about one-half of THC in marijuana smoke is absorbed when inhaled. THC is fat-soluble, is metabolized in the liver, and is excreted in the feces and urine. THC readily passes through the placental barrier to the fetus. One dose of the drug can take up to 30 days to be excreted from the body. The main effects on pregnancy and the fetus appear to be very similar to the effects of cigarette smoke and include altered fetal oxygenation, altered lean tissue growth, and possible decreased fetal growth (Frank et al., 1990). Other researchers suggest that heavy marijuana smoking in pregnancy impairs the newborn's neurophysiological integrity by affecting sleep patterns and sleep efficiency (Day and Richardson, 1991).

PRENATAL MANAGEMENT

The primary objective of prenatal management is education about marijuana use and its cessation. Specific guidelines and interventions by the care provider are the same as those used for tobacco smokers. It is common for both of these habits to be evident in the same prenatal client, and interventions are best addressed for all forms of smoking behaviors if cessation is to be successful.

MANAGEMENT OF THE NEWBORN

Newborn marijuana exposure can also occur through secondhand smoke or through breast milk. If the mother wishes to breastfeed her infant, she must be informed that fat-soluble THC is rapidly transmitted to breast milk and remains in the breast tissue for as long as 60 days (Day and Richardson, 1991; Lee, 1998; Richardson, Day, and McGauhey, 1993). Marijuana exposure does not appear to cause long-term complications (Day et al., 1992; Dreher, Nugent, and Hudgins, 1994; Fried, 1995; Zuckerman et al., 1989). Treatment for children who were prenatally exposed to marijuana is symptomatic and may involve assessing the environment and providing referrals to early intervention programs, WIC, and psychosocial services.

Barbiturates

Barbiturates are among the most frequently abused drugs in the general population. Over 15,000 deaths per year have been reported in the United States secondary to barbiturate poisoning (Chavkin and Breitbart, 1997; Coupey, 1997; Kwong and Shearer, 1998; Wheeler, 1993). Maternal barbiturate abuse can cause fetal addiction and withdrawal both in utero and during the neonatal period. Most risks associated with barbiturate abuse involve long-term addiction or acute intoxication. It is necessary to obtain blood levels of barbiturates during a comprehensive assessment to identify the addicted client and determine appropriate intervention. Acute intoxication occurs at mild, moderate, or severe levels. The higher the blood toxicity level, the more serious the immediate danger is: Mild intoxication is evident in maternal drowsiness; moderate intoxication causes a low level of consciousness, depressed or absent deep tendon reflexes, and shallow respirations; severe intoxication can result in life-threatening changes in both the pulmonary and circulatory systems of the body, with serious fetal outcomes. Depressed consciousness, severe respiratory depression, abnormal low blood pressure, pulmonary edema, cyanosis, and decreased body temperature are also associated with severe barbiturate intoxication (Botelho and Novak, 1997; Coupey, 1997).

Prenatal Management

The obstetrical client who uses barbiturates is at high risk and requires co-management protocols of care by nursing and medicine. Mild or moderate barbiturate intoxication is managed with observation and supportive measures. Cases of severe intoxication require vigilant monitoring and immediate intervention to minimize medical complications. Maintaining an open airway and providing adequate ventilation are primary concerns. An endotracheal tube may be necessary to maintain oxygenation. If the intubated client is unresponsive, gastric lavage may be necessary. Intravenous fluids should be initiated to help the kidneys excrete the drug. Long-acting barbiturates can cause coma. Hemodialysis is used as a method of detoxification and may also be necessary if kidney function is compromised. Long-term use of barbiturates leads to tolerance of the drugs and cross-tolerance to drugs of similar action.

Chronic users and their fetuses can suffer withdrawal if the drug is stopped abruptly in pregnancy or in labor and delivery. The withdrawal symptoms that the fetus experiences are those seen in other narcotic-addicted fetuses. If the addicted client is identified in pregnancy, a safe and gradual withdrawal from the drug can be accomplished. The basic protocol for treatment of barbiturate withdrawal requires the administration of 0.2 gram pentobarbital by mouth every 6 hours (Cross and Hennessey, 1993). The drug is administered and titrated downward to decrease the dangerous withdrawal effects on mother and fetus.

Labor and delivery protocols focus on the identification of the substance use and any presenting signs and symptoms of intoxication or withdrawal. Decreased affect and/or impaired motor or cognitive function should alert the APN to evaluate for drug levels. Blood values should be obtained and appropriate treatment and care implemented to facilitate maternal and fetal safety. Because withdrawal symptoms may not be manifested until 48 to 72 hours after the last dose, close observation of the client is necessary. In severe cases, the client may experience seizures, delirium, and even death.

Management of the Newborn

An infant exposed to barbiturates displays symptoms of irritability, severe tremors, excessive crying, vasomotor instability, diarrhea, increased muscle tone, vomiting, and disturbed sleep. Onset of symptoms may be as early as the first 24 hours after delivery but can be as late as 10 to 14 days postdelivery. Symptoms may last as long as 4 to 6 months even with treatment. Pharmacological treatment follows protocols for NAS; comfort measures should be initiated.

Amphetamines

Amphetamines are sympathomimetic drugs and are usually used for appetite suppression, weight loss, and treatment of narcolepsy (Bragg, 1997; Chavkin and Breitbart, 1997; Glanz and Woods, 1991; Kwong and Shearer, 1998; Plessinger, 1998). They stimulate the CNS and are abused for this stimulant property. Their use is often seen in conjunction with other drugs. Amphetamine use in pregnancy has not been shown to increase the risk of fetal anomalies, but the abusing client is at increased risk for hypertension, tachycardia, and hyperthermia. A preexisting, underlying pathology can increase the abusing client's risk for cardiac arrhythmia, cerebrovascular accident, and myocardial infarction. Toxic levels of amphetamines are manifested in symptoms of tremors, increased motor activity, restlessness, insomnia, and excessive talking.

PRENATAL AND NEWBORN MANAGEMENT

Treatment protocols for both mother and infant involve supportive and comfort care components. No specific concerns characterize labor and delivery. A multidisciplinary approach is necessary to address the client's medical, psychosocial, and environmental needs.

Over-the-Counter Medications and Prescription Drugs

The use of over-the-counter (OTC) and prescription medications is extremely common and often goes unrecognized in pregnancy. As the numbers of sophisticated OTC drugs increase, so does concern for the possible long-term effects on the developing fetus and the state of a pregnancy in general.

There is a wide range of drugs available for use, and these are taken in a variety of combinations; therefore, it is difficult to study the direct effects of these drugs in the general population. Specific risks in pregnancy have also been difficult to identify, but it is known that most pregnant women do take some types of OTC medications during their pregnancies. In a study of OTC drug use in the first trimester, only 34 percent of women studied did not use any drugs (Buitendijk and Bracken, 1991). Various studies attempting to document the numbers of drugs used at different times throughout pregnancies have reported that women often do not ask for information about the effects of these drugs on themselves or their fetuses, and they do not know the potential side effects or food and drug interactions (Buitendijk and Bracken, 1991; Garland, 1998). This basic information, available from any pharmacist and most physicians and APNs, is often included in individual product inserts.

The greatest concern about exposure to OTC and prescription drugs relates to early pregnancy and effects on organogenesis, when fetal tissue is growing at its fastest rate. Potential effects derive from the strength, frequency, and class of drug used.

Pregnancy affects the digestion, absorption, and excretion of all substances ingested by the mother. Increases or decreases in absorption may alter the excretion of drugs from the body due to physiological changes in kidney and liver function. Pregnancy changes the distribution of drugs in the body due to circulatory changes that alter intravascular and extravascular levels. These effects may, in turn, result in fetal exposure to these substances through placental circulation.

In an attempt to provide guidelines for the public regarding drug use in pregnancy, the Food and Drug Administration developed five separate categories for drug risk identification in pregnancy (Buitendijk and Bracken, 1991). They are as follows:

1. Category A—Controlled studies with these drugs show no risk in pregnancy.
2. Category B—There is no evidence of risk to humans. This may mean that animal studies did not show effects or that animal studies did show effects but that human studies did not.
3. Category C—The risk to drug exposure and risk to humans cannot be ruled out. Human studies may not be possible, and the results of animal studies are either positive for fetal risk or inconclusive.
4. Category D—There is proof of risk to the human fetus. In some circumstances, the benefits to use of the drug may outweigh the potential risks to the developing fetus.
5. Category X—These drugs are contraindicated for use in pregnancy. There is evidence that their use in pregnancy can be very harmful to the fetus and that their benefits are significantly outweighed by the risks of their use.

PRENATAL AND NEWBORN MANAGEMENT

APNs should educate clients about the potential harmful effects of OTC and prescription drugs on the developing fetus; no medication or drug can be presumed to be benign. Clients need to be educated to recognize that, after delivery, these same drugs may pass through into breast milk and can still have an adverse effect on the newborn. Incorporating a complete drug recall (including OTC and prescription drugs) at the first prenatal visit is an important part of the early screening process.

Polydrug Use

Pregnant women who abuse drugs rarely abuse only one. Heroin addicts may also use cocaine and alcohol; the marijuana user may also smoke cigarettes. Women using illegal drugs often also use OTC and prescription medications. Unfortunately, the interactions and potential synergistic effects of more than one drug are not widely known.

PRENATAL MANAGEMENT

The best means of ascertaining polydrug use is by assessment at each prenatal visit. If a mother reports use of one drug, she is likely to be using others. It is important to know the types of drugs, the amounts, and the frequencies of use by the mother so that readiness to change is assessed and rehabilitation plans can be individualized. If the type of drug is unknown, the physical response to cessation or detoxification may be unexpected. The mother in treatment for cocaine use who is also an alcoholic has responses to detoxification that pose additional risks.

MANAGEMENT OF THE NEWBORN

The newborn exposed to more than one drug may exhibit more severe symptoms. Infant toxicology may provide information on recent exposure to illegal drugs and alcohol; the use of tobacco and OTC or prescription medications must be ascertained by interview. Rating symptoms using the NAS helps to determine the need for pharmacotherapeutics. Comfort measures are necessary for symptom management. Long-term management varies with the combinations of drugs used and requires a multidisciplinary approach.

Related Issues

Prepregnancy Treatment of Substance Abuse

A recent study of 284 women at 6 weeks' postpartum found that when drug use was discontinued at least one year before delivery, the pregnancy outcome was no different than if the mother had never used drugs (Mahony, 1998). Therefore, it is worthwhile to address issues of use, treatment, and potential rehabilitation for the substance-abusing client prior to conception. As more is learned about the impact of diet, drugs, environment, and social stressors on conception and early fetal organogenesis, the importance of early intervention in optimizing positive outcomes in pregnancy is realized.

A routine gynecological examination is an opportunity to provide information about substance use and abuse, STDs, contraceptive issues, and effects of maternal drug use on the mother and the developing fetus. Education should include the general risks of substance use and abuse, the adverse effects of drugs on the developing fetus, and the maternal risks of pregnancy that can be heightened by substance abuse. Simply advising a client to stop drug use and, if necessary, to enroll in treatment may be insufficient. Suggestions for treatment must be presented with rationales that explain the desired outcomes for the mother as well as the baby. Suggestions must also consider the woman's readiness to change. Drug rehabilitation programs sensitive to the needs of women are slowly becoming available. Through early identification of substance-related problems and the early initiation of substance education, it is hoped that the substance abuser will respond more positively to the notion of treatment and rehabilitation, thus preventing later complications of fetal exposure and negative outcomes for the woman and her family.

Drug Rehabilitation for Pregnant, Drug-Using Women

In the past, there have been a limited number of drug rehabilitation facilities for pregnant and parenting women. Recommendations for treatment must consider appropriate medical management for a woman who is pregnant and who may also have dependent children. Many drug rehabilitation programs are traditionally focused on the needs of male populations and are unable to undertake the appropriate development of services to support state-approved care for pregnant women. Many agencies are unwilling to accept the liability associated with pregnancy (Chavkin, 1990). Some newly developed programs are designed for pregnant women only; others have provisions for newborns and other children. Programs that provide care for children have better postdischarge outcomes (LaFazia et al., 1996). The National Institute of Drug Abuse (NIDA) has sponsored research and program development specifically for drug-abusing pregnant and postpartum women and their drug-exposed infants. Several start-up programs are described in monograph 166, *Treatment for Drug-Exposed Women and Their Children: Advances in Research Methodology*. In this report, problems with recruitment and retention for both research projects and rehabilitation programs are described. Seven clinical factors that affect progress of treatment and that require additional staff efforts are listed (Rahdert, 1996):

1. Addiction severity level
2. Involvement with the legal system
3. Housing problems
4. Difficulties with interpersonal relations
5. Parenting responsibilities
6. Employment-related issues
7. Need for many comprehensive services

Collaboration

Substance use and abuse during pregnancy are complex problems best addressed using a multidisciplinary approach. These problems reach beyond the initial identification and treatment of the substance abuse. Coordination of care involves members of multiple health care specialties including APNs, obstetricians, neonatologists, nurses, pediatricians, child welfare case workers, social workers, and substance abuse treatment experts. Professionals who are involved in the care and treatment of these clients must refrain from judgments about substance abuse and focus on the emotional and physical needs of the woman, her child, and her family. Specialized training may be needed to effectively assess and plan treatment for these women and their infants. Social dynamics, cultural values, and family issues that influence clients' acceptance of treatment and their ability to maintain a path to recovery must be identified and addressed. Substance abuse professionals achieve better treatment outcomes by advocating for clients and navigating the complex medical and social service systems on which these clients are dependent for treatment and recovery. Necessary services include the following (Daley and Argerou, 1997; Parente, Gaines, and Lockridge, 1990; Parker, 1993; Racine, Joyce, and Anderson, 1993):

- Educational and vocational training
- Financial services to help meet basic needs
- Health and parenting education
- Dietary counseling for improved nutritional status
- Home health and visiting nurse services to help care for newborns and to provide supervision of postpartum recovery and adjustment
- Drug treatment and maintenance of continuing program involvement, including access to mental health services
- Birth control and contraceptive counseling to provide information and support for safe sexual activity postdelivery

Effective use of social services and appropriate referrals for outpatient follow-up increase the probability that long-term rehabilitation will be achieved. Continued therapy and intervention are necessary for months or years before positive outcomes are consistent for the mother and/or her family. Periodic reviews and evaluation of services provided through a multispecialty substance abuse treatment team are critical for continued monitoring of the rehabilitation of the addicted mother and the child's development.

Human Immunodeficiency Virus

Substance abuse is a major identified factor contributing to the spread of HIV. Substance abusers may be more prone to engage in risky behaviors such as shared needles, involvement with multiple sexual partners, unprotected sex, sex in exchange for drugs, and exposure to multiple STDs (including HIV). Any pregnant woman who reports any of these activities should be strongly encouraged to be tested for HIV. For some women, pregnancy may be the first time they are aware of the diagnosis of HIV. Others know they are positive but choose to continue with the pregnancy. Once the diagnosis is known, the client may have many questions and areas of concern. Common questions include the following (Abercrombie and Booth, 1997; Turner, Lichstein, and Peden, 1989):

- Should I continue with this pregnancy?
- Will my baby be infected?
- If my baby is infected, will he or she die?
- Are any of my other children already infected?
- Will the pregnancy make my HIV worse?
- Does my husband/partner have HIV?
- Can I get help? What should I do? Whom should I tell, or should I tell at all?
- If I die, who will take care of my baby and other children?

Education and social or mental health support services are essential at this time. Increased anxiety about the well-being of fetus, family, and self may trigger a client's desire to use or resume using drugs. In addition, she may leave the health care system in an effort to deny her condition. Coping mechanisms may be precarious at best and result in feelings of panic. Addressing the client's questions directly and providing a plan for care are essential to building trust for future treatment. When blood test results are positive for the virus, it is advised to start a treatment program as soon into the pregnancy as possible. Treatment involves a drug therapy program using zidovudine (AZT), which has been demonstrated to enhance fetal resistance to intrauterine exposure (Newschaffer et al., 1998; Turner, Lichstein, and Peden, 1989). Nutritional therapy includes increased calories and vitamin supplements to boost the immune system and to facilitate fetal growth and development. Ongoing maternal and fetal assessment is maintained. Due to the high-risk nature and long-term outcomes of HIV infection for the mother and fetus, comanagement of prenatal and newborn care is necessary. Medical expertise is imperative to focus on the very complex physiological issues of care. APNs, using the nursing process, can identify issues that influence treatment and compliance, provide individualized teaching, and enhance clients' participation in their care.

PRENATAL MANAGEMENT

The initial prenatal blood workup includes all standard testing as previously described. Such pregnancies are managed as high risk with increased awareness of the mother's vulnerability to opportunistic infections and the need for diligent monitoring of signs of cytomegalovirus, genital herpes virus, and pulmonary infections.

Routine labor management is standard in most cases, with continuous fetal monitoring maintained. Neonatal specialists should be in the delivery room at the time of delivery for care and assessment of the newborn.

MANAGEMENT OF THE NEWBORN

The infant is transferred to the NICU for observation, and treatment with AZT is started immediately. Maternal and infant bonding should be encouraged as soon as possible after delivery. Breastfeeding is contraindicated for any mother known to be HIV-positive because HIV transfers into the breast milk, thus presenting a significant additional risk to the newborn for acquiring the virus. The infant will be monitored closely throughout childhood, with treatment protocols designed specifically for the child's needs.

Support services should remain in place after delivery to address both substance abuse and HIV care needs. Additional counseling and services should also be made available for the testing and follow-up of the clients' children and partners as needed. Maximizing family involvement in the decision-making process throughout pregnancy, labor and delivery, and postpartal period can lead to a stronger commitment to continue participation to support a successful outcome in meeting long-term health care needs of each member of the involved family.

Ethical Considerations

Identification of Those at Risk

APNs face difficult dilemmas when treating pregnant and parenting women whom they suspect are using drugs that are harmful to the women themselves and their children. Dilemmas emerge around identification of those at risk. Who should have a toxicology screen? There are three choices:

1. Mandatory universal screening for all women who are receiving prenatal care
2. No toxicology screening for any prenatal or newborn client
3. Screening of women in prenatal care who report a positive history and who exhibit physical signs of drug use

The most equitable and best prevention is universal screening. In this case, protection of the fetus is more important than the woman's right to autonomy over her own body and behavior. This choice also avoids reinforcement of stereotypes about which women use drugs. Two major premises for mandatory reporting are (1) the belief that the mother is willingly harming the fetus and (2) the fetus will be protected from harm if the mother is being closely monitored. Even though research has shown that mothers who use drugs during pregnancy experience guilt and its effects (Kearney, Murphy, Irwin, and Rosenbaum, 1995), many nurses still have negative attitudes toward mothers of drug-affected newborns (Ludwig, Marecki, Wooldridge, and Sherman, 1996). Some health care providers believe that if the mother is either incarcerated or in mandatory drug treatment, drug use can be controlled and the effects on the fetus will be minimal. In addition, the high financial costs (approximately $500 million annually) of neonatal expenses and longer hospital stays of undiagnosed drug exposure weigh heavily on policy considerations for this population (Meadows, 1994; Phibbs, Bateman, and Schwartz, 1991; Robins and Mills, 1993). Opponents of mandatory drug screening point out that mothers who use substances, especially illicit ones, will fear the consequences of mandatory drug screening and will not seek prenatal care that can prevent other complications and minimize the harmful effects of drug use.

The choice not to screen, which protects maternal rights, may interfere with appropriate client management and denies the obligation to take all steps to ensure positive birth outcomes for mother and baby. When an infant is exposed to drugs in utero, treatment involves an individualized protocol. Pharmacotherapy, as previously described, needs to be specific to the drug or drugs used as well as the symptoms displayed. However, a decision not to use a toxicology screen as part of the prenatal, postpartum, or newborn assessment screen does take into consideration a woman's autonomy and her right to privacy and, as with universal screening, eliminates the bias of subjective assessments.

The third choice, toxicology screening based on a comprehensive medical and psychosocial history that includes specific information on maternal drug use that is part of all prenatal and newborn evaluation, is recommended by the American Academy of Pediatrics (AAP) (American Academy of Pediatrics, 1998). Toxicology screens are performed only after the comprehensive history and physical. However, due to the subjective nature of a health history, the decision to use a toxicology screen may be biased, based on the client's living conditions, socioeconomic status, marital status, race, or ethnicity. In addition, different clinics and hospitals have different policies for drug screening, especially concerning informed consent. The U.S. Preventive Services Task Force (1996) recommends informed consent before any toxicology screen.

Positive Drug Screen

A second dilemma concerns the use of positive toxicology results. What happens when a drug screen is positive? In some states, the choices are limited because reporting of a positive drug screen to legal or child protective services is mandatory. In a national survey of states' policies and practices on drug-using women, 61 percent of the 50 states reported positive maternal toxicology screens for illicit drugs; 65 percent of the states reported positive neonatal screens to the child protective services. In addition, respondents from 34 states reported criminal prosecution of pregnant women for identified illicit drug use in their states (Chavkin, Breitbart, Elman, and Wise, 1998). Criminal prosecution and/or the involvement of child protective services may deter potential users and help to protect the fetus, but it is widely believed that a punitive approach causes women to mistrust health providers and to avoid comprehensive care (DeVille and Kopelman, 1998). The AAP recommends that effective drug treatment programs be available and contends that punitive measures such as criminal prosecution and incarceration are unjustified (American Academy of Pediatrics, 1995).

A parallel concern emerges when an APN discovers that the mother is smoking cigarettes or using alcohol. The APN knows the risks associated with exposure to these two legal drugs but needs to continue to provide care. One choice is to explore treatment options as previously described, and to monitor fetal and newborn well-being. A second option is to refuse to provide care unless the mother quits her drug use, an action that has other ethical implications. If the APN chooses to provide care (the preferred option) and if the mother chooses to continue with her tobacco and alcohol use, the challenge will be to provide nonjudgmental comprehensive prenatal care.

Foster Care

In some cases, when a newborn screens positive for illicit drugs or a history of maternal drug use is reported, child protective services have either recommended or mandated that the infant be put in family or state-run foster care. This usually happens when the home situation places the child at risk for child abuse or neglect. The criteria for foster placement may vary in different states and towns, but children of mothers who use substances during pregnancy are at high risk for foster placement. In a recent study that investigated visiting nursing services to 145 drug-exposed infants over a 7-year period, 50 percent of these infants were either permanently or temporarily placed in foster care (Mahony and Murphy, 1999). Should the APN encourage foster placement of an infant who was prenatally exposed to drugs? Foster care, although a short-term resolution, is transient and can affect the infant's development. Foster care placement adds to a mother's despair and may interfere with drug rehabilitation. The fear of foster placement may also act as a barrier to comprehensive prenatal care and drug treatment. Can an infant be removed from his or her mother and placed in foster care against the mother's will for a positive toxicology screen at birth? The readiness of child protective services to use foster care and the quality of available foster care, ultimately affect an APN's management decisions.

Summary

Drug use is a public health problem evident in all communities. The prevalence of drug use, especially tobacco and alcohol, in women of childbearing age is disturbing, due to the potential effect on pregnancy. Ideally, drug use should be identified prior to pregnancy. When drug use continues into pregnancy, identification should be early and treatment-specific for the drug-using pregnant woman and her family. Treatment protocols for the mother vary according to the type, frequency, and quantity of drug used. Newborn care involves comfort measures according to the degree of symptoms and may include pharmacological intervention if symptoms are severe. Health care for women who use drugs and their families is complex and requires a multidisciplinary approach to care provision and care coordination. Most importantly, as advocates for healthy women and children, APNs have the responsibility to educate clients about the dangers of drug abuse and support nonjudgmental treatment protocols, especially during pregnancy.

Case Study

Emily arrives at the prenatal clinic at an urban medical center for her first prenatal visit. Emily is seven and one-half months pregnant and is experiencing abdominal cramping with occasional bloody discharge. A comprehensive health history reveals that Emily has been in drug rehabilitation for cocaine, heroin, and alcohol abuse three times. Her three children were placed in foster care after her apartment had been raided for drugs. Her current boyfriend and the father of her unborn child is in prison as a result of that raid. She tells you that she was unaware of the drug sales going on in her home but realizes that it caused her the temporary loss of her children and her subsidized housing. She relies on friends for food and a bed, but she states that she may have to go to a shelter as her friends are "getting on her nerves." When she is asked if she is using drugs now, she states that she had smoked coke about a week ago, but that she was also around people who smoked all the time so she may be exposed to secondhand smoke. Extensive screening reveals that Emily is positive for cocaine, that she is suffering from malnutrition, and that her 30-week male fetus is small for gestational age.

You ask Emily if she feels safe with her living arrangements; she says, "Not always." You strongly suggest that Emily be admitted to the women's substance abuse in-patient program that is offered by your medical center. She agrees with this suggestion but states that she has to return to her current apartment to get her clothing and valuables. You make arrangements for her admission to the substance abuse program; however, Emily does not return to the clinic and is not admitted to the program.

One week later, Emily is admitted to labor and delivery via the emergency room in a late stage of labor and delivers a 31-week, 3-pound infant boy who demonstrates severe withdrawal symptoms.

1. Identify the factors that put Emily at risk for drug use during pregnancy.
2. How do the results of the screening tests influence the development of Emily's treatment plan?
3. Describe the medical management plan that you would put in place for this client.
4. How would you approach Emily about her treatment plan?
5. What collaborative efforts would be part of your treatment plan?
6. Describe how you would inform Emily of the diagnosis of neonatal abstinence syndrome (NAS) for her son as evidenced by documented withdrawal signs, urine toxicology report, and physical manifestations of NAS.
7. What would the treatment plan entail for an infant with a high score on the NAS scale?
8. What would the postpartum management plan be for Emily and her child? If you are required by law to report a positive infant toxicology screen to the state, how would this factor affect your treatment plan?

CRITICAL THINKING QUESTIONS

1. Discuss specific nursing interventions that can be implemented to facilitate prepregnancy education and prevention of substance abuse during pregnancy.
2. As a nurse practitioner or certified nurse-midwife, the nurse-client relationship should be established during the initial assessment. Discuss why this is an essential component of care and the benefits to be achieved as a result of establishing this relationship.
3. Discuss common physical characteristics of a pregnant substance abuser.
4. Describe various methods of screening for specific drugs and any ethical issues related to these drug-screening options.
5. Describe the physiological pathways affected in the pregnant alcohol abuser and how these changes in turn affect fetal physiology and development.
6. Discuss the classic signs of heroin withdrawal and how the condition can affect the client. Include in the discussion screening, prenatal testing, consultations, comanagement of maternal and fetal well-being, and differences in effects during the first, second, and third trimesters of pregnancy.
7. Describe the neonatal abstinence syndrome scale and how the scoring relates to treatment protocols.
8. Describe the possible long-term effects of polydrug use on the developing child and the need for a multidisciplinary approach to treatment.
9. Develop a risk profile for a pregnant woman who is using drugs and describe its use as a screening tool in practice.
10. Discuss how the treatment protocol varies when a pregnant addict is also HIV-positive.

REFERENCES

Abel, E.L. (1988). *Fetal Alcohol Abuse Syndrome.* New York: Plenum Press.

Abercrombie, P.D., and Booth, K.M. (1997). Prevalence of human immunodeficiency virus infection and drug use in pregnant women: A critical review of the literature. *Journal of Women's Health 6*(2), 163–187.

Adams, K., and Melvin, C. (1998). Costs of maternal conditions attributable to smoking during pregnancy. *American Journal of Preventive Medicine 15,* 212–219.

Amaro, H., Zuckerman, B., and Cabral, H. (1989). Drug use among adolescent mothers: A profile of risk. *Pediatrics 84*(1), 144–151.

American Academy of Nurse Practitioners. (1993). *Nurse Practitioner as an Advanced Practice Nurse: Role Position Statement.* Washington, DC: ACNP.

American Academy of Pediatrics [AAP]. (1995). Drug-exposed infants. *Pediatrics 96*(2), 364–367.

American Academy of Pediatrics [AAP]. (1998). Neonatal drug withdrawal. *Pediatrics 101*(6), 1079–1088.

American College of Nurse Midwives. (1993). *Standards for the Practice of Nurse Midwifery.* Washington, DC: ACNM.

American College of Nurse Midwives. (1997). *The Collaborative Management in Nurse Midwifery Practice for Medical, Gynecologic, and Obstetric Problems.* Washington, DC: ACNM.

Barnet, B., Duggan, A.K., Wilson, M., and Joffe, A. (1995). Association between postpartum substance use and depressive symptoms, stress, and social support in adolescent mothers. *Pediatrics 96*(4), 659–666.

Bateman, D.A., Ng, S.K.C., Hansen, C.A., and Haegarty, M.C. (1993). The effects of intrauterine cocaine exposure in newborns. *American Journal of Public Health 83*(2), 190–193.

Bender, S.L., Word, C.O., DiClemente, R.J., Crittenden, M.R., Persaud, N.A., and Ponton, L.E. (1995). The developmental implications of prenatal and/or postnatal crack cocaine exposure in preschool children: A preliminary report. *Journal of Developmental and Behavioral Pediatrics 17*(2), 107–108.

Bibb, K.W., Stewart, D.L., Walker, J.R., Cook, V.D., and Wagener, R.E. (1995). Drug screening in newborns and mothers using meconium samples, paired urine samples, and interviews. *Journal of Perinatology 15*(3), 199–207.

Boshuizen, H., Verkerk, P., Reerink, J., Herngreen, W., Zaadsra, B., and Verloove-Vanhorick, S. (1998). Maternal smoking during lactation: Relationship to growth during the first year of life in a Dutch birth cohort. *American Journal of Epidemiology 147*, 117–126.

Botelho, R.J., and Novak, S. (1997). Dealing with substance misuse, abuse, and dependency. *Primary Care 20*(1), 51–70.

Bragg, E.J. (1997). Pregnant adolescents with addictions. *Journal of Obstetric, Gynecologic and Neonatal Nursing 26*(5S), 577–584.

Buitendijk, S., and Bracken, M.B. (1991). Medication in early pregnancy: Prevalence of use and relationships to maternal characteristics. *American Journal of Obstetrics and Gynecology 165*, 33.

Burkett, G., Yasin, S., and Palow, D. (1990). Perinatal implications of cocaine exposure. *Journal of Reproductive Medicine 35*, 35–42.

Bush, P.J., and Iannotti, R.J. (1993). Alcohol, cigarette, and marijuana use among fourth-grade urban school children in 1988/9 and 1990/91. *American Journal of Public Health 83*(1), 111–115.

Callahan, C.M., Grant, T.M., Phipps, P., Clark, G., Novack, A.H., Streissguth, A.P., and Raisys, V.A. (1992). Measurement of gestational cocaine exposure: Sensitivity of infants' hair, meconium, and urine. *Journal of Pediatrics 120*(5), 763–768.

Chang, G. (1992). Improving treatment outcome in pregnant opiate-dependent women. *Journal of Substance Abuse Treatment 9*(4), 327–330.

Chasnoff, I.J., Burns, W.J., Schroll, S.H., and Burns, K.A. (1985). Cocaine use in pregnancy. *The New England Journal of Medicine 313*(11), 666–669.

Chasnoff, I., Griffith, D., Greier, C., and Murray, J. (1992). Cocaine/polydrug use in pregnancy: Two-year follow-up. *Pediatrics 89*(2), 284–289.

Chasnoff, I.J., Landress, H.J., and Barrett, M.E. (1990). The prevalence of illicit-drug or alcohol use during pregnancy and discrepancies in mandatory reporting in Pinellas County, Florida. *New England Journal of Medicine 322*(17), 1202–1206.

Chavkin, W. (1990). Drug addiction and pregnancy: Policy crossroads. *American Journal of Public Health 80*(4), 483–487.

Chavkin, W., and Breitbart, V. (1997). Substance abuse and maternity: The United States as a case study. *Addiction 92*(9), 1201–1205.

Chavkin, W., Breitbart, V., Elman, D., and Wise, P.H. (1998). National survey of the states: Policies and practices regarding drug-using pregnant women. *American Journal of Public Health 88*(1), 117–119.

Christmas, J.T., Knisely, J.S., Dawson, K.S., Dinsmoor, M.J., Weber, S., and Schnoll, S.H. (1992). Comparison of questionnaire screening and urine toxicology for detection of pregnancy complicated by substance use. *Obstetrics and Gynecology 80*(5), 750–754.

Coles, C.D., and Smith, I.E. (1993). Maternal drug use: Issues and implications for mother and child. *International Journal of the Addictions 28*(13), 1275–1393.

Coles, C.D., Platzman, K.A., Smith, I., James, M.E., and Falek, A. (1992). Effects of cocaine and alcohol use in pregnancy on neonatal growth and neurobehavioral status. *Neurotoxicology and Teratology 14,* 23–33.

Committee on Environmental Health, American Academy of Pediatrics. (1997). Environmental tobacco smoke: A hazard to children. *Pediatrics 99,* 639–642.

Coombs, R.H., and West, L.J. (1991). *Drug Testing: Issues and Options.* New York: University Press.

Cornelius, M.D., Taylor, P.M., Geva, D., and Day, N.L. (1995). Prenatal tobacco and marijuana use among adolescents: Effects on offspring gestational age, growth, and morphology. *Pediatrics 95*(5), 738–743.

Coupey, S.M. (1997). Barbiturates. *Pediatrics in Review 18*(8), 260–264.

Cross, G.M., and Hennessey, P.T.G. (1993). Principles and practices of detoxification. *Primary Care 20*(1), 81–93.

Curry, M. (1998). The interrelationship between abuse, substance use, and psychosocial stress during pregnancy. *Journal of Obstetrical, Gynecologic, and Neonatal Nursing 27,* 692–699.

Dahl, R.E., Scher, M.S., Williamson, D.E., Robles, N., and Day, N. (1995). A longitudinal study of prenatal marijuana use. Effects on sleep and arousal at age 3 years. *Archives of Pediatric and Adolescent Medicine 149*(2), 145–150.

Daley, M., and Argeriou, M. (1997). Characteristics and treatment needs of sexually abused pregnant women in drug rehabilitation. The Massachusetts MOTHERS Project. *Journal of Substance Abuse Treatment 14*(2), 191–196.

Das, T., Moutquin, J., Lindsay, C., Parent, J., and Fraser, W. (1998). Effects of smoking cessation on maternal airway function and birth weight. *Obstetrics and Gynecology 92,* 201–205.

Day, N.L., and Richardson, G.A. (1991). Perinatal marijuana use: epidemiological issues and infant outcomes. *Clinics in Perinatology 18,* 77–90.

Day, N., Cornelius, M., Goldschmidt, L., Richardson, G., Robles, N., and Taylor, P. (1992). The effects of prenatal tobacco and marijuana use on offspring growth from birth through 3 years of age. *Neurotoxicology and Teratology 14,* 407–414.

Day, N.L., Richardson, G.A., Goldschmidt, L., Robles, N., Taylor, P.M., Stoffer, D.S., Cornelius, M.D., and Geva, D. (1994). Effect of prenatal marijuana exposure on the cognitive development of offspring at age three. *Neurotoxicology and Teratology 16*(2), 169–175.

deCubas, M.M., and Field, T. (1993). Children of methadone-dependent women: Developmental outcomes. *American Journal of Orthopsychiatry 63*(2), 266–276.

Delaney, D.B., Larrabee, K.D., and Monga, M. (1997). Preterm premature rupture of membranes associated with recent cocaine use. *American Journal of Perinatology 14*(5), 285–288.

DeVille, K.A., and Kopelman, L. (1998). Moral and social issues regarding pregnant women who use and abuse drugs. *Obstetrics and Gynecology Clinics of North America 25*(1), 237–254.

Dogra, V.S., Shyken, J.M., Menon, P.A., Poblete, J., Lewis, D., and Smeltzer, J.S. (1994). Neurosonographic abnormalities associated with maternal history of cocaine use in neonates of appropriate size for their gestational age. *American Journal of Neuroradiology 15*(4), 696–702.

Dreher, M.C., Nugent, K., and Hudgins, R. (1994). Prenatal marijuana exposure and neonatal outcomes in Jamaica: An ethnographic study. *Pediatrics 93*(2), 254–260.

Dyer, C. (1998). Addict died after rapid opiate detoxification. *British Medical Journal 316*(7126), 170.

Edwall, G.E., Hoffman, N.G., and Harrison, P.A. (1989). Psychological correlates of sexual abuse in adolescent girls in chemical dependency treatment. *Adolescence 24,* 279–288.

Ewing, J.A. (1984). Detecting alcoholism: The CAGE questionnaire. *Journal of the American Medical Association 252,* 1905–1907.

Eyler, F.D., Behnke, M., Conlon, M., Woods, N.S., and Wobie, K. (1998). Birth outcomes from a prospective, matched study of prenatal crack/cocaine use: II. Interactive and dose effects on neurobehavioral assessment. *Pediatrics 101*(2), 237–241.

Fares, I., McCulloch, K.M., and Raju, T.N. (1997). Intrauterine cocaine exposure and the risk for sudden infant death syndrome: A meta-analysis. *Journal of Perinatology 17*(3), 179–182.

Feldman, J., Minkoff, H., McCalla, S., and Salwen, M. (1992). A cohort study of the impact of perinatal drug use on prematurity in an inner-city population. *American Journal of Public Health 82,* 726–728.

Finnegan, L.P. (1981). The effects of narcotics and alcohol on pregnancy and the newborn. *Annals of New York Academy of Sciences 362,* 136–157.

Finnegan, L.P. (1991). Treatment issues for opioid-dependent women during the perinatal period. *Journal of Psychoactive Drugs 23*(2), 191–201.

Flandemeyer, A., Kenner, C., Bragg, L., and Campinha-Bacote, J. (1992). Nursing care of women who abuse alcohol. *Medical-Surgical Nursing Quarterly 1,* 122–139.

Forsyth, B.W., Leventhal, J.M., Qi, K., Johnson, L., Schroeder, D., and Votto, N. (1998). Health care and hospitalization of young children born to cocaine-using women. *Archives of Pediatric and Adolescent Medicine 152*(2), 177–184.

Frank, D.A., Zuckerman, B.S., Aboagye, K., Bauchner, H., Cabral, H., Fried, L., Hingson, R., Kayne, H., Levenson, S., Parker, S., Reece, H., and Vinci, R. (1988). Cocaine use during pregnancy: Prevalence and correlates. *Pediatrics 82,* 888–895.

Frank, D.A., Bauchner, H., Parker, S., Huber, A., Kyei-Aboagye, K., Cabral, H., and Zuckerman, B. (1990). Neonatal body proportionality and body composition after in utero exposure to cocaine and marijuana. *Journal of Pediatrics 117,* 622–626.

Fried, P.A. (1995). Prenatal exposure to marihuana and tobacco during infancy, early and middle childhood: Effects and attempts at synthesis. *Archives of Toxicology Supplement 17,* 223–260.

Garland, M. (1998). Pharmacology of drug transfer across the placenta. *Obstetrics and Gynecology Clinics of North America 25*(1), 21–41.

Gfroerer, J. (1987). Correlation between drug use by teenagers and drug use by older family members. *American Journal of Drug and Alcohol Use 13,* 95–108.

Glanz, J.C., and Woods, J.R. (1991). Obstetric issues in substance abuse. *Pediatric Annual 20,* 531–539.

Graham, K., Koren, G., Klein, J., Schneiderman, J., and Greenwald, M. (1989). Determination of gestational cocaine exposure by hair analyses. *Journal of the American Medical Association 262*(23), 3328–3331.

Grant, T.M., Ernst, C.C., and Streissquth, A.P. (1996). An intervention with high-risk mothers who abuse alcohol and drugs: The Seattle Advocacy Model. *American Journal of Public Health 86*(12), 1816–1817.

Haegerman, G., and Schnoll, S. (1991). Narcotic use in pregnancy. *Clinics in Perinatology 18*(1), 51–76.

Hanna, E., Faden, V., and Dufour, M. (1994). The motivational correlates of drinking, smoking, and illicit drug use during pregnancy. *Journal of Substance Abuse 6,* 155–167.

Hanna, E.Z., Faden, V.B., and Dufour, M.C. (1997). The effects of substance use during gestation on birth outcome, infant and maternal health. *Journal of Substance Abuse 9,* 111–125.

Hansen, W.B., Graham, J.B., Sobel, J.L., Shelton, D.R., Flay, B.R., and Johnson, C.A. (1986). The consistency of peer and parent influences on tobacco, alcohol, and marijuana use among adolescents. *Journal of Behavioral Medicine 10,* 559–579.

Hays, R.D., and Revetto, J.P. (1990). Peer cluster theory and adolescent drug use: A reanalysis. *Journal of Drug Education 20,* 191–198.

Hess, D.J., and Kenner, C. (1998). Families casing for children with fetal alcohol syndrome: The nurse's role in early identification and intervention. *Holistic Nurse Practitioner 12*(3), 47–54.

Hickey, J.E., Suess, P.E., Newlin, D.B., Spurgeon, L., and Porges, S.W. (1995). Vagal tone regulation during sustained attention in boys exposed to opiates in utero. *Addictions Behavior 20*(1), 43–59.

Hite, C., and Shannon, M. (1992). Clinical profile of apparently healthy neonates with in utero drug exposure. *Journal of Obstetric, Gynecologic, and Neonatal Nursing 21*(4), 305–309.

Hollinshead, W.H., Griffin, J.F., Scott, H.D., Burke, M.E., Coustan, D.R., and Vest, T.A. (1990). Statewide prevalence of illicit drug use by pregnant women—Rhode Island. *Mortality and Morbidity Weekly Report 30,* 225–227.

Howard, C., and Lawrence, R.A. (1993). Breast feeding and drug exposure. *Primary Care 20*(1), 210–215.

Hulse, G., English, D., Milne, E., Holman, C., and Bower, C. (1997). Maternal cocaine use and low birth weight in newborns: A meta-analysis. *Addiction 92,* 1561–1570.

Hurt, H., Malmud, E., Betancourt, L., Brodsky, N.L., and Giannetta, J. (1997). A prospective evaluation of early language development in children with in utero cocaine exposure and in control subjects. *Journal of Pediatrics 130*(2), 310–312.

Hutchins, E., and DiPietro, J. (1997). Psychosocial risk factors associated with cocaine use during pregnancy: A case control study. *Obstetrics and Gynecology 90*(1), 142–147.

Jacobson, S.W., Jacobson, J.L., Sokol, R.J., Martier, S.S., Chiodo, L.M. (1996). New evidence for neurobehavioral effects of in utero cocaine exposure. *Journal of Pediatrics 129*(4), 581–590.

Jessup, M. (1997). Addiction in women: Prevalence, profiles, and meaning. *Journal of Obstetric Gynecologic, and Neonatal Nursing 26*(4), 449–458.

Johnson, J.M., Seikel, J.A., Madison, C.L., Foose, S.M., and Rinard, K.D. (1997). Standardized test performance of children with a history of prenatal exposure to multiple drugs/cocaine. *Journal of Community Disorders 30*(1), 45–72.

Jones, K., and Smith, D.W. (1973). Recognition of the fetal alcohol syndrome in early infancy. *Lancet 2,* 999–1001.

Kaltenbach, K., and Finnegan, L.P. (1992). Methadone maintenance during pregnancy. In T. Sonderegger (ed.), *Perinatal Substance Use.* Baltimore, MD: Johns Hopkins University Press.

Kaltenbach, K., Berghalla, V., and Finnegan, L. (1998). Opioid dependence during pregnancy. *Obstetrics and Gynecology Clinics of North America 25*(1), 139–151.

Kandel, D. (1973). Adolescent marijuana use: Role of parents and peers. *Science 181,* 1067–1070.

Kandel, D.B., and Andreus, K. (1987). Process of adolescent socialization by parents and peers. *International Journal of Drug Addiction 22,* 319–342.

Kandel, D.B., Kessler, R.C., and Marguiles, R.Z. (1978). Antecedents of adolescent initiation into stages of drug use: A developmental analysis. *Journal of Youth Adolescence 7,* 13–40.

Kaplan, J.L. (1993). Effectiveness and safety of intravenous nalmefene for emergency department patients with suspected narcotic overdose, a pilot study. *Annual of Emergency Medicine 22*(2), 187–190.

Kearney, M.H. (1996). Reclaiming normal life: Mothers' stages of recovery from drug use. *Journal of Obstetric, Gynecologic, and Neonatal Nursing 25*(9), 761–768.

Kearney, M.H., Murphy, S., Irwin, K., and Rosenbaum, M. (1995). Salvaging self: A grounded theory of pregnancy and crack cocaine. *Nursing Research 44*(4), 208–213.

Kelley, S. (1998). Stress and coping behaviors of substance-using mothers. *Journal of the Society of Pediatric Nurses 3,* 103–110.

Kenner, C., and D'Apolito, K. (1997). Outcomes for children exposed to drugs in utero. *Journal of Obstetric, Gynecologic, and Neonatal Nursing 26*(5), 595–603.

King, T., Perlman, J., Laptook, A., Rollins, N., Jackson, G., and Little, B. (1995). Neurologic manifestations of in utero cocaine exposure in near-term and term infants. *Pediatrics 96,* 259–264.

Kliegman, R.M., Madura, D., Kiwi, R., Eisenberg, I., and Yamashita, T. (1994). Relation of maternal cocaine use to the risks of prematurity and low birth weight. *Journal of Pediatrics 124*(5), 751–756.

Kline, J., Ng, S.K., Schittini. M., Levin, B., and Susser, M. (1997). Cocaine use during pregnancy: Sensitive detection by hair assay. *American Journal of Public Health 87*(3), 352–358.

Kwong, T.C., and Shearer, D. (1998). Detection of drug use during pregnancy. *Obstetrics and Gynecology Clinics of North America 25*(1), 43–57.

LaFazia, M.A., Kleyn, J., Lanz, J., Hall, T., Nyrop, K., Stark, K.D., Hansen, C., and Watts, D.H. (1996). Case management: A method of addressing subject selection and recruitment issues. In E.R. Rahdert (ed.), *Treatment for Drug-Exposed Women and Their Children: Advances in Research Methodology.* Rockville, MD: National Institute on Drug Abuse Research Monograph 165. NIH Pub. No. 96-3632.

Lee, M.J. (1998). Marihuana and tobacco use in pregnancy. *Obstetrics and Gynecology 25*(1), 65–83.

Lester, B.M., Corwin, M.J., Sepkoski, C., Seifer, R., Peucker, M., McLaughlin, S., and Golub, H.L. (1991). Neurobehavioral syndromes in cocaine-exposed newborn infants. *Child Development 62*(4), 694–705.

Levy, M., and Spino, M. (1993). Neonatal withdrawal syndrome: Associated drugs and pharmacological management. *Pharmacotherapy 13*(3), 202–211.

Libscomb, G.H., Mercer, B.M., Cashion, K.C., Jackson, L.D., Devall, D.D., and Sibai, B.M. (1992). The predictive value of routine urine drug screening in a high-risk obstetric population. *Journal of Fetal Medicine 1*(3), 117–120.

Lindsay, M.K., Carmichael, S., Peterson, H., Risby, J., Williams, H., and Klein, L. (1997). Correlation between self-reported cocaine use and urine toxicology in an inner-city prenatal population. *Journal of the National Medical Association 89*(1), 57–60.

Lipshultz, S.E., Frassica, J.J., and Orav, E.J. (1991). Cardiovascular abnormalities in infants prenatally exposed to cocaine. *Journal of Pediatrics 118*, 44–51.

Lopez, S., Taeusch, H., Findlay, R., and Walther, F. (1995). Time of onset of necrotizing enterocolitis in newborn infants with known perinatal exposure. *Clinical Pediatrics 34*, 424–429.

Ludwig, M.A., Marecki, M., Wooldridge, P.J., and Sherman, L.M. (1996). Neonatal nurses' knowledge of and attitudes toward caring for cocaine-exposed infants and their mothers. *Journal of Perinatal and Neonatal Nursing 9*(4), 81–95.

Lundsberg, L.S., Bracken, M.B., and Saftless, A.F. (1997). Low-to-moderate gestational alcohol use and intrauterine growth retardation, low birth weight, and preterm delivery. *Annuals of Epidemiology 7*(7), 498–508.

Lynch, M., and McKeon, V.A. (1990). Cocaine use during pregnancy: Research findings and clinical implications. *Journal of Obstetric, Gynecologic, and Neonatal Nursing 19*(4), 285–292.

Macones, G.A., Sehdev, H.M., Parry, S., Morgan, M.A., and Berlin, J.A. (1997). The association between maternal cocaine use and placenta previa. *American Journal of Obstetrics and Gynecology 177*(5), 1097–1100.

Mahony, D. (1998). Outcomes associated with self-reported drug use during pregnancy. *Addictions Nursing 10*(3), 115–122.

Mahony, D.L., and Murphy, J.M. (1999). Neonatal drug exposure: Assessing a specific population and services provided by visiting nurses. *Pediatric Nursing 25*(1), 27–34.

Marcenko, M.O., Spence, M., and Rohweder, C. (1994). Psychosocial characteristics of pregnant women with and without a history of substance abuse. *Health and Social Work 19*(1), 17–22.

Mascola, M., Van Vanakis, H., Tager, I., Speizer, F., and Hanrahan, J. (1998). Exposure of young infants to environmental tobacco smoke: Breast-feeding among smoking mothers. *American Journal of Public Health 88*, 893–896.

Matera, C., Warren, W.B., Moomjy, M., Fink, D.J., and Fox, H.E. (1990). Prevalence of use of cocaine and other substances in the obstetric population. *American Journal of Obstetrics and Gynecology 163*(3), 797–801.

McFarlane, J., Parker, B., and Soeken, K. (1996). Physical abuse, smoking, and substance abuse during pregnancy: Prevalence, interrelationships, and effects on birth weight. *Journal of Obstetrics, Gynecology, and Neonatal Nursing 25*(4), 313–320.

Meadows, P.D. (1994). The costs of cocaine (crack) exposure: A broader perspective. In J.C. McCloskey (ed.), *Current Issues in Nursing* (4th ed., pp. 522–527). Detroit, MI: Mosby Year Book.

Medoff-Cooper, B., and Verklan, T. (1992). Substance abuse. *NAACOGS Clinical Issues in Perinatal and Women's Health Nursing 3*(1), 114–128.

Miller. J.M., Boudreaux, M.C., and Regan, F.A. (1995). A case-control study of cocaine use in pregnancy. *American Journal of Obstetrics and Gynecology 172*(1 pt 1), 180–185.

Mirochnick, M., Frank, D.A., Cabral, H., Turner, A., and Zuckerman, B. (1995). Relation between meconium concentration of the cocaine metabolite benzoylecgonine and fetal growth. *Journal of Pediatrics 125*(4), 636–638.

Mishra, A., Landzberg, B.R., and Parente, J.T. (1995). Uterine rupture in association with alkaloidal ("crack") cocaine abuse. *American Journal of Obstetrics and Gynecology 173*(1), 243–244.

Mortality and Morbidity Weekly Report [MMWR]. (1997). Surveillance for fetal alcohol syndrome using multiple sources: Atlanta, Georgia, 1981–1989. *MMWR 46*(47), 1118–1120.

Nafstad, P., Fugelseth, D., Qvistad, E., and Ershoff, D. (1997). Nicotine concentration in the hair of nonsmoking mothers and the size of their infants. *American Journal of Public Health 88,* 120–124.

National Association of Pediatric Nurse Associates and Practitioners [NAPNAP]. (1990). *Scope of Practice for Pediatric Nurse Practitioners.* Cherry Hill, NJ: NAPNAP.

National Institutes of Drug Abuse [NIDA]. (1996). *National Pregnancy and Drug Survey: Drug Use Among Women Delivering Live Births* (NIH Pub. No. 98-4297).

Neerhoff, T.E., MacGregor, S.N., Retsky, S.S., and Sullivan, T.P. (1989). Cocaine abuse during pregnancy: Peripartum prevalence and perinatal outcome. *American Journal of Obstetrics and Gynecology 161,* 633–638.

Neuspiel, D.R. (1994). Behavior in cocaine-exposed infants and children: Association versus causality. *Drug and Alcohol Dependence 36*(2), 101–107.

Newschaffer, C.J., Coroft, J., Hauck, W.W., Fanninf, T., and Turner, B.J. (1998). Improved birth outcomes associated with the enhanced Medicaid prenatal care drug using women infected with the human immunodeficiency virus. *Obstetrics and Gynecology 91*(6), 885–891.

Obel, C., Henriksen, T., Hedegaard, M., Secher, N., and Ostergaard, J. (1998). Smoking during pregnancy and babbling abilities of the 8-month-old infant. *Pediatric and Perinatal Epidemiology 12,* 37–48.

Olson, H., Streissguth, A., Sampson, P., Barr, H., Bookstein, F., and Theide, K. (1997). Association of prenatal alcohol exposure with behavioral and learning problems in early adolescence. *Journal of the American Academy of Child and Adolescent Psychiatry 36,* 1187–1194.

Oro, A.S., and Dixon, S.D. (1987). Perinatal cocaine and methamphetamine exposure: Maternal and neonatal correlates. *Journal of Pediatrics 111,* 571–578.

Osterloh, J.D., and Lee, B.L. (1989). Urine drug screening in mothers and newborns. *American Journal of the Disabled Child 143,* 791–795.

Ostrea, E.M., Brady, M., Gause, S., Raymundo, A.L., and Stevens, M. (1992). Drug screening of newborns by meconium analysis: A large-scale, prospective, epidemiologic study. *Pediatrics 89*(1), 107–113.

Ostrea, E.M., Romero, A., and Yee, H. (1993). Adaptation of meconium drug test for mass screening. *Journal of Pediatrics 122,* 152–154.

Ostrea, E.M., Ostrea, A.R., and Simpson, P.M. (1997). Mortality within the first years in infants exposed to cocaine, opiate, or cannabinoid during gestation. *Pediatrics 100*(1), 74–83.

Parente, J.T., Gaines, B., and Lockridge, R. (1990). Substance abuse during pregnancy. *New York State Journal of Medicine 90,* 336–337.

Parker, B. (1993). Abuse of adolescents: What can we learn from pregnant teenagers. *AWOHNN: Clinical Issues in Perinatal and Women's Health Nursing 4,* 363–370.

Peacock, J., Cook, D., Carey, I., Jarvis, M., Bryant, A., Anderson, H., and Bland, J. (1998). Maternal cotinine level during pregnancy and birth weight for gestational age. *International Journal of Epidemiology 27,* 647–656.

Pegues, D.A., Engelgau, M.M., and Woernle, C.H. (1994). Prevalence of illicit drugs detected in the urine of women of childbearing age in Alabama public health clinics. *Public Health Reports 109*(4), 530–538.

Perkins, S., Belcher, J., and Livesay, J. (1997). A Canadian tertiary care center study of maternal and umbilical cord cotinine levels as markers of smoking during pregnancy: Relationship to neonatal effects. *Canadian Journal of Public Health 88*(4), 232–237.

Pettiti, D.B., and Coleman, C. (1990). Cocaine and the risk of low birth weight. *American Journal of Public Health 80*, 25–28.

Phibbs, C.S., Bateman, D.A., and Schwartz, R.M. (1991). The neonatal costs of maternal cocaine use. *Journal of the American Medical Association 266*(11), 1521–1526.

Plessinger, M.A. (1998). Prenatal exposure to amphetamines. *Obstetrics and Gynecology Clinics of North America 25*(1), 119–138.

Racine, A., Joyce, T., and Anderson, R. (1993). The association between prenatal care and birth weight among women exposed to cocaine and New York City. *Journal of the American Medical Association 270*(13), 1581–1586.

Rahdert, E.R. (ed.). (1996). *Treatment for Drug-Exposed Women and Their Children: Advances in Research Methodology.* Rockville, MD: National Institute in Drug Abuse.

Richardson, G.A., Day, N.L., and McGauhey, P. (1993). The impact of perinatal marijuana and cocaine use on the infant and child. *Clinical Obstetrics and Gynecology 36*, 302–318.

Richardson, G.A., and Day, N.L. (1994). Detriment effects of prenatal cocaine exposure: Illusion or reality? *Journal of the American Academy of Child and Adolescent Psychiatry 33*(1), 28–34.

Richardson, G.A., Day, N.L., and Goldschmidt, L. (1995). Prenatal alcohol, marijuana, and tobacco use: Infant mental and motor development. *Neurotoxicology and Teratology 17*(4), 479–487.

Richardson, G.A., Conroy, M.L., and Day, N.L. (1996). Prenatal cocaine exposure: Effects on the development of school-aged children. *Neurotoxicology and Teratology 18*(6), 627–634.

Robins, L.N., and Mills, J.L (1993). Effects of in utero Exposure to Street Drugs. *American Journal of Public Health 83* (Supplement), 1–32.

Russell, M. (1994). New assessment tools for drinking during pregnancy: T-ACE, TWEAK, and others. *Alcohol Health and Research World 18*, 55–61.

Ryan, R., Wagner, C., Schultz, J., Varley, J., DiPreta, J., Shrerer, D.M., Phelps, D.L., and Kwang, T. (1994). Meconium analysis for improved identification of infants exposed to cocaine in utero. *Journal of Pediatrics 125*(3), 435–440.

Schneider, J.W., and Hans, S.L. (1996). Effects of prenatal exposure to opioids on focused attention in toddlers during free play. *Journal of Development and Behavior in Pediatrics 17*(4), 240–247.

Seoane, A. (1997). Efficacy and safety of two new methods of rapid intravenous detoxification in heroin addicts previously treated without success. *British Journal of Psychiatry 171*, 340–345.

Shutzman, D.L., Frankenfiled-Chernicoff, M., Clatterbaugh, H.E., and Singer, J. (1991). Incidence of intrauterine cocaine exposure in a suburban setting. *Pediatrics 88*, 825–827.

Singer, L.T., Yamashita, T.S., Hawkins, S., Cairns, D., Baley, J., and Kliegman, R. (1994). Increased incidence of intraventricular hemorrhage and developmental delays in cocaine-exposed, very low birth weight infants. *Journal of Pediatrics 124*(5), 765–771.

Sokol, R.J., Martier, S.S., and Ager, J.J. (1989). The T-Ace questions: Practical prenatal detection of risk drinking. *American Journal of Obstetrics and Gynecology 160*, 863–870.

Soyseth, V., Kongerud, J., and Boe, J. (1995). Postnatal maternal smoking increases the prevalence of asthma but not of bronchial hyperresponsiveness or atopy in their children. *Chest 107*, 389–394.

Spence, M.R., Facog, R.W., DiGregario, G.J., Kirby-McDonnell, A., and Polansky, M. (1991). The relationship between recent cocaine use and pregnancy outcome. *Obstetrics and Gynecology 78*, 326–329.

Sprauve, M.E., Lindsay, M.K., Herbert, S., and Graves, W. (1997). Adverse perinatal outcomes in parturients who use crack cocaine. *Obstetrics and Gynecology 82*(5), 674–678.

Stinus, L. (1998). Continuous quantitative monitoring of spontaneous opiate withdrawal: Locomotion activity and sleep disorders. *Pharmacology Biochemical Behavior 59*(1), 83–89.

Stratton, K., Howe, C., and Battaglia, F. (eds.). (1996). *Fetal Alcohol Syndrome: Diagnosis, Epidemiology, Prevention, and Treatment.* Washington, DC: National Academy Press.

Substance Abuse and Mental Health Services Administration [SAMHSA]. (1997). *Substance Use Among Women in the United States.* Rockville, MD: National Clearing House for Alcohol and Drug Information.

Substance Abuse and Mental Health Services Administration [SAMHSA]. (1998). *Preliminary Results for the 1997 National Household Survey on Drug Abuse.* Rockville, MD: National Clearing House for Alcohol and Drug Information.

Turner, R.C., Lichstein, P.R., and Peden, J.G. (1989). Alcohol withdrawal syndrome: A review of pathophysiology, clinical presentation and treatment. *Journal of General Medicine 4,* 432.

U.S. Preventive Services Task Force. (1996). *Guide to Preventive Services.* (2nd ed.). Baltimore, MD: Williams and Wilkins.

Vaughn, A.T., Carzoli, R.P., Sanches-Ramos, L., Murphy, S., Khan, N., and Chiu, T (1993). Community-wide estimation of illicit drug use in delivering women: Prevalence, demographics, and associated risk factors. *Obstetrics and Gynecology 82*(1), 92–96.

Vega, W.A., Kolody, B., Hwang, J., and Noble, A. (1993). Prevalence and magnitude of perinatal substance exposures in California. *New England Journal of Medicine 329*(17), 850–854.

Vega, W.A., Kolody, B., Porter, P., and Noble, A. (1997). Effects of age on perinatal substance abuse among whites and African Americans. *American Journal of Drug and Alcohol Abuse 23,* 431–451.

Wang, D.S. (1998). Nalmefene: A long-acting opioid antagonist, clinical applications in emergency medicine. *Journal of Emergency Medicine 16*(3), 471–475.

Waterson, E.J., and Murray-Lyons, I.M. (1990). Preventing alcohol-related birth damage: A review. *Social Science Medicine 30*(3), 349–364.

Weimann, C.M., Berenson, A.B., and San Miguel, V.V. (1994). Tobacco, alcohol, and illicit drug use among pregnant women: Age and race/ethnic differences. *Journal of Reproductive Medicine 39,* 379.

Wheeler, S.F. (1993). Substance use during pregnancy. *Primary Care 20*(1), 191–207.

Windham, G., Von Behren, J., Fenster, L., Schaefer, C., and Swan, S. (1997). Moderate maternal alcohol consumption and the risk of spontaneous abortion. *Epidemiology 8,* 309–314.

Winecker, R.E., Goldberger, B.A., Tebbett, I., Eyler, F.D., Conlon, M., Wobie, K., Karlix, J., and Bertholf, R.L. (1997). Detection of cocaine and its metabolites in amniotic fluid and umbilical cord tissue. *Journal of Analytic Toxicology 21*(2), 97–104.

Wright, L., Thorp, J., Kuller, J., Shrewsbury, R., Ananth, C., and Hartmann, K. (1997). Transdermal nicotine replacement in pregnancy: Maternal pharmokinetics and fetal effects. *American Journal of Obstetrics and Gynecology 176,* 1090–1094.

Yamaguchi, K., and Kandel, D.B. (1984). Patterns of drug use from adolescents to young adulthood: III. Predictors of progression. *American Journal of Public Health 74,* 673–681.

Yawn, B.P., Thompson, L.R., Lupo, V.R., Googins, M.K., and Yawn, R.A. (1994). Prenatal drug use in Minneapolis-St. Paul, Minn. *Archives Family Medicine 3,* 520–527.

Zebaleta, I., Jhaveri, R.C., and Rosenfield, W. (1995). Maternal use of cocaine, methadone, heroin and alcohol: Comparison of neonatal effects. *Neonatal Intensive Care 8*(3), 40–43.

Zhang, J., and Ratcliffe, J.M. (1993). Paternal smoking and birthweight in Shanghai. *American Journal of Public Health 83*(2), 207–210.

Zuckerman, B., Frank, D.A., Hanson, R., Amaro, H., Levenson, S., Kayne, H., Parker, S., Vinci, R., Aboagye, K., Fried, L.E., Cabral, H., Timpieri, R., and Bauchner, H. (1989). Effects of maternal marijuana and cocaine use on fetal growth. *New England Journal of Medicine 320,* 762–768.

10

Mental Health and Substance-Related Health Care

Madeline A. Naegle, RN, PhD, CS, FAAN

LEARNER OUTCOMES

On completion of this chapter, the learner will be able to:

1. Analyze commonly occurring substance abuse problems for mental health implications.
2. Develop evidence-based strategies for advanced practice nursing interventions with substance-related problems in the context of mental health care delivery.
3. Use principles of consultation in addressing problems of substance abuse encountered in primary care settings.
4. Determine relationships between psychiatric and substance abuse disorders in human responses, including dual diagnoses.
5. Implement appropriate advanced practice nursing interventions for the prevention of relapse.
6. Implement evidence-based interventions that promote recovery from mental health problems, including substance abuse and dependence.

KEY TERMS

antagonists	cross-tolerance	motivational interviewing
at risk	dual diagnoses	opiate substitution therapy
biopsychosocial perspective	harm reduction	primary mental health care
case management		

The belief in the complexity of human and environmental systems underlies the biopsychosocial perspective that shapes the current practice of psychiatric–mental health nursing. A **biopsychosocial perspective** connotes that psychiatric–mental health nursing theory derives from biological, cultural, environmental, psychological, and sociological sciences as well as nursing science.

A contemporary view of psychiatric–mental health nursing articulated by Haber and Billings (1995) incorporates the notion that mental health care, while traditionally considered a specialty beyond primary care, includes a primary care component that is often overlooked. The Institute of Medicine Committee (1994) defines primary care as the provision of integrated, accessible health care services by clinicians who are accountable for addressing the majority of personal health care needs, developing a sustained partnership with clients, and practicing in the context of family and community.

Primary mental health care addresses basic mental health needs through primary prevention of emotional and mental disorders, inclusive of substance abuse disorders. Using the primary care components of the mental health specialty, the nurse addresses the majority of personal health care needs through direct care provision and referral. Haber and Billings (1995) note that although psychiatric–mental health nursing has been a specialized area of nursing practice that employs theories of human behavior and purposeful use of self as its art, the primary care components of the role have been less frequently emphasized. Continuous and comprehensive primary mental health care includes the *prevention* and *treatment* of mental illness, *health maintenance,* and *rehabilitation.* It begins at or before the first point of contact with the mental health care delivery system (Bellak, 1976) and targets well populations, populations **at risk,** and individuals with disorders along the continuum of mental illness.

Primary care interventions are directed at well populations and include culturally congruent activities such as parenting education and school-based programs for building and promoting self-esteem. Selective preventive interventions are also used for populations at risk and include activities such as prevention of human immunodeficiency virus (HIV) in drug users, elder support groups, respite for caregivers, and bereavement counseling. All of these activities are equally useful in the care of clients and families who use, or may develop problems using, alcohol and other drugs.

Advanced practice psychiatric nurses (APPNs) are newly emphasizing the biological links to mental health and addiction. Not only has recent research elucidated new biological factors that influence mental-emotional illness and addiction, but consumer groups have demanded clear definitions of such diseases as biologically as well as behaviorally based. Neuroscience research that supports brain dysfunction in the diagnosis and treatment of psychiatric disorders is now widely acknowledged as necessary to the knowledge base.

Advanced Practice Psychiatric Nurses

Although advanced practice nurses (APNs) in all specialties need to be able to identify substance-related health problems, recognize their associated mental health symptoms and related nursing diagnoses, and refer clients and families to appropriate specialists for treatment, advanced practice psychiatric–mental health nurses have expertise in this domain.

Advanced practice roles in psychiatric–mental health nursing include psychiatric–mental health clinical nurse specialist (CNS) and psychiatric–mental health nurse practitioner (NP). Moller and Haber (1996) present a strong argument for blending the two roles under the title *advanced practice psychiatric–mental health nurse*. Nurses in both these roles use expert psychiatric–mental health nursing knowledge to deliver direct care to acutely ill clients, families, and groups. They provide education, care, consultation, and research perspectives for colleagues, consumers, and organizations.

Master's-degree levels of knowledge about basic health problems are essential for greater understanding of the biological components of commonly occurring health problems in psychological and physical realms. Client care approaches reflect the nurse's abilities to ascertain the client's basic health needs, as well as assess and treat mental health needs. When there are significant medical symptoms, both the CNS and the psychiatric–mental health NP make appropriate referrals to an adult health NP or physician specialist. Talley (1997) provides excellent examples of primary mental health care services that these nurses are prepared to address. These include:

- Maintenance of the medical health care record in the mental health treatment record
- Provision of selected lifetime health screening and health education in mental health settings (e.g., drug and alcohol history, blood pressure and cholesterol screening, weight checks, and education about mammography, resources for family planning, Papanicolaou [Pap] smears, and HIV and acquired immunodeficiency syndrome [AIDS])
- Evaluation of health care risks and problems secondary to psychiatric illnesses or psychopharmacologic interventions (e.g., diabetes insipidus, agranulocytosis, tardive dyskinesia, or hypothyroidism)
- Monitoring before drug treatment, during drug treatment, and during drug discontinuation as well as monitoring the laboratory and medical procedures needed to ensure safe psychopharmacological interventions

Psychiatric–mental health APNs who implement these new roles work primarily in ambulatory care; are highly autonomous; deliver care through treatment modalities formerly the domains of psychiatrists, social workers, and others; and provide mental health teaching, education, and consultation to schools, social agencies, and service centers. Nurses are often the client's first contact with the health care delivery system and can assume responsibility for continuing care. In the new primary mental health role, care necessarily includes identification, management, and referral of health problems coexisting with acute or chronic mental and substance-related illnesses and requires the use of knowledge derived from generalist and specialist preparation.

APNs implement interventions and professional role responsibilities congruent with *A Statement on Psychiatric Mental Health Clinical Nursing Practice and Standards of Psychiatric-Mental Health Clinical Nursing Practice* (American Nurses' Association, 1994) and *Standards of Addictions Nursing Practice with Selected Diagnoses and Criteria* (ANA, 1988). Direct interventions in psychiatric–mental health nursing at basic and advanced practice levels include counseling, crisis intervention, health teaching, milieu therapy, **case management,** and psychobiological interventions such as biologic assessment (including laboratory tests). Psychobiological interventions at the basic level include interpretation and implementation of prescriptions; at the advanced level, the nurse may have prescribing privileges in accord with legal statutes governing NPs in the state of practice and collaborative physician and institutional agreements and protocols.

Although nurses at both the basic and advanced practice levels function as client advocates, are involved in professional organizations, and take community-level action based on health policy, it is the APN who most clearly embodies the change agent role and assumes leadership responsibility in collaboration with intra- and interdisciplinary colleagues (Chambers, Dangel, Tripodi, and Jaeger, 1987). Nurses at generalist and advanced practice levels must use education in culturally diverse traditions, knowledge of variations among racial and ethnic groups in manifestations of health and illness, and understanding of differences in sexual preference and lifestyles to individualize care delivery. In the care of clients with substance-related problems, the nurse needs to know the specific beliefs and traditions about the use of natural and prescription drugs and alcohol; trends that vary by race, ethnicity, and gender grouping; and the needs of minority populations, such as elderly addicts and members of gay and lesbian communities. The integration of some level of primary care into psychiatric–mental health nursing practice creates a more holistic model of care for clients whose ability to attend to their own physical and mental health needs is compromised (Talley and Caverly, 1994). Given the high prevalence of physical health problems in psychiatric populations, the expansion to general care provision is especially important (Worley, Drago, and Hadley, 1990).

Professional trends emphasizing quality care, consumer advocacy, and accountability all support greater independence of practice in the psychiatric nursing role. Trends have moved psychiatric nursing away from institution-based interventions, with a focus on pathology, to nursing roles addressing mental health needs along a continuum. Roles such as *direct care provider, case manager, consultant and collaborator,* and *interdisciplinary team member* are implemented in settings that include hospitals but that also increasingly include community agencies, clinics, and long-term residences.

Direct Care Provider

The advanced practice psychiatric–mental health nurse implements the role of direct care provider for individuals, groups, and families manifesting complex problems in the community. In the climate of managed care, psychiatric hospitalization is reserved for individuals experiencing acute illness states, those with complex diagnostic profiles, and those requiring pharmacologic management, as well as individuals who are a danger to themselves and/or others. Most clients in need of secondary and tertiary psychiatric care live in the community in group homes, in halfway houses, with families, in therapeutic communities, or in single-room occupancies. Depending on the region, a significant number are homeless and sporadically seek care in general medical and psychiatric settings. Many can be maintained in these settings through crises and require hospitalization only during acute exacerbations of illness. These individuals have acute psychiatric illnesses, including **dual diagnoses** of substance abuse and exacerbations of severe and persistent mental illness. They require ongoing management of multiple diagnoses such as substance abuse, HIV, and associated psychiatric illness, as well as management of other coexisting medical conditions.

Like that of other APNs, the scope of practice of APPNs includes mental and basic health assessments; nursing diagnoses; treatment interventions, including medication prescription and monitoring; counseling and psychotherapy; and psychoeducational activities. The APPN is accountable for a caseload of clients (case management), collaborates with members of other disciplines, and is responsible for evaluating treatment outcomes. Examples of treatment settings that currently employ mental health nurses in the direct care provider role include psychiatric emergency rooms, social agencies that provide mental health care, mental health and substance abuse agencies that are expanding mental health services to include primary care, group homes for the severely and persistently mentally ill and developmentally disabled, day care settings, and centers for vocational rehabilitation counseling and client services.

Advanced practice psychiatric–mental health nurses need to be able to implement interventions with individuals with substance-related problems at the levels of primary, secondary, and tertiary care. These include substance abuse prevention activities and programs (see Chapter 8) and acute care for medical emergencies related to intoxication, overdose, withdrawal, and medical detoxification (see Chapter 7). In the role of direct care provider, the APN obtains a brief history of the use, type, amount, and frequency of all prescription, over-the-counter, and illicit drugs, tobacco, and alcohol. This type of data collection (Chapter 6) becomes part of the nursing and medical history and is a resource for anticipating health problems resulting from drug use or predicting potential problems in the presence of other coexisting conditions. For example, limited use of alcohol by the elderly woman in good health becomes important to the prevention of health problems when the client is placed on a medical regimen that includes antihypertensive drugs or is newly diagnosed with diabetes. If the data collected suggest frequent and/or heavy drug use, the nurse may use one of the screening tools described in Chapter 6 to ascertain the need, if any, for a referral to an addictions specialist.

All nurses need to know that the National Institute of Alcoholism and Alcohol Abuse has identified safe levels of alcohol consumption, that is, a level of consumption that (over time) is unlikely to be linked independently to health problems in healthy adults:

- Men: No more than two drinks daily or no more than three drinks per occasion
- Women: No more than one drink daily or no more than three drinks per occasion

The levels of alcohol consumption considered safe change when the individual suffers acute or chronic disease, is taking psychotherapeutic drugs or other medications, or is pregnant (a period when no alcohol consumption is the only guaranteed way to eliminate the potential for damage to the fetus).

CONSUMER EDUCATION AND RISK FACTORS

All APNs in the direct care provider role should have sufficient alcohol, tobacco, and other drug (ATOD) knowledge to counsel clients on constitutional factors and behaviors that place them at risk for health problems with alcohol and other drugs. Constitutional factors include (1) family histories positive for alcoholism, (2) personal history of drug dependence and/or drug abuse, and (3) an anxiety disorder or depression that is not formally treated but that provokes the use of a drug to alter mood. Behaviors that place the individual at risk include the use of illicit drugs that increases the risk for various illnesses, substance abuse, and possible addiction. Smoking marijuana, for example, poses risks similar to smoking tobacco as well as undetermined damage to the central nervous system (CNS). The use of drugs by inhalation and/or injection can result in organ damage, such as destruction of nasal mucosa, infection, exposure to the AIDS virus, and death. Social problems associated with the use of illicit drugs include risk of legal action and exposure to criminal activity with the potential for violence, injury, and homicide. The excessive use of alcohol can result in various types of accidents, including driving while intoxicated (DWI) or driving under the influence (DUI). Acts of engaging in unprotected sex or using prescription drugs that result in impaired thinking places the individual at risk for being sexually victimized or assaulted. Acute intoxication in an individual with little tolerance (a naïve drinker) can result in death. Polypharmacy in the elderly, for whom two-thirds of all drugs in this country are prescribed, places them at special risk when they are consumers of alcohol. Smoking tobacco and using chewing tobacco and snuff place individuals at risk for addiction and associated long-term health problems and death from malignancies. Facts about the risks of tobacco and all other drug use should be presented nonjudgmentally and accurately to clients.

Early Interventions

Some specialists working in drug abuse treatment advocate the use of the harm reduction model for existing drug use, which constitutes a form of secondary prevention. **Harm reduction** is based on the notion that substance use exists on a continuum of abstinence to problematic use or abuse and that reduction in the quantity/frequency of substance use can reduce the likelihood of negative consequences (Marlatt and Tapert, 1993). This approach seeks to more effectively engage and retain active substance users in treatment, works toward behavioral change in gradual and incremental steps, and recognizes alternatives to abstinence for people who are unwilling, unable, or unready to achieve abstinence (the most effective means of avoiding drug-related problems). Counseling for harm reduction is directed toward decreasing both the unhealthy circumstances of drug taking and the frequency and/or amount of drugs used.

APNs in the direct care provider role who do not specialize in addictions or psychiatric–mental health can perform early interventions in the forms of motivational interviewing and other brief interventions. **Motivational interviewing** (Miller and Rollnick, 1991) builds on the trans-theoretical model proposed by Prochaska and DiClemente (1992), which proposes that individuals move through a series of stages of change as they progress in modifying problem behaviors. The model identifies five separate stages:

1. The contemplation stage entails the individual's realizing that he or she has a problem and the feasibility and costs of changing that behavior.
2. As the individual progresses to the determination stage, a decision is made to take action and change.
3. Once the individual takes steps to change his or her behavior, the action stage begins and lasts 3 to 6 months.
4. After an individual negotiates the action stage, he or she passes to a stage of maintenance, or sustained change.
5. If these efforts fail, the individual relapses and the cycle begins again.

The goal of motivational interviewing is to "break down the client's denial" (Miller, 1989, p. 75) using empathic approaches and avoiding confrontation and argumentation. By supporting the client's belief that one can perform a particular behavior or accomplish a task (self-efficacy), both nurse and client adopt an optimistic attitude that change is possible.

Central to the motivational interviewing approach is beginning at the point where the client is in the change process. The goal is to help clients consider how much of a problem their drinking or drug use poses and how their drug use is affecting them positively and negatively. By noting the pros and cons, the clinician hopes to tip the decisional balance in the direction of decreasing or eliminating drug use. Motivation for change occurs when people perceive a discrepancy between where they are and where they want to be. Motivational interviewing is focused on increasing the client's attention to such discrepancies and reinforcing the client's belief about the ability to change. Presenting the client with laboratory data or other concrete measures of the impact of drug use on health (giving feedback), exploring the meaning of negative consequences related to drug use, and reviewing the individual's values and goals as they are affected by drug use (personal responsibility) can bring into clear focus discrepancies between aspirations and reality that the client has rationalized or denied. Raising the client's awareness assists in the development of discrepancies and, hence, increases the motivation for change.

APNs may also utilize a brief intervention in the form of counseling, which is built around core components that have been demonstrated to evoke change (Miller and Sanchez, 1993). Six elements are believed to induce positive change in people who consume excessive amounts of alcohol or who are problem drinkers; they are summarized in the acronym FRAMES (see Table 10-1).

Brief interventions can be conducted over brief periods (one to four weeks) or longer (one to six months) and have been found to be effective in initiating treatment and reducing long-term alcohol use, alcohol-related problems, and health consequences of drinking (Bien, Miller, and Tonigen, 1993). These interventions should be in the skill repertoire of all APNs. APPNs provide consultation and resources when these interventions used by colleagues indicate a need for referral to specialized treatment.

PSYCHOEDUCATION

Psychoeducation is another intervention conducted by APNs but done most frequently by APPNs. Psychoeducation is a "program of didactic and experiential learning offered in individual, group, or family contexts" directed toward educational and psychosocial goals (Williams, 1997, p. 142). Psychoeducation addresses a variety of needs and is essentially health teaching with a focus on psychological adjustment and care within the mental health/substance abuse field. Examples of psychoeducation interventions include education of the client and family (who are confronting a new mental health diagnosis) about the illness and its treatment; support and assistance offered to family caregivers of the client with psychiatric illness;

TABLE 10-1 FRAMES

- **F**eedback of personal risk or impairment
- Emphasis on personal **R**esponsibility for change
- Clear **A**dvice to change
- **M**enu of alternative change options
- Therapist **E**mpathy
- Facilitation of client **S**elf-efficacy or optimism

and support and education provided during long-term illness that requires lifestyle adjustment. This particular component is essential for the individual seeking recovery from a substance-related problem, as recovery is dependent on changing habits linked with drug use, ending friendships with heavy drug users, learning new ways to cope with stress, and mending work, family, and social relationships. Health teaching and psychoeducation overlap, inasmuch as care of psychiatric and substance-related problems should include attention to total health, which includes exercise, nutrition, sleep, elimination, and stress management.

Case Manager

The case manager role in substance abuse treatment may include elements of the direct care provider role or may be limited to case management functions. Case management focuses on meeting treatment outcomes related to an illness episode in a given period of time. Case management interventions are directed toward achieving positive outcomes of hospitalization early in illness to avoid less serious stages of illness, reducing length of stay, promoting higher functioning, improving self-care, and enhancing better access and use of medical services (Atkinson, 1996). Interventions include early recognition of medication side effects as well as early detection and intervention with relapse. As a case manager, the psychiatric–mental health nurse is responsible for coordinating care delivered to an assigned group of clients or to clients in his or her own caseload. Care is provided according to guidelines for diagnostic groups and standard-based protocols developed between the nurse and a collaborating physician or nurse colleague. It includes health teaching, psychoeducation, and health maintenance activities (Cohen and Cesta, 1994). As a case manager, the nurse focuses on stabilizing acute problems, seeking diagnostic clarification, establishing nursing diagnoses, and monitoring initiation of treatment. In addition, the nurse oversees the utilization of resources by determining the eligibility and reimbursement potential for a client in a specific program. The case manager also engages in follow-up and review of the client's care and progress. Psychiatric–mental health nurses are increasingly being employed in this role in drug and alcohol treatment facilities, by managed care companies for care of substance-related problems, and in acute care psychiatric facilities. Advanced practice nurses now function as case managers for the seriously and persistently mentally ill, with interventions directed toward improved self-care, earlier and less serious hospitalizations of reduced length, higher functioning, and improvement in obtaining and receiving medical services (Atkinson, 1996).

Consultant and Collaborator

The role of the psychiatric–mental health nurse as consultant is well described in *A Statement on Psychiatric-Mental Health Clinical Nursing Practice and Standards of Psychiatric-Mental Health Nursing Practice* (1994) and in *Standards of Addictions Nursing Practice with Selected Diagnoses and Criteria* (1987). As a consultant to other APNs, the APPN uses nursing theory, expert knowledge of substance abuse and mental health, and a broad base of biologic knowledge. An excellent example of this specialty is the use of psychiatric–mental health NPs in community-based clinics that treat the large numbers of individuals in the correctional system who have substance-related problems. Men and women arraigned in the community and evaluated for alternatives to incarceration have a prevalence of substance-related (56 percent) and/or mental health (42 percent) problems as well as being at risk for

HIV and other health problems (J.D. Fitzgerald, personal communication, July 12, 1998). The NP can implement assessment and screening that consider the basic health problems of the clients and can develop a nursing care plan that is congruent with the action ordered by the court (e.g., detoxification, community service with mental health follow-up, or psychiatric hospitalization).

Interdisciplinary Team Member

A comprehensive plan of action by the APPN involves collaboration with adult health NPs and/or physicians, social workers, or counselor coworkers. In primary care settings where individuals with mental health and substance abuse problems are seen but often undiagnosed or misdiagnosed, the nurse provides consultation for the provision of effective and appropriate mental health care.

Expansion of the Substance Abuse Knowledge Base

The APN requires an advanced level of understanding of the neurobiological aspects of addiction that have only recently been reported in the findings of basic science research. Although all findings are not definitive and there is much that remains unclear, some basic neurobiological mechanisms of addiction are described in the following paragraphs.

Drug Use and Mental Health

Substance-related illnesses constitute major mental health problems. Signs and symptoms of drug use, intoxication, and withdrawal derive from the action of various drugs on the parts of the CNS affected directly by the drug. By knowing the properties and actions of drugs, the nurse can better anticipate and respond to the behavior of the client under the influence of medications and/or drugs. All drugs of abuse act on the mesolimbic system of the brain and cause changes in mood, perception, cognition, and psychological state. The surge of dopamine in the nucleus accumbens caused by the action of a drug on the brain is the common denominator in animal responses to drug use. An additional phenomenon characterizing neurological responses to drug use is kindling. In withdrawal from selected drugs (e.g., cocaine and alcohol) and with some psychiatric illnesses, the severity of symptoms increases following repeated episodes of illness or drug withdrawal. Such exacerbations may be accounted for by a process called kindling. Kindling is a phenomenon in which weak electrical or chemical stimuli, which initially cause no overt behavioral change, result in behavioral effects such as seizures when kindling occurs repeatedly (Becker, 1999). Continuing research suggests that kindling may account for relapse by triggering conditioned withdrawal symptoms, particularly with alcohol.

The structural connections of the mesolimbic dopamine system make it the reward pathway in the ways it mediates drug action. Prolonged drug use changes the brain in fundamental and long-lasting ways. These changes are felt to be a major component of addiction;

they vary by individuals and drugs used. Adaptations occur at the neurotransmitter level, as in change in the amount of neurotransmitter released, change in the number of receptors activated, and change in the intracellular transduction signal machinery. Changes also occur in structural proteins, which affect the shape of cells, and in transcription factors, which regulate gene expression.

Neurobiological adaptations take place at many levels in the brain and along two major routes: (1) drug-associated learning, a process of reinforcement that occurs at the start of drug taking and continues through long-term use, wherein associations between drug taking and drug effects are formed in the brain (classical conditioning); and (2) direct effect of the drug on brain cells. These learning experiences are influenced by behavioral and social contexts.

Two main systems of the brain are involved in addiction: the locus caeruleus, which is a pigmented eminence in the superior angle of the floor of the brain, and the ventral tegmental area (VTA), which contains neurons that project to the nucleus accumbens. The locus caeruleus plays a central role in physical dependence on and withdrawal from opiates. The VTA is believed to be a major substrate of drug reinforcement because all drugs of abuse activate the release of dopamine. Neuroadaptations to all drugs take place at both the presynaptic and postsynaptic sites. When an individual takes drugs, certain changes precipitated in inhibitory and disinhibitory proteins at synaptic sites are believed to explain the differences between addicted and normal populations.

To some degree, research with animal models helps to explain the phenomena of craving and relapse. With repeated drug taking, the chemical balance of activating proteins is altered. Three events appear to cause relapse to drug-seeking behavior: stress, low doses of drugs of abuse, and drug-associated stimuli (condition cues). In each case, relapse into drug-seeking behaviors is associated with an increase in dopamine release in the nucleus accumbens (Self, 1997). Drugs that stimulate dopamine receptors D1 and D2 are known to induce relapse.

Specific drugs influence brain structures in different ways. Cocaine blocks the uptake of dopamine, increasing the amount of dopamine at the synapse. For opiate drugs and alcohol, there are multiple neurotransmitter systems and neurotransmitters involved in their reinforcing effects. The mesolimbic dopamine system is central. Opiate peptide systems (endorphins) also appear to function in reinforcement. Alcohol reacts with GABAnergic receptors, opioid peptides, dopamine serotonin, and glutamate. Nicotine, both neurochemically and pharmacologically, has been implicated in activating dopamine and opioid peptide systems, thereby influencing multiple sources of neurotransmitters (Koob, 1997).

Drug Abuse and Mental Health

Other ways in which drug use influences mental health derive from the intrapersonal, interpersonal, social, and legal consequences of abusive or excessive use. Self-concept and self-esteem, for example, are negatively impacted by social stigma, the lack of social and economic productivity, and the compulsion and dependence associated with drug use. Interpersonal relations in the workplace and at home are negatively influenced when drug use results in the misappropriation of financial resources, marital discord, domestic violence, and repeated problems with meeting interpersonal responsibilities and role expectations. *The Diagnostic and Statistical Manual of Mental Disorders, Fourth Edition* (DSM-IV), details diagnoses for acute and chronic states induced directly by substance use and links disturbances in other major bodily functions, such as the sexual response cycle, to substance use/misuse.

Alcohol, Tobacco, and Other Drug-Related Problems Addressed by Advanced Practice Nurses

Nurses in general care settings treat the largest number of health problems and illnesses because these result from the use of nicotine (primarily) and alcohol (secondarily), as well as the results of infections, vehicular accidents, firearms, sexual behavior, illicit drugs, diet/activity patterns, and toxic agents (SAMHSA, 1997a). Regarded for many years as an unhealthy habit, nicotine dependence is now classified as an addiction in DSM-IV; it has been found to be closely associated with the presence of psychiatric diagnoses (Madden et al., 1995). Alcohol accounts for 9.4 percent, or 100,000, of all deaths; illicit drug use accounts for 1.9 percent, or 20,000, of all deaths in the United States.

Mental health disorders afflict around 30 percent of the general population, and 4.7 percent experience both mental health and substance-related disorders. The coexistence of psychiatric disorders with substance use, abuse, and dependence poses complicated clinical problems that are encountered with increasing frequency in general care settings and the community. Co-occurring mental health problems that derive from substance use, abuse, and dependence include symptoms such as anxiety and depression, which are precipitated by use or withdrawal from a drug, mild to moderate depression, suicide attempts and completions, and post-traumatic stress disorder (30 percent to 59 percent) (Coffey et al., 1998; Najavits, Weiss, and Shaw, 1997). Substance use is often a factor in violence, child abuse, spousal abuse, and sexual assault and abuse, linking it directly with consequent mental health problems for both perpetrator and victim (Downs and Harrison, 1998; Walker, Scott, and Koppersmith, 1998). Similarly, traumatic life events may play an etiologic role in the development of substance-related problems; as high as 90 percent of men and women (Dansky et al., 1996) and 68 percent of women (Goldberg, 1995; Teets, 1995) treated for substance-related problems, for example, report childhood sexual abuse. Limited research findings suggest the presence of alcohol in 10 percent to 57 percent of incidents of marital violence, 13 percent of incidents of child abuse, and 32 percent to 54 percent of child molestation cases (Roizen, 1992). In rape cases, alcohol was found to be present in 13 percent to 50 percent of offenders and in 6 percent to 36 percent of victims. The interface of life experiences with trauma, substance abuse, and psychiatric disorders results in phenomena that are antecedent to substance abuse, that cooccur with substance abuse, and that are consequent to substance abuse.

The use of tobacco is widespread, with 75.3 percent of men and 66.1 percent of women reporting having ever used it (SAMHSA, 1997b). Although perhaps only 1 in 10 men and fewer women will become alcohol-dependent, initiation of use places the individual, depending on his or her constitutional characteristics, at risk for health problems. Of men reporting cigarette use, 31.2 percent report smoking in the last month, only slightly above the percentage of women engaging in the same activity (28.2 percent) (SAMHSA, 1997b). Of all substances used, tobacco correlates most closely with the development of cancers and respiratory and cardiac problems (U.S. Department of Health and Human Services, 1992). When tobacco and alcohol are both used, the incidence of these disorders expands significantly. Primary prevention of excessive alcohol and prescription drug use and the prevention of smoking and illicit drug use are activities that APNs can implement using basic principles that are broadly applicable to all drugs and to the use or misuse of prescription drugs.

Primary Prevention

Interventions and strategies that APNs can use by expanding their knowledge of substance-related syndromes and diagnoses fall into categories of primary, secondary, and tertiary prevention. Primary prevention approaches are described in detail in Chapter 6. Strategies for smoking cessation, which constitute a secondary prevention intervention, are also detailed in Chapter 6. In the role of direct care provider, the APN educates the client and family about the risks associated with both the initiation of drug use and the excessive use of alcohol and prescription drugs. The content of health teaching is determined by health status, including pregnancy, ages of the client and family members, and existing patterns of drug use in the nuclear and extended family. Health teaching evolves from an assessment of need for information, guidance, and interpretation of existing situations that compromise or support health. Education about the physical and psychological effects of drugs is particularly important because of the actions of drugs on the cognitive and emotional states of the individual. The psychological effects of drugs evolve from the chemical nature of the drug, the interaction of the drug with existing cognitive and mood states, and the basic personality of the individual user. The potential changes that occur with drug use serve as deterrents to use for many individuals but should be particular deterrents for women anticipating or planning pregnancy, persons suffering mental and emotional problems, families and individuals who highly value health, and elderly persons.

EXCESSIVE BEHAVIORS AS PSYCHOLOGICAL ADDICTIONS

Orford has discussed the similarities among alcoholism, drug dependence, compulsive gambling, excessive eating, and excessive sexuality (Orford, Oppenheimer, and Edwards, 1976). He notes the commonality among these behaviors in their potential for producing pleasure or, at least, providing relief from painful states. Although neurochemical mechanisms characteristic of drug dependence have not been demonstrated in relation to these excessive behaviors, many people regard them as addictions.

Gambling is perhaps the most widely recognized of these behaviors. Pathological gambling, identified in the DSM-IV, has as its defining characteristic persistent and recurrent maladaptive gambling that compromises, disrupts, or damages personal, family, or vocational pursuits (APA, 1994). It is estimated that as much as $586.5 billion was spent in legal gambling in the United States in 1996 (Pasternak, 1997), and pathological gambling is prevalent in 1 percent to 3 percent of the population in a gender ratio of 3 men to 1 woman (APA, 1994). Pathological gambling develops in four phases characterized by increasing activity and negative outcomes of the activity, such as increasing debt and involvement in criminal activity to obtain funds. Physiological changes accompany the high or euphoric state associated with gambling and include a physiological rush: sweaty palms, tachycardia, and a sense of anticipation (Lesieur and Rosenthal, 1991). Pathological gambling has been observed to begin following major life events, such as losses, and to be associated with childhood abuse, incarceration, and criminal activity. Problem gambling frequently coexists with other addictions (such as alcoholism), other drug abuse, overspending, eating disorders, and sexual addictions (Lesieur and Rosenthal, 1991). Associated health problems arise from exposure to environments with high levels of secondhand smoke and excessive noise. In addition, pathological gamblers report stress-related symptoms such as hypertension, gastrointestinal problems, headaches, and skin problems (Sibbald, 1997). Depression and suicide are also prevalent, with as many as 24 percent of study populations completing suicide (DeCaria et al., 1996). Treatment parallels that of the other addictions and includes psychoanalytic, cognitive, and pharmacologic therapies, as well as referrals to self-help.

Secondary Prevention

Secondary prevention is an important intervention for APNs when the client history indicates that the individual uses drugs and has experienced problems related to use such as respiratory illness, gastrointestinal problems, psychological and/or emotional problems, trauma secondary to vehicular or work-related accidents, or treatment for acute intoxication of withdrawal from a drug. The goal of secondary intervention is to arrest the progress of an addiction and to prevent negative health outcomes, such as disabilities, that are associated with continued use. For the APN unfamiliar with the management of substance-related problems, secondary prevention may begin with referral to a peer with specialist-level information or consultation with a peer or colleague familiar with the diagnosis of a substance-related problem.

The advanced practice role in mental health nursing also includes acute and long-term care of individuals who are abusing and/or dependent on substances. The APPN incorporates primary care skills together with a specialty focus in the care provided. The nurse completes the history and physical examination, including the mental status exam and an assessment for ATOD use and abuse, formulates medical and nursing diagnoses, and develops a care plan in the form of care mapping and outcomes for the evaluation of interventions. When the APN lacks NP skills, a comprehensive profile, including diagnoses and related medical treatment, is assembled by obtaining information about the client's health status from the physician or NP primary care provider. This comprehensive approach is essential as psychiatric clients have a high prevalence of medical problems and limited access to primary care. They are also at specific risk for certain medical problems, such as skin problems related to environmental exposure while on psychotropic medications, trauma, and side effects of medications that disturb gastrointestinal function. Clients who abuse drugs have many associated medical problems related to the type of drug used, the route by which it is taken, and the length of time of the abuse or addiction. When individuals inject drugs, damage to the vascular system can be extensive and infections are frequent; individuals are also at risk for development of HIV and hepatitis A, B, and C. Excessive alcohol intake damages organ systems and results in nutritional and immunological compromise. The first line of secondary interventions, therefore, should address comprehensive health status and interventions that address the client's immediate health problems through the provision of direct care or referral to acute or ambulatory services.

The APPN plans nursing interventions based on the identification of health and drug-related problems and client readiness to address changes linked with interventions for health problems such as nutrition, weight control, exercise, and stress management that should be planned and implemented as appropriate. These draw on the APPN's advanced level of knowledge about health promotion.

Treatment Modalities for Substance Abuse and Dependence

Psychotherapeutic nursing interventions vary in their effectiveness with substance-abusing and -dependent individuals. Individual treatment, group counseling, psychotherapy, and family therapy modified in consideration of the addictive process, have all been used with some degree of success. Recent study findings suggest that cognitive-behavioral models and interpersonal approaches produce the most successful outcomes. Success is often determined by the extent to which the choice of treatment modality is made with the client's individual characteristics and treatment needs in mind, and when treatment maintains the drug-related problem as a central focus. Addressing individual needs is increasingly possible as recent research on approaches to care delivery to subpopulations of drug users continues to emerge. Groups who respond best to treatment that is individualized but that considers their shared characteristics are women, gay and lesbian persons, persons with disabilities, and the elderly. Approaches to family treatment are described in Chapter 11.

APPNs employed in in-patient settings, ambulatory care clinics, and community practice use a range of modalities that are found to be increasingly helpful with the substance-abusing client because of their evidence-supported efficacy and short-term nature. Psychodynamic models, such as ego psychological approaches, are used with modifications such as limit setting, contracts about drug use, and straightforward suggestions regarding efforts to achieve and maintain sobriety. One general consideration when implementing these modalities is that the talking psychotherapies are not effective when clients actively using drugs attend treatment sessions under the influence of a drug. Approaches directed toward achieving insight are most effective once sobriety is established. The best use of the client's cognitive capacities and potential for learning can then be brought to bear on goals for behavioral change.

In all forms of therapy, anxiety must be monitored closely because the uncovering of painful memories and conflicts of which the client was not previously conscious may provoke the client's return to drug use. Client denial of the severity of the drug-related problem is common and appears adaptive; confronting the losses, destructive acts, and damaged interpersonal relations that result from drug abuse has the potential to overwhelm the individual. It is with this in mind that the nurse works sensitively to build a trusting relationship, never ignoring the links between drug use and negative outcomes but maintaining a factual, nonjudgmental approach to the client's drug use patterns. Traditional strategies, such as empathy, limit setting, and role modeling, are key. Drug and alcohol abusers are generally ambivalent about seeking treatment and often only obtain treatment at the urging of family members or employers, thus making the establishment of a helping relationship difficult. Providers must attend to the importance of constancy, accessibility, and commitment, especially in the early stages of the relationship. Because slips and relapses are common, the nurse should establish a contract about how these will be dealt with, and assurance that the nurse will not abandon the client should these occur.

Models for individual counseling include supportive-expressive therapy (Center for Substance Abuse Treatment, 1997) and cognitive-behavioral therapy. Supportive-expressive therapy attempts to create safe and supportive therapeutic alliances. This approach is present-oriented rather than focused on past history or developmental issues; it seems to be most effective with substance-dependent individuals without dual diagnoses and limited psychopathology. Problem solving, confronting and handling of stresses of daily living, interpersonal relationships, and compliance with abstinence or controlled drinking are primary treatment themes.

The cognitive-behavioral model of treatment, originally developed as a structured, short-term, present-oriented psychotherapy for the treatment of depression, is used in individual or group therapy approaches (Beck, 1964). All forms of cognitive therapy are based on both a cognitive formulation of a specific disorder and its application to understanding the individual. Therapy is directed toward producing change in the individual's thinking and belief systems in order to bring about emotional and behavioral change (Beck, 1995). In treatment of drug abuse, the primary goal of this model is the mastery of skills that help to maintain total abstinence from alcohol and all nonprescribed psychoactive drugs. These skills may include the management of feelings; awareness of negative thinking; handling of criticism and negative moods; assertiveness training; improved interpersonal relations and communication; expansion of the social network; coping with triggers, cravings, and urges to use drugs; problem solving; drink/drug refusal skills; planning for emergencies; and coping with relapse. The development of job skills and marital or family involvement may also be addressed. This approach requires active participation; clients are expected to complete homework and engage in behavioral rehearsal and other activities.

TREATMENT SETTINGS

The choice of treatment settings is determined by the acute nature of alcohol and/or drug dependence, as described in Chapter 7. The need for in-patient treatment is generally indicated when the individual (APA, 1995):

- Is in severe overdose or respiratory coma
- Has severe withdrawal symptoms and a history of delirium tremens
- Has an acute, chronic medical condition that could complicate withdrawal
- Has marked psychiatric comorbidity and is a danger to self or others
- Has acute substance dependence and a history of nonresponse to less intensive forms of treatment

Additional factors may include lack of motivation and the inability to abstain from using because of environmental circumstances such as high accessibility of the drug or other users in the family.

Many general hospitals and most psychiatric hospitals have detoxification units; uncomplicated detoxification takes 3 to 5 days. Detoxification is considered a medical emergency, and clients generally comply with the recommendation. Continuation of treatment in a rehabilitation setting or acute psychiatric hospital, however, requires some motivation to change drug use habits and is voluntary. If the client is suicidal or homicidal, admission can be accomplished through two physician certificates or similar legal procedures. For the APPN, this can be done with the collaborating physician.

Nursing interventions in treatment settings are determined in protocols and by the credentials and preparation of the nurse. Increasingly, APPNs are being employed in psychiatric in-patient settings as well as alcohol and drug rehabilitation settings that introduce the client to rehabilitation based on the traditional 12-step model or the therapeutic community model. The Minnesota model of residential chemical dependency treatment incorporates a biopsychosocial disease model of addiction that focuses on abstinence as the primary goal and that uses the Alcoholics Anonymous (AA) 12-step model as a tool for recovery and relapse prevention. Originally, this model required 28 days of in-patient treatment followed by extensive community-based care. Newer models in both public and private sectors have modified the length of stay and combined medical and nursing care with 12-step approaches. Skilled chemical dependency counselors are members of teams of physicians, nurses, social workers, and psychologists, and all participate in a variety of behavioral, reality-oriented approaches. The nursing roles range from staff nurse to advanced practice nurse.

Outpatient treatment is provided in partial hospitalization or through a variety of approaches that vary in intensity from 9 hours weekly to 3 to 8 hours a day for 5 to 7 weeks (Center for Substance Abuse Treatment, 1997). Day, evening, and weekend programs provide group, marital, and individual therapy and counseling, pharmacotherapy as indicated, psychoeducation, and other services including vocational counseling and social services. Clients attending outpatient treatment should have appropriate social support networks including housing, transportation, and source of income. Outpatient treatment is most effective for individuals who have good social support networks, are highly motivated, and are employed or otherwise engaged in activities. Public and private facilities as well as practitioners in private practice offer resources for aftercare and follow-up (Institute of Medicine, 1994).

Methadone maintenance, or opioid substitution treatment for chronic heroin or opioid addicts, does not focus on abstinence but on rehabilitation and development of a productive lifestyle. Clients are required to appear daily for methadone distribution, and programs that have been observed to be most effective are those that combine group or individual counseling and social services with methadone maintenance.

Therapeutic community residential treatment is generally recommended for individuals with substance dependence and serious psychosocial adjustment problems. The community is a highly structured social setting designed to resocialize the addict through the maintenance of behavioral norms. Treatment is focused on changing negative behaviors through reality-oriented groups and individual therapy, intensive peer group encounters, and participation in a therapeutic milieu with hierarchical roles, responsibilities, and privileges. Daily work assignments and remedial or formal education are central to efforts to promote behavioral change, increase self-control, and build self-discipline. Clients must agree to minimum stays of 3 to 9 months of residential living and a gradual return to the community, through halfway houses and partial residence.

SELF-HELP

Recovery for substance-related disorders can occur through a variety of means including discontinuing drug use altogether without formal treatment and involvement in self-help. Most individuals, however, need assistance to terminate destructive drug use and to develop healthy lifestyles. Self-help is an important adjunct to formal treatment programs; it is recommended by health care providers and often incorporated into program activities. Self-help reinforces the client's responsibility to address recovery by recognizing the relationship of drug use to mental and physical health problems, as well as interpersonal, economic, and legal problems, and treating the illness of addiction. Self-help groups provide opportunities to solve problems with peer support and build self-esteem by personally taking charge of the recovery process.

Two self-help approaches have long been associated with addiction: AA and Narcotics Anonymous. Founded by men seeking to recover from addiction, they are based on 12 steps to recovery that form the framework for living a drug-free life by surrendering to a higher power and meeting together to discuss and support each other through their experiences with drugs (see Appendix IV). Al-Anon, an associated resource, is a fellowship of relatives and friends of alcoholics who share their experiences, strengths, and hopes. Nar-Anon and Gam-Anon function similarly. All of these organizations are supported by contributions and provide referrals to treatment and written materials about 12 step–based self-help programs. At any given time, there are about 2 million Americans active in AA, although membership is constantly rotating for many. Meetings are designed for participation in different levels of the program, which is totally self-supporting and anonymous. Sobriety is a goal for 12-step program involvement, but it is not a requirement for attendance at open meetings. Therefore, it is also a helpful resource for individuals who are unsure of the existence of an alcohol or other drug problem. Members abide by agreements to remain anonymous, and personal disclosures in closed meetings are respected. Additional self-help programs include Adult Children of Alcoholics (ACOA), Overeaters Anonymous, Gamblers Anonymous, and Recovery, the latter based on Abraham Lowe's self-help approach to mental health problems.

There are other self-help programs, including Rational Recovery, based on Albert Ellis's theory of rational emotive therapy and women for sobriety. Treatment interventions should always include information about self-help resources as well as information on local chapters, available meetings, and resources for family members.

Pharmacotherapeutic Interventions and the Advanced Practice Psychiatric–Mental Health Nurse

All APNs should know the actions, side effects, therapeutic outcomes, and dosing and administration of psychotropic drugs. APNs prepared as NPs will most likely also have prescribing privileges, as 78 percent of states now have some degree of prescriptive authority for APNs (Bailey and Snyder, 1995). Prescribing privileges expand the role of the nurse in treatment of all psychiatric and substance-related disorders, including intoxication, withdrawal, and detoxification from alcohol and other drugs. Protocols for acute care situations related to drugs are described in Chapter 7. APPNs with prescribing privileges need to know essential elements of biological psychiatry, including assessment of target symptoms, diagnosis, tests to prescreen and monitor client response to medications, and knowledge of each class of commonly used medications, psychotropic medications, and illicit drugs (Bailey and Snyder, 1995). The nurse should be familiar with the pharmacologic properties of alcohol, nicotine, and common drugs of abuse. The 15 basic principles of effective psychopharmacologic management delineated by the ANA (1994) provide excellent guidelines for the APPN:

1. Identify target symptoms.
2. Obtain a detailed history of illness and of past medications.
3. Screen for medical problems, organicity, substance abuse, and drug interactions.
4. Be clear about diagnosis.
5. Always talk to other treaters involved (past and present), and request past medical records.
6. Take the time and effort to form a therapeutic alliance with the client and (if permitted by the client and if appropriate) with family members, health care providers, or significant others who are invested in the client's well-being.
7. Concentrate on knowing well one or two drugs per class.
8. Administer a full trial with adequate doses and duration of treatment.
9. Keep regimens as simple as possible.

10. Be aware of different drugs' financial cost to the client.
11. Be aware of side effects, and warn clients of risks and benefits.
12. Know which adverse reactions require reassurance versus treatment or drug discontinuation, and know which ones may mimic treatment.
13. Learn to identify the client's unique signs of impending relapse; enlist family or significant other(s) to monitor the client's status.
14. Know and adhere to adequate standards of documentation, including informed consent.
15. When in doubt, seek a consultation and document.

Medications Used in the Treatment of Addiction

In addition to the psychiatric nursing modalities used in substance abuse treatment, the APPN incorporates the use of pharmacological approaches in care for the individual addicted to alcohol and other drugs. Most of the pharmacological approaches are recommended for use in conjunction with self-help and/or other types of treatment, with the exception of disulfiram, which has been helpful as the major intervention in chronic alcoholism. Prescribing considerations for clients with patterns of abuse or dependence on drugs require knowledge of the addictive potential of certain medications; the potential interactions with drugs of abuse (because abstinence is inconsistent, and recovery includes slips and relapses); and the extensive education about, and monitoring of, medications. The APPN should be familiar with the common drugs prescribed to directly treat the addiction, which include the drugs to decrease or impact craving and/or deter use **(antagonists),** and the drugs to treat psychiatric disorders that coexist with abuse or addiction, which include antianxiety, antipsychotic, and antidepressant medications.

Medications that assist in decreased craving for alcohol include calcium acetylchromotaurinate (acamprosate) and naltrexone (ReVia). Calcium acetylchromotaurinate is a synthetic drug recently introduced to alcoholism treatment in Europe and anticipated for future use in the United States. It is thought to act on several neurotransmitter networks to reduce the craving for alcohol in alcohol-dependent individuals who have been detoxified (Pelu et al., 1997; Poldrugo, 1997). Given three divided doses of 1.32 grams daily for 3 to 12 months, men and women show abstinence rates superior to individuals given placebos (Wilde and Wagstaff, 1997). When used in combination with disulfiram, this drug appears to be even more effective (Besson et al., 1998; Carroll et al., 1998).

ReVia is naltrexone in oral form. It reduces craving for alcohol by blocking its pleasurable effects by binding with opiate receptors that are dependent on alcohol. Clients who are alcohol-dependent and who are not abusers or users of opiates can be given the drug as soon as alcohol withdrawal has ceased. Initial dose is 25 mg (one-half tablet) once a day with a meal. If no side effects occur, the dose can be raised to 50 mg daily (Wesson, 1997). Clients who are abusers and committed to reducing their intake should have had abstinence time before beginning naltrexone treatment and do best when highly motivated to change drinking patterns. Naltrexone is also used to deter the use of opiates with highly motivated, drug-free opioid addicts to block the effects of street heroin or morphine derivatives. It has been used with some success with health professionals recovering from synthetic opioids and opioid derivatives use. Naltrexone keeps opioids from occupying receptor sites, thereby inhibiting their euphoric effects. The use of naltrexone is contraindicated for clients who:

- Have SGOT or SGPT levels greater than five times the upper normal limit
- Have acute hepatitis
- Are dependent on opiates
- Have stopped opioid use in the last two weeks
- May require intermittent opioid treatment for pain
- Are pregnant or trying to get pregnant

Disulfiram creates an aversion to alcohol consumption by producing unpleasant physical symptoms for 1 to 3 hours if alcohol is taken while the client is being medicated with this drug. Disulfiram blocks the metabolism of acetaldehyde, an intermediary in the oxidation of alcohol. Consuming alcohol within 12 hours of taking disulfiram results in facial flushing, intense vasodilatation of the face and neck, diaphoresis, tachycardia, and hyperpnea. Nausea and vomiting may follow in 30 to 65 minutes and may be so intense as to cause hypotension, dizziness, and syncope (Wesson, 1997); disulfiram has been known to lead to respiratory and cardiac collapse in unusual cases. Disulfiram therapy can be initiated after the client is free of alcohol for 4 to 5 days; the initial dose is 0.5 g orally once daily for 1 to 3 weeks. A maintenance dosage, 0.25 g to 0.50 g orally daily, can be adjusted individually. The client's willingness to adhere to medication routines and the education of the client and family are key to the successful use of disulfiram. Education should include the following areas:

- The need to take the prescribed dose and the need to have adequate hydration and nutrition
- The avoidance of all medications containing alcohol, such as tinctures and over-the-counter cold medications
- Signs and symptoms that will appear should the client ingest alcohol
- The importance of daily adherence to the prescribed dose

The use of disulfiram is contraindicated for clients experiencing the following (Wesson, 1997):

- Acute hepatitis
- Significant heart disease
- Pregnancy or desire for pregnancy
- Severe chronic lung disease or asthma
- Schizophrenia or manic-depressive illness (disulfiram may precipitate psychosis)
- Suicidal ideation or intent
- Allergy to rubber
- Jobs including handling of alcohol or solvents

Opiate substitution therapy remains the major pharmacological treatment for opioid addiction; it is predicated on the view of opiate dependence as a medical illness caused by opiate exposure through a variety of mechanisms. Opiate substitution therapy replaces illicit opioids with a prescribed medication that both prevents withdrawal symptoms from emerging and reduces craving. This therapy has been effective in reducing illicit opiate use and crime and enhancing social productivity as well as reducing the spread of viral diseases such as HIV and hepatitis (NIH, 1997). A drug-free state represents the optimum treatment goal, but research indicates that this state cannot be achieved or sustained by the majority of opiate addicts. The two leading substitution therapies are methadone and levo-alpha acetylmethadol (LAAM). LAAM is a longer-acting drug that can be taken three times weekly rather than daily (as for methadone). Dosage and prescribing recommendations are not yet fully available on this drug as it is not yet released for prescribing outside of federally sponsored programs.

Both methadone and LAAM dispensation are limited to federally controlled clinics and selected treatment providers; however, persons engaged in either of these therapies are frequently treated in medical and psychiatric settings by APNs. Methadone is the most frequently used agent in medically supervised opiate withdrawal and maintenance. The effectiveness of methadone is dependent on many factors, including adequate dosage, duration and continuity of treatment, and accompanying social services, which have been shown to increase the effectiveness of treatment. Stable employment is an excellent indicator of clinical outcome. The average methadone maintenance dose is 60 mg daily, but many clients require more (NIH, 1997). It has a half-life of 24 hours, and detoxification should be accomplished over several weeks. If detoxification is too rapid, abstinence symptoms are likely, prompting the individual to return to illicit drug use. This is especially relevant for emergency room treatment of opiate addicts.

Buprenorphine (Buprenex), a partial opioid agonist, is also effective in decreasing opioid dependence. Rapid detoxification, as in situations of opioid overdose, is accomplished with naltrexone, which blocks the cognitive and behavioral effects of opioids. When used with actively using opioid addicts, however, it produces immediate withdrawal symptoms with potentially serious side effects. Clonidine (Catapres) used in combination with naltrexone reduces many symptoms of withdrawal. Used in medically supervised in-patient and outpatient settings, this combination can accomplish methadone detoxification in 3 days. All APPNs should be aware of the indicators of rapid opioid and methadone withdrawal and should be prepared to serve as consultants to colleagues regarding opiate substitution therapy.

Interventions with Dual Diagnosis as an Example of Tertiary Intervention

With new medications providing an increase in psychopharmacologic options and the movement of clients to the community, contact with and care of clients who have dual diagnoses have increased for nurses in all specialties. The complexity of the interface among various diagnoses is challenging to providers, making the management of the dually diagnosed client an excellent example of advanced practice nursing activities. APNs in all specialties care for these clients, although it is generally necessary to seek consultation from an APPN or psychiatrist if an APN does not have mental health expertise.

Clients frequently have co-occurring conditions, in addition to those previously discussed in this chapter; they include mental retardation, physical disabilities, and conditions that affect learning, such as attention deficit disorders. These will not be addressed in this chapter, but resources to assist in their management are listed in Appendix V. The existence of substance abuse with other conditions is known as comorbidity; its presence complicates both treatment initiatives and prognosis. Individuals with severe and persistent mental illness who abuse or are dependent on alcohol and/or other drugs are a vulnerable population that manifests rates above that of the general population's for violence, reduced adherence to HIV regimens, accidents, and illnesses (Gournay, Sandford, Johnson, and Thornicroft, 1997). The term *dual diagnosis* is most widely used to refer to the coexistence of a psychiatric disorder and a diagnosis of an alcohol or other drug disorder (Ries, Mullen, and Cox, 1994). Although the prevalence of these coexisting disorders is estimated to be 39 percent over a lifetime in the general population, it is estimated that as high as 51 percent of individuals with serious mental illness are dependent on alcohol or illicit drugs (Kessler et al., 1996).

Comorbidity of alcohol use disorders and major depression is pervasive in the general population, with the association of alcohol dependence rather than alcohol abuse being more commonly associated with depression (Grant and Harford, 1995). The most common drug problems among the seriously and persistently mentally ill are linked to alcohol, the drug most frequently abused (Breakey, Calabrese, Rosenblatt, and Crum, 1998; Kirchner, Owen, Nordquist, and Fischer, 1998), as well as marijuana and cocaine abuse (Comtois, Reis, and Armstrong, 1994). The wide range of prevalence reported for dual diagnosis is attributed to the use of different criteria, various screening devices, and timing of assessment (Boyd and Hauenstein, 1997). Originally, dual diagnosis was applied only when the psychiatric diagnosis was a major one, such as schizophrenia and bipolar or unipolar depression. More recently, additional diagnoses, such as borderline personality and dissociative disorders, are being identified and discussed in relation to dual diagnoses (Kolodner and Frances, 1993). Substance-related diagnoses alone are more prevalent among men; recent population research suggests that the existence of alcoholism with other psychiatric disorders is more common among women. For example, 44 percent of men with alcoholism have a second diagnosis, whereas 65 percent of women do (Helzer and Pryzbeck, 1988). National surveys indicate that among those with a mental disorder and a substance abuse/dependence problem, men are most frequently diagnosed as having an antisocial personality disorder and women are more frequently diagnosed as suffering depression (Helzer and Pryzbeck, 1988).

As this population has many health-related problems, APNs in mental health and other specialties treat dually diagnosed clients in both institutional and ambulatory care settings (Gafoor and Rasool, 1998). Nursing care is enhanced by knowledge of the pharmacological action of drugs of abuse and the relationship between substance abuse/dependence and psychiatric disorders. Recognition of these co-occurring problems increases when the nurse knows the DSM-IV criteria for substance-related disorders and major psychiatric disorders. Methods described in Table 10-2 assist the clinician in evaluating the client with dual diagnoses.

In attempting to understand dual diagnosis, three relationships can be postulated between psychiatric and substance-induced symptoms (First and Gladis, 1993):

1. There is a primary psychiatric disorder resulting in a secondary substance use disorder.
2. There is a primary substance use disorder with resulting secondary psychiatric symptomatology.
3. Both the psychiatric symptomatology and substance use/abuse are primary and must be addressed with equal emphasis.

In each circumstance, psychiatric symptoms may be induced, exacerbated, or obscured by the use of one or more substances. Anthenelli and Schuckit (1994) suggest that the primary disorder is the symptom cluster that appeared first in the client's clinical history.

The existence of major psychiatric and substance abuse disorders creates a clinical picture that, although less frequent than singular disorders, poses challenges to both client and care provider. Individuals with both of these disorders often have poor clinical courses, are

TABLE 10-2 Methods of Assessment of Dual Diagnosis.

1. History, physical examination, and lab tests (e.g., liver tests, blood count for screening for STDs, HIV) to confirm medical indicators related to substance disorders and to rule out medical disorders with psychiatric presentations.

2. Substance use history and severity of consequences, including physical symptoms.

3. Mental status exam and severity of symptoms.

4. Interview with family members and assessment of family constellation to verify or determine accuracy of self-reported substance abuse and mental history and sequential development of illness and treatment.

5. Interviews with partners, other care providers, friends, and persons identified as significant to the client.

6. Review of records from other systems, medical, correctional, social, and previous mental health and substance abuse treatment.

7. Urine and blood toxicity screens; use of Breathalyzer to evaluate BAC p.r.n.

8. Revision of initial assessment by observation of the client in the clinical setting; full assessment of psychiatric problems may be delayed for up to six months.

9. Observation for the reappearance of psychiatric symptoms during periods of sobriety.

10. Assessment of client's motivation to seek treatment, desire to change behavior, and understanding of diagnosis.

Source: Modified from Faltz, B.G. (1998). Special care concerns for persons with dual diagnosis. In M.A. Boyd and M.A. Nihart (eds.), *Psychiatric Nursing: Contemporary Practice.* Philadelphia: Lippincott.

difficult to properly diagnose, are likely to need treatment that emphasizes both support and confrontation, require services that are typically provided in different sectors of the mental health system (Greenfield, Weiss, and Cohen, 1995), and show poor adherence to posthospitalization aftercare (Wolpe, Gorton, Serota, and Sanford, 1993). Study findings further suggest that dually diagnosed clients experience more severe symptomatology, more unstable living situations, and more treatment complications, including being more prone to relapse than individuals who do not have a concurrent psychiatric diagnosis (Drake and Wallach, 1989; Kay, Kalanthra, and Meinzer, 1989; Talbott, Bachrach, and Ross, 1986). They have poor short-term outcomes in traditional mental health programs and do not readily fit into traditional substance abuse programs (Noordsy, Schwab, Fox, and Drake, 1996).

Management of client care for dually diagnosed individuals requires the coordination of multiple social, medical, nursing, and rehabilitation services as well as ongoing contact among families, providers, and agencies. Therapeutic approaches that appear to be linked to the most favorable outcomes are those that include the use of coercive leverage to facilitate compliance with traditional approaches to care. The integrated approach, first introduced in 1984, differs from traditional substance abuse treatment programs in its less confrontational approach to denial and resistance and its acceptance and treatment of all symptoms (Sciacca, 1996). This approach to treatment blends elements of mental health and substance abuse treatment services; its care components include intensive case management, direct care provision, substance abuse treatment groups, and linkage with self-help groups in the community.

One approach to group treatment for persons with substance-related disorders and personality disorders describes the integration of the disease-recovery model and the cognitive-behavioral model and notes that each is effective for brief group therapy interventions, depending on whether treatment was occurring in in-patient or outpatient settings (Fischer and Bentley, 1996).

For the APPN case manager or nurse therapist, five components of models for outpatient treatment appear to support successful treatment (Carey, 1996):

1. Establishing a working alliance
2. Evaluating the cost/benefit ratio of continued substance use
3. Individualizing goals for changes in substance use
4. Building an environment and lifestyle supportive of abstinence
5. Anticipating and coping with crises

Establishing a trusting relationship can require many months or even years, yet it is the most essential step in the client's successful initiation and continuation of treatment. It serves to establish the nurse as a credible and sincere caretaker and delineates a safe environment that supports the client's expression of fears and his or her honest reporting of concerns and behavior. Cost/benefit ratio discussions are directed toward enhancing the client's motivation for change. By discussing the pros and cons of substance use, the decisional balance can be shifted to permit the client to acknowledge the negative outcomes of continuing use. Accurate information about the long- and short-term effects of substance use and their effects on cognitive and emotional function, as well as behavior, provides education and opportunities to discuss concerns. A supportive environment and a lifestyle supportive of abstinence are achieved through supporting client efforts and the coordination of environmental support in the family, the work setting, and religious or community groups. Involvement of the client's family and significant others must be negotiated with the individual, but the creation of a network is very helpful in resolving crises and acute illness episodes. Crises are frequent in the lives of dually diagnosed individuals and are precipitated by numerous biological, psychological, and social factors. These factors and their links to the client's life need to be explored in relapse prevention counseling, with efforts by the client and therapist directed toward anticipating responses to stressful situations.

Approaches to care need to be modified in consideration of the special needs of these clients for structure, monitoring, and close follow-up. Structure is an important element at all phases of treatment, but its importance is decreased as the client achieves long periods of abstinence from drug use and indicates motivation and behaviors for recovery (Comtois, Reis, and Armstrong, 1994). Studies indicate that an impasse in treatment often occurs when clinicians do not explore or share explanations or meanings that clients attribute to their problems (Kleinman, 1983). Findings suggest that consumers of psychiatric services have many ideas about their illnesses and how medications affect their symptoms. Clinicians are encouraged to listen to clients' explanatory models of distress rather than to try and impose a specific model of addiction treatment on them. This approach is also applied in dealing with clients' substance use. Rather than requiring and expecting that abstinence from drugs be a treatment goal, the therapist more realistically may work from a model of harm reduction in the early stages of treatment, modifying the goals as the client progresses (Carey, 1996).

Although it is generally assumed that abstinence from nonprescribed drugs is the safest outcome for psychiatrically ill substance users, this goal is realistically achieved over time. A plan developed collaboratively is suggested to help the abuser begin decreasing the amount and frequency of drug use, including increasing the number of sober days. Feelings of self-efficacy are central to changing behavior, so identifying and reinforcing successes is essential (Marlatt and Gordon, 1985). Self-help is viewed as an important adjunct to treatment of individuals with substance-related problems, but only a small percentage of individuals with severe mental illness attend self-help programs regularly, despite extensive efforts by care providers to create linkages (Noordsy, Schwab, Fox, and Drake, 1996). Vigorous efforts to promote self-help interventions seem to alienate clients; positive connections appear linked to clients' diagnoses and associated social skills (Samson, Simpson, and Tsuang, 1988). Noordsy and colleagues (1996) suggest the following four guidelines in relation to self-help:

1. Introduce self-help programs as one treatment option, and make other options available.
2. Help clients to sample self-help by accompanying them to meetings and easing social entry.
3. Promote independent function by treating the addiction, mental illness, and underlying social skills deficit aggressively.
4. Do not insist on self-help involvement, but reintroduce the option as treatment progresses.

Some consumers have found self-help groups very useful in recovery. One such resource is Double Trouble, a 12-step self-help group designed as a special forum in which dually diagnosed clients can discuss their psychiatric disabilities, medications, and substance use. Findings on the use of this model in the New York metropolitan area indicate that clients can discuss their dual recovery and that attendance and decreased use of substances are positive trends. Other helpful resources include clinician-run groups available to dually diagnosed individuals.

Problems with the use of psychotherapeutic medications still occur within the health care delivery system, as many health care providers still advocate total drug-free recovery. Such clashes in philosophy can confuse the client, who may require advocacy by the nurse provider to resolve concerns. Although the need for psychotherapeutic medication may be clear, prescribing medications for dually diagnosed clients should be undertaken with caution. It is important that an accurate differential diagnosis be made, which can be difficult. A second consideration is that the client who has abused drugs in the past may be inclined to combine medications with abused substances or take more than the prescribed dose, increasing the likelihood of accidental or intentional overdose (Center for Substance Abuse Treatment, 1997). Pharmacologic interventions that generally include the use of both psychotropic drugs specific to the mental health diagnosis and appropriate medications to address and support controlled drinking or abstinence from all drugs, appear to be most effective in individuals who are abusing rather than dependent on alcohol.

Medications with a high potential for the development of dependence should be avoided with dually diagnosed clients and persons with substance-related diagnoses. The largest group of psychotropic medications in this category is the benzodiazepines, which are usually prescribed for anxiety reactions and phobias. With frequent use, tolerance develops to the antianxiety effects of these drugs. In addition, cross-tolerance to other CNS depressants often develops. **Cross-tolerance** is defined as tolerance induced by repeated administration of one psychoactive substance that is manifested toward another substance to which the individual has been recently exposed (Steindler, 1994). When chemically dependent clients manifest anxiety disorders or sleep disturbances, it is recommended that benzodiazepines not be prescribed, that the client and family members be referred to 12-step programs, and that the therapist and client explore nonpharmacologic means of managing anxiety and insomnia (Dupont and Saylor, 1991). Other pharmacological options for the management of anxiety can also be explored. One alternative is buspirone (BuSpar), which carries a low potential for abuse and is not associated with withdrawal phenomena, sedation, and cognitive impairment. A 12-week regimen of buspirone (5 mg three times daily, increasing every 3 or 4 days to a maximum dose of 40 to 60 mg/day) can be prescribed (Kranzler et al., 1994).

A second group of psychotropic drugs is the sedative-hypnotics, which frequently includes barbiturates and benzodiazepines. Barbiturates are commonly used to induce anesthesia and muscle relaxation and to avoid seizures. The problems associated with their use include the rapid development of tolerance and the danger of overdose from CNS depression. Benzodiazepines are widely prescribed for insomnia and rapidly induce sedative effects that dissipate when the person no longer needs to sleep. Problems associated with using benzodiazepines as hypnotics include the development of tolerance, with resulting lack of therapeutic effect, and rebound insomnia, which occurs with termination of long-term treatment. These associated problems tend to support excessive use of the drug by clients and the development of dependence. Some tricyclic antidepressants have sedative properties and may be considered for use with the depressed individual who is abstaining from alcohol and suffering from insomnia.

Among clients diagnosed with anxiety disorders (up to 8 percent of this population, with more women [23 percent] than men [12 percent]), alcohol dependence or abuse is a common problem (Mirin and Weiss, 1991). As many as 25 percent to 45 percent of alcoholic clients are diagnosed with anxiety disorders (Chambless, Cherney, Caputo, and Rheinstein, 1987; Ross, Glazer, and Germanson, 1988). The relationships between anxiety and alcohol or depressant drug use are complex. Symptoms of anxiety are common and well documented in acute and protracted cases of withdrawal from alcohol and other depressant drugs; symptoms can persist for three to six months after abstinence has been achieved (Schuckit, 1990). Intoxication with stimulants such as cocaine or amphetamines can also produce marked symptoms and signs of anxiety. When anxiety is secondary to alcohol abuse/dependence or the use of other drugs, anxiety generally diminishes with abstinence. When anxiety disorders are identified before the onset of alcohol-related life problems or during an abstinence period of two to three months, it is likely that the client has two disorders. Psychotropic medications should be used minimally, although tricyclic antidepressants have demonstrated some success. Nonmedical efforts to manage anxiety, such as cognitive-behavioral approaches or supportive-expressive therapy, are recommended. Nursing techniques used with primary anxiety disorders include teaching clients anxiety management skills such as imagery and relaxation techniques and desensitization of stressors and triggers for anxiety. Clients with a primary anxiety disorder should be educated that alcohol or other drug use only worsens their symptomatology.

Mood disorders, including major depressive disorder, dysthymic disorder (particularly bipolar I and bipolar II disorders), and cyclothymic disorder, are among the common comorbid disorders in men and women. It is estimated that 32 percent of clients with mood disorders have comorbid substance abuse disorders and that 56 percent of individuals diagnosed with bipolar disorder have a substance abuse problem (Regier et al., 1990). When the co-occurring disorder is alcoholism, two factors contribute to frequent reports of depression: the depressant nature of alcohol on mood and the depressing effects of events associated with alcohol abuse and its effects on relationships, job performance, and legal problems. The depression produced by heavy and prolonged use of alcohol is generally alleviated with abstinence. The individual with a drug problem and a primary depression will manifest symptoms of depression during an abstinence phase following withdrawal from the drugs of abuse. Symptoms of depression that are drug-related, such as those seen in approximately 50 percent of cocaine abusers and in alcoholics, diminish with abstinence and a supportive treatment environment within two to four weeks (Anthenelli and Schuckit, 1994). Approximately 5 percent of men and 10 percent of women treated for alcoholism warrant the diagnosis of major depression after two to four weeks of abstinence.

Although suicide is often correlated with primary depression, the depressed feelings induced by substance dependence, coupled with the impaired judgment of the user, place substance abusers at high risk for successful suicide. Alcohol abuse is a factor in 25 percent of suicides, even among nonalcoholics, and substance abuse is believed to be a factor in 50 percent of successful suicides. A comprehensive suicide assessment should be part of the history and physical examination for all individuals with a substance-related problem. Suicide assessment consists of determining the following client information:

- History of previous suicide attempts; family history of suicide
- Current thoughts about self-harm and/or suicide
- Suicide intent and existence of a plan
- Lethality of means
- Availability of means to accomplish suicide

Treatment of depression coexisting with substance dependence or abuse depends on the primacy of depression versus its presence secondary to substance dependence. Effective outcomes can be achieved using psychotherapeutic models such as cognitive-behavioral therapy and individual or group interventions. Within the context of the therapeutic relationship, it is useful to develop a contract with the client about attempts of suicide. By discussing the risk openly and working with the client to achieve agreement about disclosure of suicidal thoughts to others, successful suicide can be averted. Depression, when it is primary, may require the use of antidepressants in the classes of serotonin-sensitive reuptake inhibitors, tricylic antidepressants, or monoamine oxidase inhibitors. Tricyclic antidepressants must be used with caution because their combination with alcohol or other depressant drugs often results in coma and death. Opiate dependence is also associated with high rates of depressive disorders; Anthetelli and Schuckit (1994) note that 50 percent to 70 percent of clients seeking treatment for opiate dependence have depression. Management of opiate dependence is often dependent on the client's successful use of a methadone maintenance program and/or movement into a therapeutic program directed toward abstinence. Antidepressants are sometimes used with this population when close monitoring of their drug use is possible.

Long-term or maintenance nursing care is essential for all clients with mental health diagnoses (Haber and Billings, 1995). It is a particularly challenging phase of care for dually diagnosed individuals because the rate of participation in aftercare is poor for this group. These clients frequently discontinue prescribed medications and return to the use of alcohol and illicit drugs, exacerbating symptoms and/or precipitating relapse. Factors that appear to influence nonadherence to aftercare regimens are numerous, and no one clear picture emerges (Pollack, Stuebben, Kouzekanani, and Krajewski, 1998). Some reasons cited by clients included poor support services, such as housing, employment, families, and transportation, which complicate attending sessions; the observation that alcohol decreases symptoms of the disorder; and denial of a substance-related problem, the psychiatric disorder, and the need for medication. Control and the wish to be normal often emerge as psychological themes. The best treatment outcomes have been observed to emerge from integrated substance abuse treatment/mental health programs characterized by systematic motivational interventions (Mercer-McFadden, Drake, Brown, and Fox, 1997). Mercer-McFadden and colleagues (1997) studied 13 integrated treatment programs nationwide that implemented approaches of integrated treatment, including engagement, persuasion/motivation, active treatment, and relapse prevention. Additional services were case management, outreach, and service planning/coordination. Retention rates ranged from 59 percent to 87 percent for up to one year (El-Mallakh, 1998).

Individualized approaches to care are recommended with advanced practice nursing approaches in programs and in independent practice. Psychoeducation about the nature of their mental health disorder and the effects of substance use on brain function can help to promote clients' self-understanding. When depression, schizophrenia, or bipolar disorders are explained as biochemical imbalances over which the client has little control, the guilt and stigma of such disorders may be reduced. Although clients may make the decision to use a mind-altering substance, for the dependent person, the decision to continue use after the first few tokes of marijuana or alcoholic drink is no longer a rational one. Simple explanations of the effects of chemicals on the brain, both therapeutic and recreational, must be included in the early phases of the nurse-client relationship.

Common patterns of recovery should also be discussed and explored with the client. Both substance dependence and psychiatric illness are chronic illnesses, characterized by relapse. Relapse prevention, then, is an important component of maintenance care. Lapses, defined as "falling back; a single mistake, an error" (Marlatt and Gordon, 1985), often occur as the individual considers a commitment to a recovery based on abstinence. Goals for treatment include preventing lapses, and preventing lapses from becoming relapses, that is, the return of full-blown symptoms of addiction. Relapse prevention, generally defined, is a collaborative process in which the client tries to identify and cope with difficult events, and the health care provider offers early intervention to reduce harm should a relapse occur (Carey, 1996). An assessment of client characteristics and the client's coping skills should be undertaken in the early days of recovery. Some individuals will have greater dispositions to relapse than others. Gorski (1988) identified these individuals as those with unstable or conflictual social situations; persons with stressful lifestyles or inadequate treatment resources; and those who exhibit symptoms that characterize the dually diagnosed client or person with psychiatric illness. Factors that often precipitate relapses are biological, psychological, and social. Biological factors that may trigger relapses include withdrawal symptoms, poor response to psychotherapeutic medications, and extreme physiological states captured in the acronym HALTS (Hungry, Angry, Lonely, Tired, or Sick) (Carey, 1996). Negative mood states are a frequent psychological factor in relapse, with the positive expectation that alcohol or a drug of abuse will change depressed or anxious feelings. Social factors include association with former friends and/or associates who are users, lack of support from friends or family, interpersonal conflict, or social occasions and holidays where alcohol and drug use has occurred in the past.

Tertiary or long-term care involves the full range of comprehensive health interventions by the direct provider, case management, and psychopharmacotherapeutic treatment and monitoring. Outreach and community follow-up are essential for these clients, who may cancel appointments or maintain infrequent therapeutic contact as a function of their ambivalence about treating either or both disorders. The APPN, whether direct provider or consultant to colleagues, must maintain a position of availability, client advocacy, and acceptance of the client's efforts at recovery.

Case Study

Mr. Malcolm T. is a 34-year-old single male of Native American and Chinese heritage. He is admitted to the partial care treatment program following a hospitalization of 10 days on the medical center's in-patient unit. Mr. T. was intoxicated with alcohol and marijuana on his admission to the in-patient unit and required detoxification with benzodiazepine therapy prior to medical and nursing assessment. Mr. T. had been living in a rooming house and has been on social assistance (SSI) since his last hospitalization 14 months ago. At that time, his parents, who reside in the same town, refused to allow him to live at home because of a previous arrest for driving while intoxicated and a police detention for purchasing marijuana. He received sentences of community service and mandated enrollment in a DWI program. He is currently unemployed, but until 6 weeks ago he worked weekends in a small grocery store as a cashier. He has completed high school and 2 years of community college. Mr. T. was first hospitalized at the age of 23; his symptoms at that time included grandiose delusions, hyperactivity, assaultive behavior, irritability, insomnia, and agitation. Since then he has experienced three additional hospitalizations lasting 10 days to 3 weeks, each of which was precipitated by his return to the use of marijuana or other illicit drugs. His initiation of illicit drug use and a pattern of regular alcohol consumption correspond to his gradual decline in taking the medications prescribed for him: lithium, paroxetine, and olanzapine. Following each hospitalization, Mr. T. was referred to a Nar-Anon group in his community but attended for only a few weeks and then dropped out. His attendance at the mental health clinic has been sporadic. Mr. T. was also diagnosed earlier this year with adult-onset asthma and obesity.

1. Using your knowledge of dual diagnosis, prioritize and outline the steps you would include in an advanced practice nursing assessment for Mr. T.
2. Identify areas needing further assessment about which you would gather additional information in formulating medical and nursing diagnoses and planning nursing interventions.
3. Analyze the correspondence between Mr. T.'s symptoms and findings derived from research on dual diagnosis. What data on evaluation and treatment should form the rationale for nurse–client interactions? For interdisciplinary team care?
4. Identify content areas and evaluation outcome criteria for health promotion for this client.
5. Discuss some therapeutic modalities that have been demonstrated to produce the best treatment outcomes with individuals with Mr. T.'s symptom profile.

CRITICAL THINKING QUESTIONS

1. Consider the need for expansion of the psychiatric–mental health nursing role. Identify four ways in which the traditional activities of the psychiatric–mental health nurse must change to better address substance-related illness.

2. The psychiatric–mental health advanced practice nurse is prepared to administer a range of therapeutic interpersonal interventions. What are some outcome measures appropriate to assess the client's behavioral change resulting from these interventions?

3. When the advanced practice psychiatric–mental health nurse is an expert in substance-related problems, consultation can be provided by the nurse to other health care providers. Describe three situations in which the APPN substance abuse expert may consult to improve management of client problems.

4. When the client manifests signs and symptoms of both a psychiatric disorder and a substance-related disorder, several principles can guide the clinician's decision making about client assessment. Discuss at least five principles that relate to the assessment of coexisting conditions.

5. The psychopharmacologic management of the client in recovery from substance dependence poses challenges for the APN in all specialties. What are some behavioral indicators of impending relapse that can be addressed with medicinal approaches? What are some indicators that the medications being prescribed are resulting in nontherapeutic responses? Discuss the components of psychopharmacologic assessment and ongoing monitoring of client behavior.

REFERENCES

American Nurses' Association. (1987). *Standards of Addictions Nursing Practice with Selected Diagnoses and Criteria*. Washington, DC: American Nurses' Association.

American Nurses' Association. (1994). *A Statement on Psychiatric-Mental Health Clinical Nursing Practice and Standards of Psychiatric-Mental Health Clinical Nursing Practice*. Washington, DC: American Nurses' Association.

American Nurses' Association Task Force on Psychopharmacology. (1994). *Psychiatric-Mental Health Nursing Psychopharmacology Project*. Washington, DC: American Nurses' Association.

American Psychiatric Association. (1994). *Diagnostic and Statistical Manual of Mental Disorders* (4th ed.). Washington, DC: American Psychiatric Association.

American Psychiatric Association. (1995). *Practice Guidelines for Treatment of Patients with Substance Use Disorders: Alcohol, Cocaine, Opioids*. Washington, DC: American Psychiatric Association.

Anthenelli, R.M., and Schuckit, A. (1994). Psychiatric disorders in the addicted patient. In *Principles of Addiction Medicine*. Chevy Chase, MD: American Society of Addiction Medicine.

Atkinson, M.M. (1996). Psychiatric clinical specialists as case managers for the seriously and persistently mentally ill. *Seminars in Nurse Management 4*(2), 130–136.

Bailey, K.P., and Snyder, M.E. (1995). The implementation of advanced practice psychiatric nurse prescriber: A comprehensive model. *Journal of the American Psychiatric Nurses Association 1*(6), 183–189.

Beck, A. (1964). Thinking and depression: II. Theory and therapy. *Archives of General Psychiatry 10*, 561–571.

Beck, J.S. (1995). *Cognitive Therapy: Basics and Beyond*. New York: Guilford Press.

Becker, H.C. (1999). Kindling in alcohol withdrawal. *Alcohol, Health and Research World 22*(1), 25–32.

Bellack, L. (1976). Geriatric psychiatry as comprehensive health care. In L. Bellak and T.B. Karasu (eds.), *Geriatric Psychiatry: A Handbook for Psychiatrists and Primary Care Physicians*. New York: Grune and Stratton.

Besson, J., Aeby, F., Kasa, A., Lehert, P., and Polgreiter, A. (1998). Combined efficacy of acamprosate and disulfiram in the treatment of alcoholism: A controlled study. *Alcoholism, Clinical and Experimental Research 22*(3), 573–579.

Bien, T.H., Miller, W.R., and Tonigen, J.S. (1993). Brief interventions for alcohol problems: A review. *Addiction 88,* 315–336.

Boyd, M.R. (1998). Substance abuse in rural women. *Nursing Connections 11*(2), 33–45.

Boyd, M., and Hauenstein, E.J. (1997). Psychiatric assessment and confirmation of dual disorders in rural substance abusing women. *Archives of Psychiatric Nursing 11*(4), 74–81.

Breakey, W.R., Calabrese, L., Rosenblatt, A., and Crum, R.M. (1998). Detecting alcohol use disorders in the severely mentally ill. *Community Mental Health Journal 34*(2), 165–174.

Carey, K. (1996). Substance use reduction in the context of outpatient psychiatric treatment: A collaborative, motivational, harm reduction approach. *Community Mental Health Journal 32*(3), 291–306.

Carroll, K.M., Nich, M., Boll, S.A., McCance, E., and Rounsaville, B.J. (1998). Treatment of cocaine and alcohol dependence with psychotherapy and disulfiram. *Addiction 93*(5), 713–727.

Center for Substance Abuse Treatment (1997). *A Guide to Substance Abuse Services for Primary Care Clinicians.* Rockville, MD: U.S. Department of Health and Human Services.

Chambers, J.K., Dangel, R.B., Tripodi, V., and Jaeger, C. (1987). Clinical nurse specialist collaboration: Development of a generic job description and standards of performance. *Journal of Clinical Nurse Specialists 1,* 124–127.

Chambless, D.L., Cherney, J., Caputo, G.C., and Rheinstein, N.J.G. (1987). Anxiety disorders and alcoholism: A study with inpatient alcoholics. *Journal of Anxiety Disorders 1,* 29–40.

Coffey, S., Dansky, B., Falsetti, S., Saladin, M., and Brady, K. (1998). Screening for PTSD in a substance abuse sample: Psychometric properties of a modified version of the PTSD Symptom Scale Self-Report. Post traumatic stress disorder. *Journal of Traumatic Stress 11*(2), 393–399.

Cohen, E., and Cesta, T. (1994). Case management in the acute care setting: A model for health care reform. *Journal of Case Management 3*(3), 110–116.

Comtois, K.A., Reis, R., and Armstrong, H.E. (1994). Case manager ratings of the clinical status of dually diagnosed outpatients. *Hospital and Community Psychiatry 45*(6), 568–573.

Dansky, B., Brady, K., Saladin, M., Killeen, T., Becker, S., and Roitzsch, J. (1996). Victimization and PTSD in individuals with substance use disorders: Gender and racial differences. *American Journal of Drug and Alcohol Abuse 22*(1), 75–93.

DeCaria, C.M., Hollander, E., Grossman, R., Wong, C.M., Mosovich, S.A., and Cherkasky, S. (1996). Diagnosis, neurobiology and treatment of pathological gambling. *Journal of Clinical Psychiatry 57*(Supplement 8), 80–84.

Downs, W.R., and Harrison, L. (1998). Childhood maltreatment and the risk of substance problems in later life. *Health and Social Care in the Community 6*(1), 35–46.

Drake, R.E., and Wallach, M.A. (1989). Substance abuse among the chronic mentally ill. *Hospital and Community Psychiatry 40,* 1041–1045.

Dupont, R.L., and Saylor, K.E. (1991). Sedative/hypnotics and benzodiazepines. In R.J. Frances and S.I. Miller (eds), *Clinical Textbook of Addictive Disorders.* New York: Guilford Press.

El-Mallakh, P. (1998). Treatment models for clients with co-occurring addictive and mental disorders. *Archives of Psychiatric Nursing 12*(2), 71–80.

First, M.B., and Gladis, M.M. (1993). Diagnosis and differential diagnosis of psychiatric and substance use disorders. In J. Solomon, S. Zimberg, and E. Shollar (eds.), *Dual Diagnosis: Evaluation, Treatment, Training and Program Development.* New York: Plenum Press.

Fischer, M.S., and Bentley, K.J. (1996). Two group therapy models for clients with dual diagnoses of substance abuse and personality disorder. *Psychiatric Services 47*(11), 1244–1249.

Gafoor, M., and Rasool, G.H. (1998). The co-existence of psychiatric disorders and substance misuse: Working with dual diagnosis patients. *Journal of Advanced Nursing 27*(3), 497–502.

Goldberg, M.E. (1995). Substance abusing women: False stereotypes and real needs. *Social Work 40*(960), 789–798.

Gorski, T.T. (1988). *The Staying Sober Workbook Exercise Manual.* Independence, MO: Independence Press.

Gournay, K., Sandford, T., Johnson, S., and Thornicroft, G. (1997). Dual diagnosis of severe mental health problems and substance abuse/dependence: A major priority for mental health nursing. *Journal of Psychiatric and Mental Health Nursing 4*(2), 89–95.

Grant, B.F., and Harford, T.C. (1995). Co-morbidity between DSM-IV alcohol use disorders and major depression: Results of a national survey. *Drug and Alcohol Dependence 39*(3), 197–206.

Greenfield, S.F., Weiss, R.D., and Cohen, M. (1995). Substance abuse and the chronically mentally ill: A description of dual diagnosis treatment. *Community Mental Health Journal 31*(3), 265–277.

Haber, J., and Billings, C. (1995). Primary mental health care: A model for psychiatric–mental health nursing. *Journal of the American Psychiatric Nurses Association 1*(5), 154–163.

Helzer, J.E., and Pryzbeck, T. (1988). The co-occurrence of alcoholism with other psychiatric disorders in the general population and its impact on treatment. *Journal of Studies on Alcohol 43,* 219–224.

Institute of Medicine. (1994). *Reducing Risks for Mental Disorders.* Washington, DC: National Academy of Medicine.

Kay, S.R., Kalanthra, M., and Meinzer, M.E. (1989). Diagnostic and behavioral characteristics of Psychiatric patients who abuse substances. *Hospital and Community Psychiatry 40,* 1062–1064.

Kessler, R.C., Nelson, C.B., McGonagle, K.A., Edlund, M.J., Frank, K.G., and Leaf, P.J. (1996). The epidemiology of co-occurring addictive and mental disorders: Implications for prevention and service utilization. *American Journal of Orthopsychiatry 66*(10), 17–31.

Kirchner, J.E., Owen, R.R., Nordquist, C., and Fischer, E.P. (1998). Diagnosis and management of substance abuse disorders among inpatients with schizophrenia. *Psychiatric Services 49*(1), 82–85.

Kleinman, A. (1983). The cultural meanings and social uses of illness. A role for medical anthropology and clinically oriented science in the development of primary care therapy and research. *Journal of Family Practice 16*(3), 539–545.

Kolodner, G., and Frances, R. (1993). Recognizing dissociative disorders in patients with chemical dependency. *Hospital and Community Psychiatry 44*(11), 1041–1043.

Koob, G. (1997). Neurochemical explanation for addiction. In W.D. Roberts (ed.), *New Understanding of Drug Addiction. Hospital Practice.* Minneapolis, MN: McGraw-Hill.

Kranzler, H.R., Burleson, J.A., Del Boca, F.K., Babor, T.K., Korner, P., Brown, J., and Bohn, M.J. (1994). Buspirone treatment of anxious alcoholics. *Archives of General Psychiatry 51,* 720–731.

Lesieur, H.R., and Rosenthal, R.J. (1991). Pathological gambling: A review of the literature. *Journal of Gambling Studies 7*(1), 5–39.

Madden, P.A., Heath, A.C., Starmer, G.A., Whitfield, J.B., and Martin, N.G. (1995). Alcohol sensitivity and smoking history in men and women. *Alcoholism, Clinical and Experimental Research 19*(5), 1111–1120.

Marlatt, G.A., and Gordon, J.R. (1985). *Relapse Prevention: Maintenance Strategies in the Treatment of Addictive Behaviors.* New York: Guilford Press.

Marlatt, G.A., and Tapert, S.F. (1993). Harm reduction: Reducing the risks of addictive behaviors. In J.S. Baer, G.A. Marlatt, and R.J. McMahon (eds.), *Addictive Behaviors Across the Life Span: Prevention, Treatment, and Policy Issues.* Newbury Park, CA: Sage.

Mercer-McFadden, C., Drake, R.E., Brown, N.B., and Fox, R.S. (1997). The community support program demonstrations of services for young adults with severe mental illness and substance use disorders. *Psychiatric Rehabilitation Journal 20*(3), 13–24.

Miller, W. (1989). Increasing motivation for change. In R.K. Hester and W.R. Miller (eds.), *Handbook of Alcoholism Treatment Approaches.* Boston, MA: Allyn and Bacon.

Miller, W., and Rollnick, S. (1991). *Motivational Interviewing: Preparing People to Change Addictive Behavior.* New York: Guilford Press.

Miller, W., and Sanchez, V.C. (1993). Motivating young adults for treatment and lifestyle change. In G. Howard (ed.), *Issues in Alcohol Use and Misuse in Young Adults*. South Bend, IN: Notre Dame University Press.

Mirin, S.M., and Weiss, R.D. (1991). Substance abuse and mental illness. In R.J. Frances and S.I. Miller (eds.), *Clinical textbook of Addictive Disorders*. New York: Guilford Press.

Moller, M., and Haber, J. Advanced practice psychiatric nursing: The need for a blended role. *Online Journal of Issues in Nursing*, August 1, 1996.

Najavits, L.M., Weiss, R.D., and Shaw, S.R. (1997). The link between substance abuse and posttraumatic stress disorder in women. *American Journal of Addictions 6*(4), 273–283.

National Institutes of Health. (1997). *Effective Medical Treatment of Opiate Addiction: NIH Consensus Statement*. Rockville, MD: U.S. Department of Health and Human Services.

Noordsy, D.L., Schwab, B., Fox, L., and Drake, R.E. (1996). The role of self-help programs in the rehabilitation of persons with severe mental illness and substance use disorders. *Community Mental Health Journal 32*(1), 71–81.

Orford, J., Oppenheimer, E., and Edwards, G. (1976). Abstinence or control: The outcome for excessive drinkers two years after consultation. *Behavior Research and Therapy 14*, 409–418.

Pasternak, A.V. (1997). Pathologic gambling: America's newest addiction? *American Family Physician 56*, 1293–1296.

Pelu, I., Verbanck, P., LeBon, O., Gavrilovic, M., Lion, K., and Lehert, P. (1997). Efficacy and safety of acamprosate in the treatment of detoxified alcohol dependent patients: A 90 day placebo-controlled dose-finding study. *British Journal of Psychiatry 171*, 73–77.

Poldrugo, F. (1997). Acamprosate treatment in a long-term community-based alcohol rehabilitation programme. *Addiction 93*(11), 1537–1546.

Pollack, L.E., Stuebben, G., Kouzekanani, K., and Krajewski, K. (1988). Aftercare compliance: Perceptions of people with dual diagnosis. *Substance Abuse 19*(1), 33–44.

Prochaska, J.O., and DiClemente, C.C. (1992). In search of how people change: Application to addictive behaviors. *American Psychologist 47*, 1102–1114.

Regier, D.A., Farmer, M.E., Rae, D.S., Locke, B.Z., Keith, S.J., Judd, L.L., Goodwin, F.X. (1990). Co-morbidity of mental disorders with alcohol and other drug abuse. *Journal of the American Medical Association 264*, 3511–3518.

Ries, R., Mullen, M., and Cox, G. (1994). Symptom severity and utilization of treatment resources among dually diagnosed inpatients. *Hospital and Community Psychiatry 45*(6), 562–568.

Roizen, J. (ed.) (1992). Issues in the epidemiology of alcohol and violence. In *Alcohol and Interpersonal Violence: Fostering Multidisciplinary Perspectives*. Rockville, MD: U.S. Department of Health and Human Services.

Ross, H.E., Glazer, F.B., and Germanson, T. (1988). The prevalence of psychiatric disorders in patients with alcohol and other drug problems. *Archives of General Psychiatry 45*, 1023–1031.

Samson, J.A., Simpson, J.C., and Tsuang, M.T. (1988). Outcome studies of schizoaffective disorders. *Schizophrenia Bulletin 14*, 542–554.

Sciacca, K. (1996). Letter to the editor. *American Journal of Orthopsychiatry 66*(3).

Schuckit, M.A. (1990). Populations genetically at high risk of developing alcohol abuse or dependence. *Current Opinion in Psychiatry 3*(3), 375–379.

Self, D.W. (1997). Neurobiological adaptations to drug use. In W.D. Roberts (ed.), *New Understanding of Drug Addiction. Hospital Practice*. Minneapolis, MN: McGraw-Hill.

Sibbald, B. (1997). Gambling can be hazardous to your health. *Canadian Nurse 93*(4), 24–25.

Steindler, E. (1994). Addiction terminology. In *Topics in Addiction Medicine*. Chevy Chase, MD: American Society of Addiction Medicine.

Substance Abuse and Mental Health Services Administration (SAMHSA). (1997a). *National Household Survey on Drug Abuse: Main Findings 1995*. Rockville, MD: U.S. Department of Health and Human Services.

Substance Abuse and Mental Health Services Administration (SAMHSA). (1997b). *National Household Survey on Drug Abuse: Population Estimates 1997*. Rockville, MD: Author.

Talbott, J.A., Bachrach, L., and Ross, L. (1986). Non-compliance and mental health systems. *Psychiatric Annals 16*, 596–599.

Talley, S. (1997). Physical diagnoses for advanced psychiatric nurse practitioners: Part I: Assessment and differential diagnosis. *Journal of the American Psychiatric Nurses Association 3*(5), 146–154.

Talley, S., and Caverly, S. (1994). Advanced practice psychiatric nursing and health care reform. *Hospital and Community Psychiatry 45*, 545–547.

Teets, J.M. (1995). Childhood sexual trauma and chemically dependent women. *Journal of Psychoactive Drugs 27*(3), 231–238.

U.S. Department of Health and Human Services. (1992). *Healthy People 2000: National Health Promotion and Disease Prevention Objectives*. Washington, DC: USDHHS.

Walker, G.C., Scott, P.S., and Koppersmith, G. (1998). The impact of child sexual abuse on addiction severity: An analysis of trauma processing. *Journal of Psychosocial Nursing and Mental Health Services 36*(3), 8–10, 40–41.

Wesson, D. (1997). Appendix A: Pharmacotherapy. In E. Sullivan and M. Fleming (eds.), *A Guide to Substance Abuse Services for Primary Clinicians*. Rockville, MD: U.S. Department of Health and Human Services.

Wilde, M.I., and Wagstaff, A.J. (1997). Acamprosate: A review of its pharmacology and clinical potential in the management of alcohol dependence after detoxification. *Drugs 53*(6), 1038–1053.

Williams, C.A. (1997). Psychoeducation. In N. Worley (ed.), *Mental Health Nursing in the Community*. St. Louis, MO: Mosby-Yearbook.

Wolpe, P.R., Gorton, G., Serota, R., and Sanford, B. (1993). Predicting compliance of dual diagnosis inpatients with aftercare treatment. *Hospital and Community Psychiatry 44*, 45–49.

Worley, N., Drago, L., and Hadley, T. (1990). Improving the physical health-mental health interface for the chronically mentally ill: Could nurse managers make a difference? *Archives of General Psychiatry 4*, 108–113.

11

Management of Substance Abuse and Dependence Problems in Families

Judith Haber, PhD, APRN, CS, FAAN

LEARNER OUTCOMES

On completion of this chapter, the learner will be able to:

1. Discuss the impact of substance abuse on the family system.
2. Compare and contrast biological, psychosocial, cultural, and family frameworks as they relate to understanding substance abuse.
3. Complete a family assessment for a family with a substance abuse problem.
4. Analyze the impact of substance abuse on family interaction patterns and community relationships.
5. Differentiate among family treatment strategies used in specific phases of the substance abuse recovery process.

KEY TERMS

codependence	family projection process	setup
craving	genogram	societal regression
destruction	multigenerational transmission process	substitution
differentiation of self	parentified	tolerance
emotional cutoff	process addiction	triangles

All advanced practice nurses (APNs), whether clinical nurse specialists (CNSs), nurse practitioners (NPs), or certified registered nurse anesthetists (CRNAs), encounter individuals and families for whom substance abuse/dependence is an acute or recurring problem. Primary care, especially practices or clinics, or mental health settings are the most common clinical sites in which APNs are likely to need expert substance-related assessment, diagnosis, and management skills; however, acute care, including critical care and perioperative settings, also require similar expertise. Clients with substance abuse problems require treatment and/or referral for substance-related problems. This process often involves treatment, including referral to community resources, of more than the identified client in a particular family. Thus, it is extremely useful for APNs to conceptualize treatment of substance abuse problems from a family systems perspective.

The purpose of this chapter is to provide a resource for APNs in all specialties that supplies a knowledge base of substance-related issues encountered in working with families in primary, acute, mental health, specialty, and home care settings.

Epidemiology

Substance abuse is one of the top three public health problems in the United States. Approximately 18 million people have a substance-related problem of some type (Naegle, 1997). Historically, 70 percent of all alcoholics were estimated to be males. However, the number of known female alcoholics is rising; possibly 50 percent, or 6 million, of the alcoholics in the United States are women. Such health problems not only affect the person who abuses alcohol or other substances but impacts the lives of at least four to five other people, usually family members. For example, the problems of alcoholics potentially adversely affect the physical and mental health of approximately 30 million relatives and friends (NIDA, 1993). The costs of substance abuse for the individual, the family, and the society are evident in the high rates of drug- and/or alcohol-related automobile fatalities (implicated in 42 percent), child abuse cases (implicated in 67 percent), spouse abuse (implicated in 49 percent), and addicted newborns (11 percent to 22 percent of infants are born to mothers who have used drugs during pregnancy) (NIDA, 1994). In addition, absenteeism and accidents on the job resulting from the effects of alcohol and use of other drugs affect industry and business. It is estimated that the medical, psychological, and psychiatric costs of alcoholism alone drain at least $15 billion per year from corporate earnings, with total economic costs for individuals, families, and industries potentially reaching $166 billion annually (SAMHSA, 1994).

Theoretical Base of Substance Abuse/Dependence

Numerous factors contribute to the development of substance abuse/dependence. Several theories suggest that no single perspective is sufficient to explain the emergence of substance abuse in a family system. The most credible theories relate to biological, psychosocial, cultural, and family variables.

Biological Context

Biological explanations of substance abuse/dependence include genetic factors and neurotransmitter functioning, as well as craving (with its reward mechanisms).

GENETIC INFLUENCE

It is proposed that there is a genetic or familial predisposition to dependence and that although the substance of choice may vary from generation to generation, the pattern of substance abuse is evident. Findings of family, twin, and adoption studies, as well as genetic research, suggest that genetically determined traits, not a specific gene, decide the type of dependence an individual may develop. A commitment to this perspective highlights the belief that an individual is born with a genetically determined protection from or predisposition to dependence; however, the complex nature of the symptoms of dependence suggests that the genetic predisposition to alcohol is polygenetic and that the genes related to alcoholism (alcogens) are interactive and may exert influence across symptoms and subtypes (Crabbe and Goldman, 1992). Conclusive identification of biological genetic markers will facilitate early identification of the disease, diagnostic specificity of subtypes, matching of treatments to subtype specificity, and biochemical dysfunction such as neurotransmitter imbalance.

NEUROTRANSMITTER INFLUENCE

There is no definitive evidence related to familial inheritance of neurotransmitter functioning, but there are familial patterns of mood disorders and other psychiatric disorders that suggest multigenerational risk patterns for neurotransmitter dysfunction in families as one explanation predisposing individuals to substance abuse/dependence occurring over several generations (Frances and Miller, 1991; Stanton, 1999). The neurotransmitter model proposes that drugs stimulate, inhibit, or change the release or action of neurotransmitters in the brain. Neurotransmitters involved in dependence include norepinephrine, serotonin, dopamine, and acetylcholine. Normally, neurotransmitter function involves the release of neurotransmitters by presynaptic cells into the synaptic cleft where they exert specific effects on postsynaptic receptor sites, followed by reuptake into presynaptic cells or a breakdown of these neurotransmitters by enzymes (Harris, 1997).

Stimulant drugs such as cocaine and amphetamines produce an excitatory response by increasing the production of norepinephrine, serotonin, dopamine, and acetylcholine. Increased excitation of the central nervous system (CNS) produces psychological effects such as heightened energy, increased cognitive performance, and increased tolerance for pain. Increased amounts of the drug result in an overabundance of these neurotransmitters, accompanied by development of additional neurotransmitter receptor sites. If a decrease in the drug occurs, neurotransmitter levels decrease, causing understimulation of the CNS. Craving for the drug or withdrawal symptoms may then occur.

CRAVING

The three-phase model of **craving,** a desire to use substances at any time, proposed by Blum and Payne (1991) is one example of this multigenerational biological predisposition. The model consists of three phases: setup, substitution, and destruction. **Setup** refers to the genetic predisposition an individual has to dependence. Genetically predisposed individuals are believed to have a reduced supply of enkephalins or a reduced ability to release these neurotransmitters in the hypothalamus. A predisposed individual may have an increased number of opioid receptors and a reduced number of dopamine receptors in the nucleus accumbens (the reward center of the brain). Feelings of well-being are therefore reduced. The setup is that alcohol and other drugs cause dopamine release, thereby reversing the deficit and leading to strong feelings of well-being. Once alcohol rewards the brain receptors, **substitution** occurs, whereby alcohol and other drugs are substituted and cause a release of dopamine, temporarily causing an offset of the genetic dopamine deficiency. The **destruction** phase involves increased intake of the substance to achieve the desired CNS effects (**tolerance**). Damage to the reward center results in intensified craving. The chronic use of drugs, either alcohol or other substances, to satisfy craving also slows the rate of neurotransmitter production and release, resulting in withdrawal symptoms or tolerance.

Psychosocial Context

Alcohol and drug problems may be regarded as learned maladaptive behaviors developed in response to external stimuli such as involvement in a drug subculture or exposure to heavy alcohol use by family members. The underlying causes are less important than the immediate rewards experienced by the user, which are often delivered or expressed in a variety of ways. Positive reinforcement might be expressed as praise for "being able to hold your liquor" or being a "chip off the old block" like all the men in the family. It may also be reflected by the rewards of heightened affective expressiveness, escape or avoidance of negative feelings, indirect expression of anger, and rebellion.

When significant components of family system functioning are organized around alcohol and drug use, family members learn about the important role the substance plays in creating and reinforcing the family identity, providing a regulatory mechanism for handling internal and external conflicts via intoxication and highlighting an organizing focus for the enactment of family rituals. For example, rituals are the mechanisms by which important components of family identity, including alcoholism, are conveyed to family members. If alcoholism is an important component of these family rituals, the message to children growing up in such families presumably is that the continuance of family identity in subsequent generations can only be ensured if alcoholism is itself perpetuated (Steinglass, Bennett, Wolin, and Reiss, 1987). The underlying assumption is that, by choosing to continue the ritual pattern of one's family of origin, children, adolescents, and adults indicate that they have learned, incorporated, and accepted the underlying family identity that these rituals reflect. Failure to continue the same pattern of family behavior means that the lesson has never been learned, has somehow gotten lost, or has been deliberately rejected perhaps due to inadequate positive reinforcement or overwhelmingly negative reinforcement (Krestan and Bepko, 1989; Steinglass, Bennett, Wolin, and Reiss, 1987).

Cultural Context

The use and abuse of alcohol and other drugs in families vary with culture, race, and ethnicity (see Chapter 5). For example, the rankings of racial/ethnic subgroups with respect to past-year illicit drug use indicate a relatively high prevalence rate among Native Americans (20 percent), Mexicans (13 percent), Puerto Ricans (13 percent), and non-Hispanic blacks (13 percent). A relatively low prevalence rate of past-year illicit drug use was found among Asian/Pacific Islanders (6.5 percent), Caribbeans (7.6 percent), Central Americans (5.7 percent), and Cubans (8.3 percent). The prevalence rate was intermediate among South Americans, other Hispanics, and non-Hispanic whites. The rankings of racial/ethnic subgroups for heavy alcohol use and alcohol dependence differ among specific groups. Specifically, the prevalence of dependence on alcohol was relatively high among Native Americans (5.6 percent) and Mexicans (5.6 percent), and relatively low among Asian/Pacific Islanders (1.8 percent), Caribbeans (1.9 percent), and Cubans (0.9 percent), whereas the prevalence of heavy alcohol use was relatively high among non-Hispanic whites (5.3 percent) (USDHHS, 1993).

Cultural trends exist, but definitive cause-and-effect relationships between cultural and family variables are difficult to establish. Community-based ethnographic studies, cross-sectional surveys, and longitudinal research studies are needed to determine the extent of alcohol and other drug use and related social and health problems among and within various cultural, racial, and ethnic subgroups (Krestan and Bepko, 1998). Five research areas to be investigated might include (Krestan and Bepko, 1998):

1. The role of individual and family socioeconomic status
2. The role played by cultural values and factors
3. The role of religious affiliation and family attitudes toward drug use in determining drug use behavior in cultural, racial, and ethnic subgroups
4. The role of acculturation-related stress in the drug use of cultural, racial, and ethnic subgroups
5. The role of social support systems (family, religious, and friendship subsystems)

For example, in the Hispanic subculture, what is the effect of the value of factors such as "machismo," "respeto," "dignidad," and "confianza" on substance abuse? Consider the Irish culture and the effect of variables such as religion, gender, socioeconomic status, and familial patterns related to coping with and expressing feelings on the high prevalence of alcoholism (McGoldrick, Pearce, and Giordano, 1982).

Family Context

Bowen (1978) locates family process in a general systems theory framework that employs a biologic evolutionary approach to describe the dynamics of a family. Two fundamental principles underlie the theory: (1) A system is a fluid, ever-changing system; and (2) a change in one part of the system is followed by a corresponding change in other parts of the system. The family is viewed as a web of parts, or subsystems, that can be understood only as a whole that is more than and different from the sum of its parts. Bowen (1978) views the family as a multigenerational system characterized by patterns of emotional interaction. Eight interlocking concepts, all of which are summarized in Table 11-1, describe the emotional patterns and interactions of the family systems approach:

1. **Differentiation of self**
2. **Triangles**

TABLE 11-1 Family Systems Concepts

Concept	Definition	Example
Differentiation of self	The degree to which a person defines the self as being separate from others	When Terry's father was drinking, she could feel her mother's emotional upset even though it was never verbalized.
Triangles	A three-sided emotional configuration present in families that describes the relational patterns of interaction among families	Alcohol abuse created an issue triangle in the P. family that provided the organizing focus for the dysfunctional relationship patterns related to closeness, distance, and conflict.
Nuclear family emotional system	An emotional system in which what happens to one family member influences other family members of the system	The stability of the marital dyad in a family with an alcoholic family member can influence the degree to which the marriage is able to sustain the stress imposed on the family system by Michael's drinking. The fact that he and his brothers, all of whom abuse one substance or another, are all still in first marriages indicates the high family tolerance for this symptom.
Multigenerational transmission process	The process by which patterns of interaction are passed from generation to generation through family relationships	Alcoholism has been a pattern in three generations of males of the P. family on both the maternal and paternal sides.
Family projection process	A process through which parental undifferentiation is transmitted to one or more children and operates within a mother-father-child triangle	Mickey, the youngest of five children in the P. family, has been a temperamentally difficult child from birth and is identified as being the spitting image of his dad, who is an alcoholic. It is no surprise to the family when Mickey, at age 13, begins to fail in school and gets drunk every weekend.
Sibling position	The place or role one assumes or learns in a family, often established by birth order and gender	Robin's role as the parental child (the caretaker of her mother with multiple sclerosis) contributed to her role as caretaker of her alcoholic husband. It was an overfunctioning role with which she was familiar and comfortable.
Emotional cutoff	The process of becoming physically or emotionally separated or isolated from one's family of origin or of denying its importance; a dysfunctional response to fusional forces within a family	John P., the third oldest of the P. family children, vowed that he would leave the family home in New York, attend college in California, and never return to the East Coast. John, age 30, has never had a drink and has only returned home once (for his mother's funeral).
Societal regression	Emotional problems in families that are similar to emotional problems in society	An alcohol- and drug-abusing society negatively influences the stability of families, including specific families such as the P. family.

Source: Adapted from Bowen, M. (1976). Theory in practice of psychotherapy. In P. Guerin (ed.), *Family Therapy: Theory and Practice* (pp. 42–90). New York: Gardner Press.

3. Nuclear family emotional system
4. **Multigenerational transmission process**
5. **Family projection process**
6. Sibling position
7. **Emotional cutoff**
8. **Societal regression**

Family Assessment

Family assessment is a holistic, comprehensive process that involves evaluation of the structural, functional, and developmental aspects of a family system, as illustrated in Figure 11-1. Family assessment is a map of the family system over at least two generations, together with information relevant to the identified client's presenting problem. A family assessment is completed during the initial session(s) but is developed over time as family relationship and interaction patterns are examined. Family assessment provides a great deal of data for the therapist and is also therapeutic for family members who invariably discover information about each other that was not known before (Leach-McMahon, 1992; Pendagast and Sherman, 1977).

The six general purposes of family assessment are:
1. To collect data about structural aspects of the family system over at least two generations
2. To observe and collect data about family relationship and interaction patterns
3. To observe and collect data about the identified client or clients in relation to the family system as a whole
4. To identify functional and dysfunctional aspects of the family system
5. To formulate a working hypothesis(es) to explain the family's dysfunction
6. To assist the family in understanding the relationship and interaction patterns operating to generate and maintain problem behaviors by the family as a whole and by any individual family members

The Genogram

A **genogram** is a diagrammatic historical map of a family over two or more generations. The genogram illustrates internal and external family structure data, including family demographic information (see Figure 11-1). It is also a starting point for assessing family function. The genogram data are connected to the identified client's presenting problem when the therapist says, "The information I am asking you about will help me to understand how the problem you are describing developed." Preparing a genogram begins at the initial session with one or more family members. Universally recognized symbols that are used to note facts about a family are illustrated in Figure 11-2. The advantage of a genogram is that it visually organizes complex data, which then become a living map that is never complete. New information is uncovered and reviewed by the therapist and family as data collection continues and the family system evolves (Leach-McMahon, 1992). Organization of the

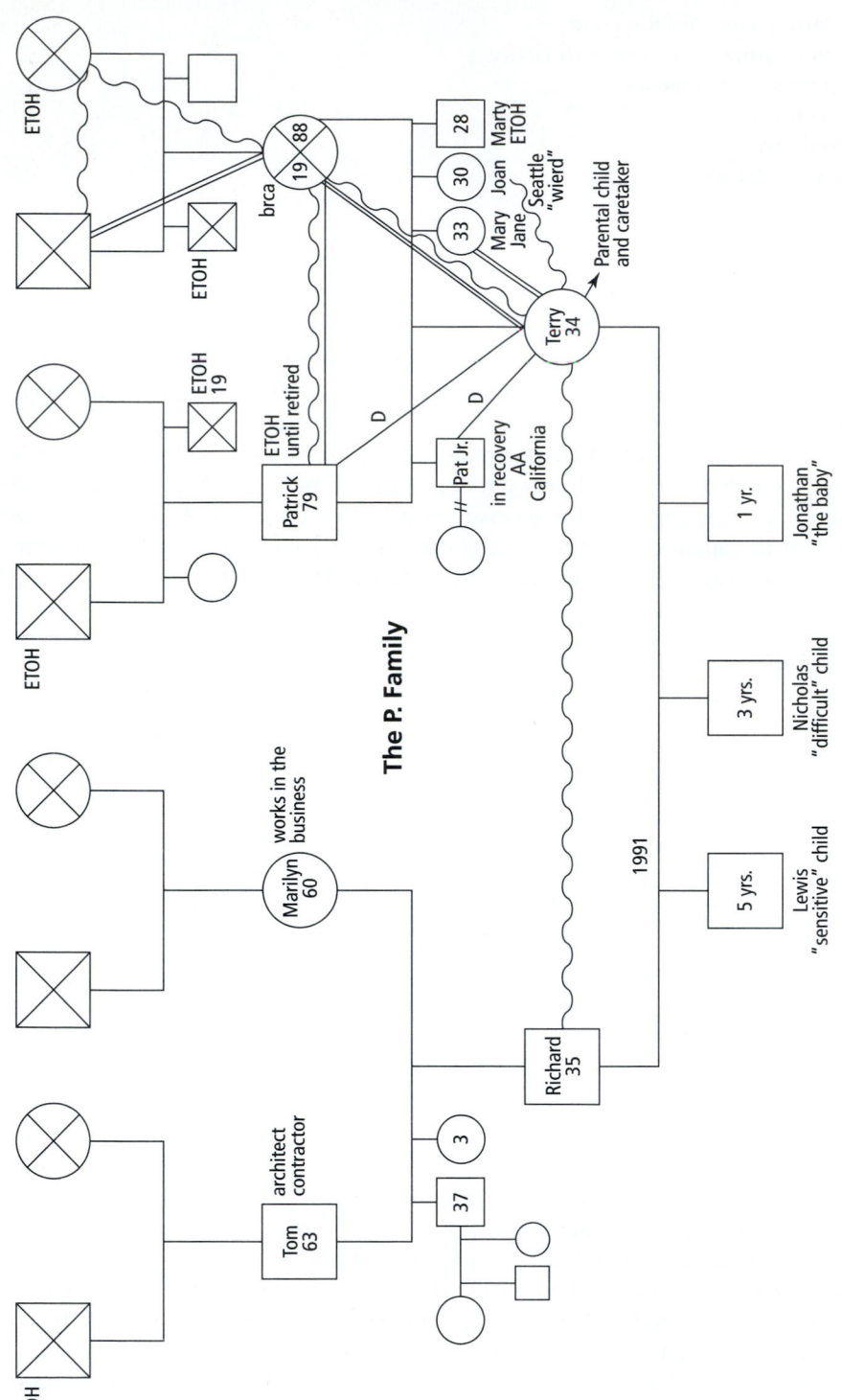

FIGURE 11-1 Components of a Genogram Family Assessment—The P. Family

*ETOH: Alcoholism or problem drinking is a factor for this individual.

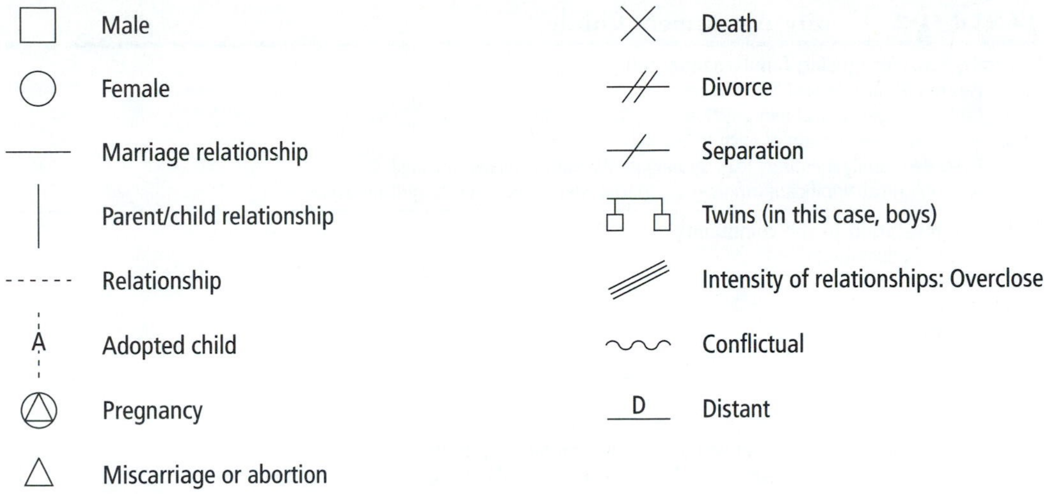

☐	Male	✕	Death
◯	Female	─//─	Divorce
────	Marriage relationship	─/─	Separation
│	Parent/child relationship	☐ ☐	Twins (in this case, boys)
- - - - - -	Relationship	⫽	Intensity of relationships: Overclose
A	Adopted child	∿∿∿	Conflictual
⟁	Pregnancy	_D_	Distant
△	Miscarriage or abortion		

FIGURE 11-2 Genogram Symbols

genogram in Figure 11-1 uses an example that illustrates multigenerational family patterns of alcoholism in the P. family.

The family assessment guide presented in Table 11-2 is a conceptual outline used to organize the data collection process to facilitate the systemic identification of internal and external family structural information (Pendagast and Sherman, 1977). The assessment questions are also designed to elicit data about multigenerational functional and dysfunctional developmental, communication, behavior, and relationship patterns. Questions related to the presenting problem of the family, such as alcohol or other drug abuse, are also included. Table 11-3 provides a set of assessment questions that can be used to appropriately assess alcoholism and to facilitate staging of treatment. Data about the presenting problem are often connected to family data that emerge in other areas of the family assessment.

Other assessment tools used to complete the comprehensive family assessment include screening tools such as the CAGE (Ewing, 1984), the brief MAST (Pokorny, Miller, and Kaplan, 1972), and the DAST (Skinner, 1982), which are discussed more extensively in Chapter 6. In addition, a complete history and physical (H&P), including blood and urine tests, are performed to expand or validate family assessment findings. Whether the H&P is completed by the APN or a physician, the findings are very important because comorbid physical health problems will be identified. Among the more common comorbidities associated with substance abuse are pancreatitis, cirrhosis, hypertension, nausea, vomiting, diarrhea, ulcers, tuberculosis, human immunodeficiency virus (HIV) positivity, malnutrition, stasis ulcers, abscesses, and dental caries.

Among the blood tests ordered are blood alcohol levels, liver function tests, hemoglobin and hematocrit levels, and HIV screening. Urine tests are more commonly ordered to detect the presence of drugs other than alcohol (see Chapter 6).

TABLE 11-2 Family Assessment Guide

A. Family structure (using family genogram)
1. Parents of nuclear family members
2. Children: ages and sibling position
3. Personality description of each individual
4. Extended family members (e.g., grandparents, aunts, uncles, cousins)
5. Nonbiological significant others (e.g., special friends, boyfriends, girlfriends)

B. Family in relation to the community
1. Level of education
2. Ethnicity
3. Religion
4. Socioeconomic status
5. Geographic location of family members

C. Presenting problem
1. Each family member's perception of the problem
2. Each family member's perception of his or her contribution to the problem
3. Each family member's perception of how he or she would like to see things change
4. Each family member's perception of the positive aspects of the family

D. Communication patterns
1. Who speaks to whom, when, and in what manner or tone
2. Emotional climate
3. Family themes and values
4. Manner in which anger and hostility are expressed
5. Frequency (e.g., daily, weekly, monthly, holidays only, annually) and type (letters, phone calls, tapes, videos, visits) of contact between family members
6. Conflict resolution style and skills
7. Triangles

E. Family roles
1. Family members who are supportive, antagonistic, critical, blaming, rescuers, victims, or codependent
2. Family coalitions, alliances, cutoffs, triangles, or pairings
3. Power structure
4. Nature of family boundaries (e.g., rigid, blurred, enmeshed, fused)
5. Each family member's feelings about his or her relationship with other members of the family

F. Family behavior patterns
1. Level of differentiation
2. Strengths
3. Coping style
4. Task allocation
5. Daily routine

G. Developmental history
1. Family's life cycle stage
2. Family's genealogy
   a. History of family of origin of each parent
   b. History of courtship of parents
   c. History of birth and rearing of each child in nuclear family
3. Developmental history of the presenting problem
   a. Early behavioral symptoms of the problem
   b. Persons involved in the problem
   c. Behavioral problems involved in the problem

H. Family's expectations of therapy

TABLE 11-3 Family Assessment of Alcoholism: Questions

1. In which life cycle stage is the individual who is drinking?

2. In which generation of the family is the individual who drinks (grandparent, parent, child), and in which life cycle stage in the family is this drinker affecting?

3. What is the multigenerational family pattern of alcohol use and/or abuse, and is there any other drug use or addiction by family members?

4. What is the time lapse between the onset of early warning signals of alcoholism and the presentation of the family for treatment?

5. How many life cycle phases have occurred since the drinking began, and how have the related life cycle issues been or not been resolved?

6. In which stage of alcoholism is the problem drinker?

7. In which phase of adjustment or adaptive response to drinking is the family (e.g., strained marital interaction, increasing social isolation of the family, over- and underfunctioning of family members)?

8. What are the key triangles within and across generations, especially those related to alcohol abuse (e.g., interlocking triangles of mothers-in-law and daughters-in-law concerned about alcoholic sons and husbands over two or more generations)?

9. Trace the projection process and examples of fusion triangles (e.g., codependencies, overfunctioning/underfunctioning patterns, marital conflicts, projections to a child) across three generations. Note defenses of choice in each member of the family, and observe how family members' defense mechanisms interface.

10. What are the maturational and situational cluster stress events that have occurred in each generation of this family? How do family members cope with stress (e.g., emotional cutoffs, projections to a child)?

11. What are the episodes of violence and/or incest in the three-generation family system?

12. Note patterns related to other addictions (e.g., shopping, gambling, spending, eating, work)

13. Is anybody in the family in recovery? Is anyone in treatment or self-help groups (e.g., AA, Al-Anon, Alateen, ACOA, GA, NA, OA)?

14. Identify problems with the extended family, community, employers, or the law.

15. Using psychometric scales, assess family members.

Impact of Substance Abuse/Dependence on Family Interaction Patterns

Alcohol or other substance abuse is a systemic process that affects and is affected by the interaction that occurs between the person who abuses alcohol or another drug, the drug itself, the person and the drug, and others such as colleagues, friends, and family members (Krestan and Bepko, 1989). The effects of substance abuse result in adaptive changes at all systemic levels and reflect an imbalance in the functioning in the total family system (Bowen, 1978). It is evident that there are interrelated alterations in management of feelings, role structures, communication, and need fulfillment within the family system.

Management of Feelings

Psychoactive drugs produce highly predictable effects that, over time, distort patterns of interpersonal feedback within the family system; as such, emotional processes are altered and emotional growth is thwarted. Denial and both the family projection process and the multi-generational transmission process are key defense mechanisms (Bowen, 1978). Emotional processes, especially those related to conflict and emotional intimacy, are repressed, suppressed, or denied so that they remain underground or are avoided. Family members are out of touch with their feelings. Distrust of inner self develops, and distress about the expression of feelings reduces initiation and use of resources for emotional problem solving. Difficulty experienced in accepting and integrating feelings leads to problems handling anger, which may result in the assumption of a victim position or inappropriate outbursts of anger.

Emotional bonds between family members as well as with others outside the family are frequently weak. Members of the nuclear family are often disconnected from extended family and from the larger community in which the family lives. In this context, the achievement of intimacy is difficult, emotionally charged issues are suppressed or avoided, and family secrets (e.g., addiction) are common. For example, sexuality is conflictual, especially when the system is "dry," making emotional expressiveness that much more difficult. Inhibited sexual desire is frequent (Steinglass, Bennett, Wolin, and Reiss, 1987). Similarly, death is a conflictual issue, and grieving may be thwarted through generations of unresolved losses. As such, emotional growth and development of the family system is disrupted. For example, Terry P. (see Figure 11-1) was unable to recognize and deal with unresolved grief about the loss of her mother from breast cancer until she addressed feelings of abandonment she felt in relation to her husband.

Within the family system, there is difficulty with emotional self-regulation. There are problems separating and integrating intellectual and emotional functioning, that is, family members are either highly rational ("dry") or highly emotional ("wet"). It is not uncommon, for example, that the excessive use of alcohol is tolerated in families because it is a vehicle that makes emotions more accessible to family members, thereby achieving greater proximity to intimacy that is so difficult to access when the family is "dry." Because emotional self-regulation and effective management of feelings are dysfunctional, limited integration of thoughts and feelings exists (Steinglass, Bennett, Wolin, and Reiss, 1987). Bowen (1978) suggests that the level of differentiation is low, which is manifested by the ineffective integration of thoughts and feelings. For example, emotional crises are common and reflect another vehicle that facilitates emotional expressiveness. In fact, family members may become addicted to emotional crises because crises are the only route to getting in touch with and expressing otherwise repressed or suppressed feelings.

Role Structures

Characteristic alterations in role structures and patterns, reflecting low levels of differentiation and fusion, are also evident in families with alcoholism and other drug dependence. Typically, there is a pattern of over- and underfunctioning, in which one partner or sibling overfunctions while the other underfunctions. For example, Robin H. had abused alcohol and benzodiazepines since she was 18 years old. Her daily episodes of intoxication created a level of dysfunction that precluded her, as the primary custodial parent, from fulfilling her parenting role. Her ex-husband, who lived down the street, would arrive at her house every morning prepared to get the children, ages 6 and 8, dressed, fed, and off to school if Robin was not fit to do so herself. He would return later in the day prepared to be in charge of dinner, homework, baths, and bedtime. He enabled her dysfunctional and underresponsible behavior with his overresponsible role assumptions rather than setting limits on it and seeking primary custody of the children himself.

Rigid role assumptions that reflect the multigenerational transmission process are also evident. Family members assume designated roles in the family system, roles from which they find it difficult to extricate themselves. Implicitly agreed-upon titles reflect special family role assignments. The family member as the hero, mascot, old faithful, prodigal son, or troublemaker enacts this role assignment that may be inherited from previous generations or that is passed on to future generations of same-gender and birth-order children. For example, Joseph B. III was the third generation of eldest-son children in the B. family, each of whom was an alcoholic "devil." The family story is that all eldest sons in this family had "devil" written into their destiny; as such, all proceeded to live up to their reputation and ensure that there was a "devil" in each generation. In contrast, wives and mothers of alcoholic husbands and sons often enact the role of "saint" or "angel."

Children of alcoholic parents are often **parentified,** that is, they act in an adult manner and perform an adult role out of phase with their chronological life cycle stage. For example, an eldest son might be inducted as an emotional spouse to his mother because of distance in the marital relationship, or a daughter might be inducted into the role of a mother who cooks, cleans, shops for food, and watches the younger brothers and sisters after school because her mother is high on heroin or crack (Krestan and Bepko, 1989).

Communication

Communication patterns are characteristically developed using triangular interaction patterns. Family members communicate through others, not directly. Alcohol or other drug abuse is frequently the third leg of the triangle, hindering intimacy (Bowen, 1978). As a result, communication is unclear, inconsistent, indirect, and closed. In Chuck D.'s family, his wife discussed his heavy drinking in an angry, resentful way with their eldest daughter, but not with Chuck. When Terry P.'s father did not show up at home after work, she and her mother would get in the car and anxiously drive from one suburban train station to another looking for him because he was having one of his spells. They would find him sleeping on a bench or wandering around a train station and would bring him home, telling the other children that their dad was having one of his forgetful spells again.

Often, a covert communication rule is that feelings are not to be shared and family dynamics are not to be discussed outside the family. For example, as Marty G.'s cocaine addiction escalated, his work performance became impaired; eventually his employment was terminated. The family maintained a pact of silence about this to the extent of doing their food shopping out of town in order to conceal the fact that they now used food stamps. This rule perpetuates the illusion of normalcy, maintains the use of denial and projection of blame, and enables families to support the status quo and resist change. For example, for 20 years, Paula B.'s parents (her father was a Lutheran church educator) denied that four of their seven children were alcoholics. The denial was facilitated by the fact that these four adult children lived in different states or countries from their parents and had distant relationships with them, visiting only infrequently.

Need Fulfillment

Rigid family rules inhibit emotional and social growth of family members. In Amy's family, emotions were considered dangerous because they were only expressed when her dad was drunk and likely to be explosive. The ensuing fights between her parents made the expression of feelings anxiety-provoking. As the adult child of an alcoholic (ACOA), Amy found herself re-creating the same patterns in peer and other intimate relationships, in which she avoided the disclosure of feelings, even in the absence of a realistic threat.

The reluctance to express feelings also may reduce the possibility of meeting age-specific emotional needs of family members. For example, parentification of a targeted child minimizes or precludes opportunities for him or her to receive age-appropriate nurturing or to engage in peer group socialization activities. Derek, whose alcoholic father was frequently out of work, was never able to participate in after-school athletics because he had to rush off to his two jobs that helped his mother make ends meet financially.

Boundary management problems are derived from dysfunctional need fulfillment issues. For example, there is a high percentage of ACOAs in the helping professions (e.g., nursing, medicine, social work, and psychology), professions that emphasize the needs of others and minimize self-care needs. The tendency to overextend the self and to have difficulty saying no facilitates a focus on others that is consistent with boundary management problems, as well as the related reduced introspection and desensitization to inner emotional cues. This may result in overwork, exhaustion, physical and emotional distress, lack of play and fun, and disconnection from the bodily and spiritual self.

This pattern is often described as one of **codependence,** in which there is physical, emotional, or social dependence on another person or object (Beattie, 1989; Mellody, 1989). The core manifestations of codependence include these areas of difficulty:

- Experiencing appropriate levels of self-esteem
- Setting functional boundaries
- Owning and expressing one's own reality
- Taking care of one's adult needs and wants
- Experiencing and expressing one's reality moderately

Codependence emerges from dysfunctionally nurturing and/or abusive family systems in which parenting practices tend to impair the growth and development of children who, as adults, are attracted to relationships that repeat the same dysfunctional patterns.

Other boundary management problems may include incest, which occurs because of boundary violations and reduced intergenerational boundaries that, in turn, reduce protective boundaries and heighten vulnerability. Incest is more likely to occur when the perpetrator is drunk or high. Debbie R.'s father only drank at night and on weekends. When drunk, he would enter her room at night, climb into her bed, and fondle her. In order to cope with the trauma of these episodes, she would dissociate her feelings and pretend that she was at an amusement park. Debbie was the recipient of the family projection process that served to bind the family's anxiety about the father's substance abuse and the parents' conflictual marriage. She was a nervous, high-strung, and shy child who had academic and social problems that provided a triangular organizing focus for the family and diverted their attention from the family's genuine problems. Profiles of incest survivors such as Debbie can also include eating disorders; self-medication; problems with anger, shame, low self-esteem, and intimacy; flashbacks; and hallucinatory-like voices. All of these can be reflected in a post-traumatic stress syndrome, even if the manifestations of these symptoms do not emerge until years later (Bradshaw, 1988, 1990).

Impact of Substance Abuse on the Family System and Community Relationships

Intergenerational patterns related to substance abuse are considered to be the foundation for those addictive behaviors most commonly noted to have a public or private impact on the community and society at large. For example, **process addictions,** those compulsive behaviors manifested in activity that act to bind and thereby reduce anxiety, include the following:

- *Workaholism*. Though socially sanctioned, workaholism may result from or lead to substance abuse that is embedded in stress-related physical or emotional illness. It ultimately creates annual workplace costs related to absenteeism, reduced productivity, and employee replacement and retraining expenses, as well as treatment and rehabilitation costs.
- *Gambling*. Gambling may or may not be comorbid with substance abuse; may be a way to emphasize intellectual manipulation and control; and seems common in high-energy, intelligent families. It results in social, economic, and legal problems.
- *Shopping, spending, and indebtedness*. Spending or indebtedness may be socially sanctioned in our credit card society, but it reflects a compulsive activity that binds anxiety or lifts depression. It may cause emotional processes to go underground to avoid dealing with feelings in a direct manner. Unfortunately, the financial impact on an individual or a family can be considerable. The results are widespread: The banking and credit card industry become involved in the situation with consolidation loans that provide fresh starts; the workplace becomes involved when salary liens occur; and the legal system becomes involved when shoplifting, embezzlement, or cashing of fraudulently signed or insufficient-balance checks are cashed to maintain the addiction.
- *Eating disorders*. Eating disorders are common in alcoholic families and may include obesity, anorexia, and bulimia. Intergenerational issues that involve being in control or out of control, having low self-esteem, and feeling shame impact the community in terms of the loss of workplace productivity and the health care treatment costs.
- *Sexual addictions*. Sexual addictions have corresponding disturbances in relationships that may be private or public. Early stages may begin with compulsive masturbation, pornography, or extramarital affairs; shame about the activity may indicate an addictive process. Middle stages often include exhibitionism or voyeurism, and late stages may include sexual abuse of others. The extent to which this behavior pattern impacts the community (e.g., other adults and children) and occurs in public locations (e.g., movies, parks, train stations, and rest rooms), will influence the extent to which social, economic, and legal systems will be involved in addressing the consequences of this addictive behavior.

Change in these behaviors is limited by the establishment of rigid patterns that serve to bind anxiety, lift depression, mask suicidality or the manic phase of bipolar disorder, dissociate painful emotions, and meet dependency needs.

Family Treatment Modalities

Treatment of families presenting with substance abuse issues is a clinical challenge for advanced practice psychiatric nurses (APPNs). Complex treatment issues require that APPNs simultaneously maintain an individual, family, and environmental systemic intervention focus (Brown and Lewis, 1999). Phases of recovery from addiction and associated treatment approaches are identified as follows:

- Early recovery (first 90 days)
- Early middle phase (90 days–1 year)
- Middle phase (1–3 years)
- Later phase (3 years and beyond)

Early Recovery

PRESOBRIETY

Early recovery begins with presobriety, at which time it is essential to deal with individual and/or family denial. The APPN must be attentive to the individual as well as the family's need to deny the seriousness of the problem. Therapist gullibility in terms of believing the family's reports about the extent of drinking and/or drug use and related dysfunction can be the most significant block to effective treatment. Therefore, it is important for the APPN to open the system up as much as possible by tracking the degree to which drinking or other drug use is a secret from other family members. Collection of genogram information during the family assessment is an excellent vehicle for tracking this pattern and determining triangular relationships that sustain denial and secrecy. All family members should be encouraged to participate in the use of outside resources available in the community for drug-involved families. At this time, decisions about detoxification, residential treatment, or rehabilitation may need to be made by family members, employers, or the legal system. Education of the family about alcoholism or other drug abuse is very important; the family needs information to correct misperceptions and break through their denial (Falloon, 1991; Keefler and Koritar, 1994; McFarlane, 1991). There is an abundance of educational materials available to family members from a variety of print and Internet sources; these are listed in Appendix V.

If drinking alcohol and/or abuse of other drugs is a current problem in the family and is the primary focus of interaction, abstinence is crucial to success of the treatment. Abstinence is best achieved through the user's participation in organizations such as Alcoholics Anonymous (AA) or other 12-step programs, with the other family members attending related programs such as Al-Anon or Al-Ateen. Each family member should be asked to make a commitment to attend at least six such meetings. Coaching the client to obtain a sponsor is a key to effective engagement in a 12-step program (Bepko and Krestan, 1985; Brown and Lewis, 1999).

In crisis situations in which the family member who is an alcoholic and/or abuses other drugs is in denial and creating havoc in the family system, at work, or in the community, the Johnson intervention approach may be effective for the whole nuclear family system (Edwards, 1994). This intervention can be described as an orchestrated confrontation that challenges family members to abandon denial, stop enabling, perceive chemical dependency as a family disease, and facilitate the transition of the family member to a treatment program.

During the presobriety phase of treatment, it is important to have the major overfunctioner in the family either remove himself or herself from the situation or give up the over-responsible role in both the functional and emotional dimensions. The partner should be coached to accomplish this objective by strategizing who he or she functionally can move toward and how to begin dwelling in his or her own activity zone. The APPN should track this behavior carefully and note whether the overfunctioning partner is giving up that role only to triangle in a child, typically the oldest child, who steps in and assumes this role. Resistance to reversing the process of overresponsibility should be anticipated; the family often has to be convinced of the importance of this action. For example, Lucille, an enabling wife, had to be convinced that the problem of her husband's alcoholism was not located solely in him. Rather, it was a case of each family member having his or her own set of emotional, behavioral, school, or work problems and that everyone was contributing to the family misery in a self-maintaining fashion. She needed to be coached as to how to assume a self-focus that enabled her to stop critically pursuing her husband about his drinking and focus on her own issues while resisting the temptation to turn her focus to her son, who was underperforming in school. If the family member who abuses alcohol or other drugs does not achieve abstinence and leaves treatment, the APPN continues to work with other family members on issues of under- and overresponsibility.

ADJUSTMENT TO SOBRIETY

The APPN's role in this phase is to stabilize the family around sobriety. The prior organization and role behaviors that the family assumed are no longer effective. Because sobriety is very tenuous at this point, it is important to keep conflict at a low level, for example, by not encouraging family members to focus on emotionally charged issues while encouraging self-focus for each family member. Conflict-laden issues, such as marital conflict, have the potential to divide family members and deter them from the priority objectives of achieving abstinence and conceptualizing substance abuse as a family problem rather than as an individual problem. It is equally important for the APPN to establish alliances with the senior nonabusing members of the family. This alliance provides leverage in initiating change in family interaction regarding the substance abuse. The APPN starts working with the most motivated family member or members (Stanton, 1992).

Family members should be coached to operate in ways that promote their ability to work together to address basic tasks of family functioning. For some families, parenting issues may be important; for others, economic issues may be of greater importance. Consider the situation of Sherry L., whose husband had just lost his third job in two years. For this family, economic issues related to accumulated debt, a past-due mortgage, no income, and an about-to-be repossessed car were major problems to be addressed. Sherry had not worked for the past 20 years and had to be coached about obtaining a job and prioritizing solutions to debt repayment, housing, and transportation. In general, marital issues should be avoided because the potential intensity of emotions that are likely to be unleashed may overload a vulnerable family system (Bowen, 1978). It is important for the APPN to help family members anticipate resentment, disappointed expectations of sobriety, and loss of hope that early sobriety may represent.

Frequency of therapy may be decreased during this phase, particularly if a strong involvement with AA or Al-Anon exists. More intensive therapy is indicated if one or more of the following are present:

- Drug or alcohol involvement of a child
- Severe depression in any family member
- Physical abuse
- Incest
- Insistence of either spouse to deal with marital issues

In any of these cases, the APPN should predict to the family that relapse is likely to occur. Without concurrent family treatment for nonabusing members, families have been known to sabotage treatment efforts when those efforts begin to succeed (Stanton, 1992). Examples of this have been commonly reported in the literature; they range from the spouse who gives a bottle of liquor to a recovering alcoholic partner on a holiday to the parents who refuse to work together in maintaining rules for their out-of-control adolescent.

In early recovery, education, communication, and validation are essential. Education involves learning about chemical dependency. The educational resources listed in Appendix V are very useful for all family members who need to develop a knowledge base about alcohol, drug abuse, community resources, and family involvement. Family members also need education about self-care activities that promote self-focus and stress reduction. Teaching about and encouragement of participation in activities such as massage, body building, exercise, sports, and dance may promote a feeling of general well-being. Encourage development of the senses by smelling incense, listening to music, touching fabrics, gardening, or attending art exhibits. The APPN is well prepared to teach family members alternative anxiety reduction strategies such as meditation, warm baths and showers, guided imagery, progressive relaxation, breath work, and yoga. Care of the physical self is often not a priority in addictive families; therefore, the APPN can teach the importance of scheduling regular physical, gynecological, dental, and visual exams and encouraging follow-through activities.

APPNs need to teach problem-solving skills related to dealing with and communicating with friends, family, school, workplace colleagues, employers, and community organizations. For example, spouses and children often scurry to hide advancing drinking problems from their neighbors and employers, finding it difficult to arrive at a socially acceptable explanation for their relative's dysfunction. They should be encouraged, if necessary, to develop scripts that provide acceptable explanations about their relative's substance abuse and treatment. For example, one teenager was able, without going into details, to tell his peers that his dad was in an out-of-state rehabilitation program for a health problem. In another situation, a spouse was able to inform her employer that her husband was in a five-week alcohol treatment program and that she anticipated this would have a positive effect on her productivity at work.

In early recovery, it is important to assume a validating, nonblaming position toward the entire family. Confrontational strategies tend to fan the fires of resistance and to inspire counterattack when dealing with families. Challenges can still be offered to families, but they must be expressed in validating ways. One strategy is to use positive interpretations when commenting on family members' behavior. Stanton and Todd (1979) have referred to this as ascribing noble intentions. Examples of positive interpretation include statements such as "He's defending the family like any good son would" and "You're trying your best to be a good mother." Such statements tune into both the caring and the frustration that most family members experience, and they seem to lessen client resistance and promote adherence, thereby facilitating the therapeutic process (Frances and Miller, 1991). Another strategy involves suggesting that family members use positive affirmations such as "I am loved" or "I can take care of myself." Affirmations are vocalized out loud 3 to 5 times or 5 to 10 times daily. This approach is designed to begin cognitive reprogramming, which combats earlier programming based on shame, guilt, and low self-esteem. As such, affirmations should be designed on an individual basis to reflect and combat the predominant scripts embedded in each person's consciousness.

Early Middle Phase

During the early middle phase of treatment, a context for sobriety has been established. The APPN needs to be prepared to deal with a new set of family issues presented by a clean and sober family system (Frances and Miller, 1991; Steinglass, Bennett, Wolin, and Reiss, 1987). Families that have been organized around drinking or other substance abuse, especially over many years, experience a profound sense of emptiness when the substance abuse stops. Family members sometimes describe feelings that they are cut adrift and are without familiar landmarks to help them regain their bearings. Once the initial relief associated with the immediate cessation of abuse recedes, they often are stunned and frightened by the unfamiliar behavior of the "new" family member. They may even make irrational statements such as "I liked you better when you were drinking." Although the primary goal of this phase is to maintain abstinence, the potential for relapse is understandably high.

Couples often describe a feeling of walking on eggshells at home and drift into what can be described as an emotional divorce. Both partners want to preserve sobriety or abstinence and keep the peace. In doing so, they interact sparingly and hesitantly, unwittingly reenacting the same patterns of closeness and distance they enacted previously. For example, a recently abstinent cocaine abuser who wanted to talk to his wife about his feelings approached her late at night and awakened her from a sound sleep, just as he used to do when he was high. She, in turn, rebuffed his awkward attempt at communication, leaving him to go off alone to sulk (whereas he once went off to get high). It is not surprising that as recovering couples get reacquainted with each other, they often find themselves bored, irrationally angry, and unable to resolve or escape from problems that were once avoided with the help of drugs.

In families with addicted young people, a family crisis can be anticipated within the first three to four months of treatment (Edwards, 1994). Most commonly, the crisis occurs in the marital relationship of the parents; long-standing marital conflict that has been underground because of the system focus on the addicted child now floats to the surface and erupts. Steps may be taken toward separation or divorce. Such a crisis puts tremendous pressure on the child in recovery to become "dirty" again in order to restore the family homeostasis and reunite his or her family (Frances and Miller, 1991).

Pressure to restore the previous status quo can inadvertently be provided by siblings and children of recovering substance abusers. Family problems are recognized that previously went unnoticed because they were hidden by the magnitude of drug or alcohol problems. As the haze of intoxication clears, parental children who were once considered very helpful may suddenly seem withdrawn and depressed. Marijuana-smoking adolescents may be discovered for the first time.

Different schools of thought exist about how quickly to move to resolve family issues at this stage. Berenson (1992) suggests that it is advisable to begin this stage with a family treatment hiatus during which the family system can calm down, and regular appointments are not scheduled at this time. He encourages families to continue their 12-step activities and resume family treatment after a 6- to 12-month period of sobriety. Others (Krestan and Bepko, 1989; Edwards and Steinglass, 1995; McCrady and Epstein, 1995; Steinglass, Bennett, Wolin, and Reiss, 1987) believe that regularly scheduled family therapy sessions can be very helpful at this time, especially if they focus on structural or behavioral approaches to solving problems that continue to recur in families and wear them down emotionally.

Family treatment strategies need to focus on these actions:
- Keeping family members connected to and attending their 12-step program
- Promoting their relationship with their 12-step program sponsor
- Using a specific structural problem-solving approach for parenting issues
- Developing conflict management strategies
- Using stress management strategies
- Implementing self-care strategies
- Promoting family education through the provision of psychoeducation materials and discussion about addiction that predicts and addresses common difficulties in recovery and fears about relapse
- Initiating behavioral couples therapy that promotes functional marital interactions, boundary management, and role flexibility
- Acting as a liaison with the primary health care providers
- Acting as a liaison with community agencies
- Providing relapse prevention education and strategies:
  - Identifying relapse risk factors
  - Identifying trigger events
  - Developing coping strategies for dealing with trigger events (e.g., high-stress thoughts, feelings and interactions or painful memories and emotions)

Examples of behavioral couples strategies that the APPN might use include positive reinforcement behaviors by the partner when the drinker abstains and negative ones (e.g., indifference) when he or she does not. It may also include assignment of positive (fun), usually conjoint, activities that compete in time and space with the prior drinking pattern (McCrady and Epstein, 1995; O'Farrell, 1993). Other positive techniques include caring days to catch the partner doing something nice!

Middle Phase

The middle stage of therapy takes place after year one of recovery and through year three. The focus of family treatment is helping families move away from family interactions organized around substance abuse issues and toward addressing multigenerational, marital, and other family issues. With sobriety and the recovery process stabilized, family therapy now shifts to developing a better marriage and more effective parent-child relationships, as well as confronting long-standing family-of-origin issues. Steinglass and associates (1987) have referred to this process as family reorganization. This rebalancing is an important process; otherwise, a family can stabilize but remain organized around alcoholism or other drug-related issues. In families in which alcoholism has been a problem, this phenomenon is called the dry alcoholic family.

The following are therapeutic goals for the APPN who continues or begins to provide family treatment during the middle stage:

- Shift extremes of reciprocal role behavior from rigid complementarity to more symmetrical and flexible complementarity.
- Promote expression of feelings and behavior previously expressible only when drinking or high on drugs.
- Facilitate the couple/family's competence in resolving issues of pride, power, and control.
- Facilitate development of functional closeness and intimacy between family members.
- Facilitate the family's ability to address multigenerational issues related to substance abuse.

During family sessions, the APPN works with a variety of family subsystem configurations. For example, sessions may be conducted with the couple dyad to address marital issues; other sessions may include the parents and specific members of the sibling subsystem, depending on the parent-child issues to be resolved. In other sessions, the entire nuclear family and its issues may be the focus. Ongoing assessment data may be used by the APPN to engage family members and provide the treatment focus. Or, by this time, the family may be engaged in treatment to the extent that they present intervention issues themselves.

Establishment of a nonjudgmental climate in which family members are encouraged to speak from an "I" position and to separate thinking from feeling is essential. For example, family members are coached to (1) specify their thoughts, ideas, and emotions, (2) locate thoughts or feelings in the appropriate category, and (3) communicate thoughts or feelings using "I" statements. These strategies decrease fusion, minimize projection and blaming, and promote a self-focus and assumption of personal responsibility for thoughts, words, and actions (Bowen, 1978). The expression of feelings also becomes safer in this therapeutic environment.

In this context, the APPN helps family members track, identify, reconsider, and redefine dysfunctional expectations, role behaviors, and communication patterns in the family system that were based on living with the addiction. For example, the T. family became accustomed to withdrawing every time the alcoholic husband/father showed a hint of anger, fearing that it was the warning cue for an explosive rage that customarily followed. In addition, they left him out of family decisions and disregarded his parenting efforts. In this phase of family therapy, he must learn to deal with his anger, to participate in making responsible decisions, and to function as a father. Other family members must test their hypothesis as to whether their fear of his anger and their perception of his irresponsibility are based on old or current, invalid or valid, expectations and allow him to change. Similarly, the spouse and children need to assume a self-focus in determining their contribution to this pattern and consider the changes they must make to restructure family expectations, role behaviors, and communication patterns in a more symmetrical, flexible fashion. Figure 11-3 provides a model for the APPN to use in facilitating family members' efforts to engage in this restructuring process.

Another important intervention focus is the couple's relationship, that is, decreasing the emotional distance and lack of intimacy so common in such marriages (Edwards and Steinglass, 1995). Priority relationship issues are pride and perfectionism, power, control, dependence versus independence, intimacy, and forgiveness (Avis, 1991; Berenson, 1976; Bowen, 1978; Frances and Miller, 1991; Krestan and Bepko, 1989). Couples who have had relationship and interaction patterns characterized by denial, distance, and repression have to be coached how to connect gradually with their emotions, how not to experience them as threatening or overwhelming, and how to express them effectively. Role play, sculpting, psychodrama, displacement media, and behavioral assignments are strategies designed to accomplish these objectives.

Couples should be encouraged to use "I" statements to express emotions and feelings in a nonblaming manner. Jasmine, for example, used a model suggested by the APPN as a template ("I feel _____ when you _____") to begin expressing feelings she had not dared to bring to the surface in years. When she realized that there were positive outcomes linked to direct communication and emotional expressiveness, she became more comfortable with spontaneously interacting with her partner. Another strategy used to explore underground emotional processes and facilitate their overt expression by focusing on the functional facts

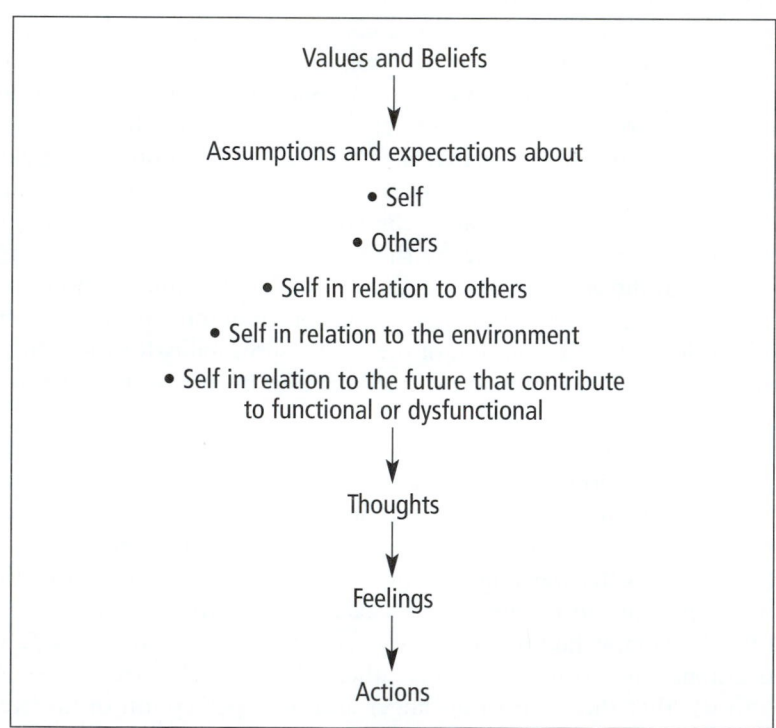

FIGURE 11-3 Model for Restructuring Expectations, Roles, and Communication Patterns

of the relationship without activating emotional triggers is to ask the questions Who? What? Where? When? and How?

Triangular relationships must be explored and tracked; they play a major role in maintaining indirect and inconsistent communication (Bowen, 1978). There is a positive correlation between the level of anxiety in the family system and the presence of triangles (Bowen, 1974). As mentioned earlier, couples benefit from learning anxiety reduction strategies; this process will decrease their vulnerability to triangulation. Couples, as well as other family members, must be taught how to identify triangles, understand their link to dysfunctional communication and relationship patterns, and learn how to detriangle by forming one-to-one relationships with members of the triangle, especially with the person in the distant, outside position (Bowen, 1976a, 1976b; Fogarty, 1975). An example of a common triangle in substance abuse families is illustrated in Figure 11-4, wherein a couple avoids intimate communication/relationship by triangulation of a child into an overclose relationship with the overfunctioning, sober spouse/parent, which leaves the addicted spouse/parent in the distant position. The intervention strategy is to coach the overclose members of the triangle how to move toward the distant member so that each establishes a more personal one-to-one relationship with that relative. The distant member of the triangle is coached on how to maintain his or her position and move toward functional relationships.

Another common triangle is an issue triangle (see Figure 11-4), in which alcohol or another substance becomes the third leg of the triangle, serving the dysfunctional purpose of providing an organizing focus for interactions and projection of blame. Couples then have a natural focus for their conflict rather than having to deal with their own vulnerability, upset, and direct expression of pain. The APPN coaches partners on how to address directly relevant personal issues rather than use the emotional detour of issue triangles. When an issue triangle has been dismantled, it is not uncommon for severe sexual problems that have plagued the marriage for years to emerge. This problem can now be addressed overtly either in couples therapy or by referral to a sex therapist.

The genogram (see Figure 11-1) is used to assess and track multigenerational patterns of alcohol and drug abuse within the family over at least three generations. Locating the origin

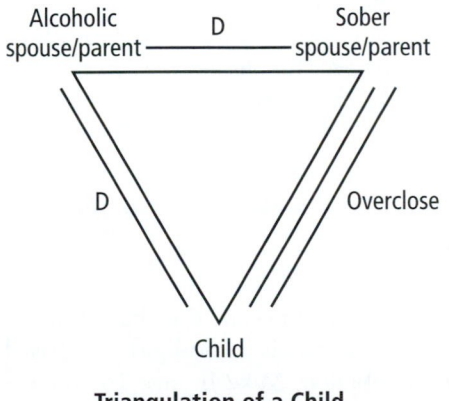
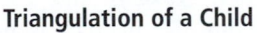
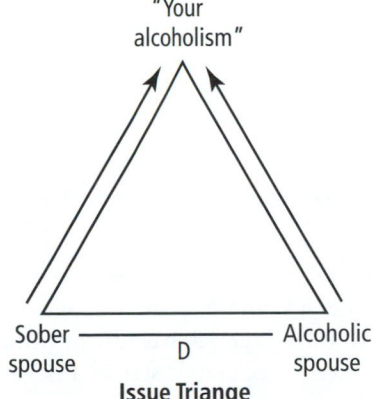

FIGURE 11-4 Common Triangles in Families with Substance Abuse

of this pattern in the family's history is extremely important. The APPN takes family members back through time on a family fact-finding mission to discover the earliest known substance abusers and to learn about what was going on in their lives and the lives of their relatives. It is very common to find that the family had experienced one or more life cycle stressors—such as unexpected or multiple critical illnesses/deaths (perhaps of children), forced immigration, prolonged unemployment, or a major natural catastrophe—prior to the onset of alcohol or other drug abuse. The result is unresolved grief that is projected onto someone in the next generation, who then becomes at risk for substance abuse. Over several generations, it can also become a learned way of coping with anxiety, stress, grief, and loss. Coleman, Kaplan, and Downing (1986) suggest that it is not necessary to address these issues in order to achieve abstinence; however, unresolved grief can erode progress. Family grief work is indicated to maintain long-term change.

Later Phase

Ideally, termination of family therapy occurs when the APPN and family members determine that the following treatment outcomes have been achieved, as follows:

- Abstinence is maintained.
- Substance abuse has not been replaced with other addictive behaviors.
- Twelve-step involvement has been maintained.
- Role complementarity is more flexible and symmetrical.
- Interaction patterns are more personal and reflect flexible and functional boundary management.
- Communication is more direct and open.
- Self-focus is maintained in communication and relationship patterns.

Families who discontinue regularly scheduled sessions can be offered the PRNs (family sessions as needed) that may include one or more booster follow-up sessions scheduled one at a time or at intervals of two to six months. Frances and Miller (1991) suggest that a primary care analogy be used with family members to guide the ongoing nature of family therapy as a process of lifelong learning. The APPN or physician becomes the provider to whom family members turn for assistance with a variety of concerns over the decades, concerns that may or may not be directly related to substance abuse in the family system.

Case Study

Robin, age 44, and Michael H., age 46, have been married for 20 years; they have three children. Ellen, age 18, has just begun her first year of college and is a good girl who has always been an academic star and her mother's rock of Gibraltar. Mike Jr., age 16 and a high school junior, has been an average student academically but, like his dad, is an outstanding athlete. Margaret, age 10 and the baby in the family, is in fourth grade; she has severe asthma, requiring frequent trips to the emergency room and hospitalizations.

Michael, a self-employed accountant, is the middle child in a chaotic family that has a three-generation history of alcoholism on the paternal side of his family, including Michael's father, grandfather, and great-uncle. Michael's youngest brother Frank, age 39, has abused drugs (primarily cocaine and benzodiazepines) since he was 16. Michael began binge drinking in high school; over the past 30 years, Michael has escalated to monthly drinking binges that last 3 or 4 days that are now beginning to affect his work productivity. Although each of these men is married to his original wife, the marriages have been characterized by cycles of overt conflict and/or fixed distance that coincide with periods of drunkenness and sobriety.

Robin, a physical therapist, is also a middle child who has an older and a younger brother. Her family has no history of alcoholism or other substance abuse. However, her mother was diagnosed with multiple sclerosis when Robin was 10 years old and died when Robin was 21. As the only daughter, Robin was a parental child and her mother's primary caregiver throughout high school and college Her father and brothers coped with her mother's illness by distancing themselves through work, sports, and school. Robin attended a local college and lived at home so she could dutifully provide or coordinate her mother's care until her death. She and Michael, who met during college, got married 6 months after her mother's death. Her father remarried 1 year later to a woman 15 years younger than he whom Robin detested from the moment she met her. He and his wife moved to another state, had two children, and never returned home to visit. Robin has not spoken to or seen her father in 15 years. She speaks to her brothers infrequently and sees them annually at the family Christmas gathering.

Robin expects Michael home for dinner on a Friday night, after which they will attend Mike Jr.'s basketball game. Robin came home from work to a quiet house: Ellen was away at college, young Mike was at practice, and Margaret was at Girl Scouts. As she prepared dinner, Robin thought about how much she missed Ellen, who, before she left for college, would help Robin with dinner preparation. Robin remembered how much she had enjoyed those moments together, moments she was never able to share with her own progressively ill mother. Robin looks at her watch and realizes that Michael is 30 minutes late; her heart begins to race, she becomes diaphoretic, and she feels that awful black cloud descend over her head. In her gut, she knows that Michael is out drinking, which signals another binge. She sits down at the table, rests her head on her arms, and sobs, "I have had it; I cannot take one more drunken weekend. What did I ever do to deserve this misery? Haven't I had enough of it in my life?"

1. What are the variables that contribute to Michael's multigenerational risk pattern for alcohol abuse?
2. How does Robin's nuclear family role as parental child contribute to maintaining Michael's alcoholism?
3. Analyze the relationship between Ellen's departure for college and Robin's apparent lack of tolerance for another drunken binge.
4. As the APPN, if Robin called you for treatment, what would your initial action be?
5. What would be the differential diagnosis?
6. What would be the four major components of the treatment plan be to manage the family and substance issues?

CRITICAL THINKING QUESTIONS

1. Explore ways in which familial biological predispositions to alcoholism can be used with families for prevention.
2. How can crises that emerge when a family member is addicted be utilized toward constructive change?
3. From the perspective of the Bowen model, discuss potential changes that occur in the family structure when a parent enters recovery.
4. Describe ways that families can address concerns of social isolation and criticism when a family member is treated for addiction.
5. What are some approaches to family therapy that can be utilized when the addicted client and/or family members are in denial of the problem?

REFERENCES

Avis, J.M. (1991). Power politics in therapy with women. In T.J. Goodrich (ed.), *Women and Power: Perspectives for Family Therapy*. New York: W.W. Norton and Company.

Beattie, M. (1989). *Beyond Codependency*. New York: Harper and Row.

Bepko, C., and Krestan, J.A. (1985). *The Responsibility Trap: A Blueprint for Treating the Alcoholic Family*. New York: Free Press.

Berenson, D. (1976). Alcohol and the family system. In P. Guerin (ed.), *Family Therapy: Theory and Practice*. New York: Gardner Press.

Berenson, D. (1992). The therapist's relationship with couples with an alcoholic member. In E. Kaufman and P. Kaufman (eds.), *Family Therapy of Drug and Alcohol Abuse* (2nd ed.). Boston: Allyn and Bacon.

Blum, K., and Payne, J.E. (1991). *Alcohol and the Addicted Brain*. New York: Macmillan.

Bowen, M. (1974). Bowen on triangles—March 1974 workshop. *The Family 1*(2), 45–48.

Bowen, M. (1976a). Theory in the practice of psychotherapy. In P. Guerin (ed.), *Family Therapy: Theory and Practice*. New York: Gardner Press.

Bowen, M. (1976b). Family reaction to death. In P. Guerin (ed.), *Family Therapy: Theory and Practice*. New York: Gardner Press.

Bowen, M. (1978). Alcoholism and the family. In M. Bowen (ed.), *Family Therapy in Clinical Practice*. New York: Jason Aronson.

Bradshaw, J. (1988). *Healing the Shame That Binds You*. Deerfield Beach, FL: Health Communications.

Bradshaw, J. (1990). *Homecoming: Reclaiming and Championing Your Inner Child*. New York: Bantam Books.

Brown, S., and Lewis, V. (1999). *The Alcoholic Family in Recovery*. New York: Guilford Press.

Coleman, S., Kaplan, J., and Downing, R. (1986). Life cycle and loss: The spiritual vacuum of heroin addiction. *Family Process 25*(1), 5–23.

Crabbe, J.C., and Goldman, D. (1992). Alcoholism: A complex genetic disease. *Alcohol Health and Research World 16*(4), 297–303.

Edwards, J.T. (1994). *Treating Chemically Dependent Families*. Minneapolis, MN: Johnson Institute.

Edwards, M.E., and Steinglass, P. (1995). Family treatment outcomes for alcoholism. *Journal of Marriage and the Family 21*(4), 475–509.

Ewing, J.A. (1984). Detecting alcoholism: The CAGE questionnaire. *Journal of the American Medical Association 252*(14), 1905–1907.

Falloon, I.R.H. (1991). Behavioral family therapy. In A.S. Gurman and D.P. Kniskern (eds.), *Handbook of Family Therapy* (Vol. 2). New York: Brunner/Mazel.

Fogarty, T. (1975). Triangles. *The Family*, Spring/Summer, 11–20.

Frances, R.J., and Miller, S. (1991). *Clinical Textbook of Addictive Disorders*. New York: Guilford Press.

Harris, B. (1997). Psychopharmacology. In J. Haber, B. Krainovich-Miller, A. Leach-McMahon, and P. Price-Hoskins (eds.), *Comprehensive Psychiatric Nursing* (5th ed.). St. Louis, MO: Mosby.

Keefler, J., and Koritar, E. (1994). Essential elements of a family psychoeducation program in the aftercare of schizophrenia. *Journal of Marriage and the Family 20*(4), 368–380.

Krestan, M.A., and Bepko, C. (1989). Alcohol problems and the family life cycle. In B. Carter and M. McGoldrick (eds.), *The Changing Family Life Cycle* (2nd ed.). Boston: Allyn and Bacon.

Leach-McMahon, A. (1992). Family theory and intervention. In J. Haber, A. Leach-McMahon, P. Price-Hoskins, and B.F. Sideleau (eds.), *Comprehensive Psychiatric Nursing* (4th ed.), St. Louis, MO: Mosby.

McCrady, B.S., and Epstein, E.E. (1995). Marital therapy in the treatment of alcoholism. In A.S. Gurman and N.S. Jacobson (eds.), *Clinical Handbook of Marital Therapy* (2nd ed.). New York: Guilford Press.

McFarlane, W.R. (1991). Family psychoeducational treatment. In A.S. Gurman and D.P. Kniskern (eds.), *Handbook of Family Therapy* (Vol. 2). New York: Brunner/Mazel.

McGoldrick, M., Pearce, J.K., and Giordano, J. (1982). *Ethnicity and Family Therapy*. New York: Guilford Press.

Mellody, P. (1989). *Facing Codependence*. New York: Harper and Row.

Naegle, M.A. (1997). Substance-related disorders. In J. Haber, B. Krainovich-Miller, A. Leach-McMahon, and P. Price Hoskins (eds.), *Comprehensive Psychiatric Nursing* (5th ed.). St. Louis, MO: Mosby.

National Institute on Drug Abuse. (1993). National survey results on drug use. In *Monitoring the Future Study, 1975–1992. Vol. 1: Secondary School Students*. NIH Pub. No. 93-9597. Rockville, MD: Author.

National Institute on Drug Abuse. (1994). *The National Household Survey on Drug Abuse: Population Estimates, 1993*. Rockville, MD: Author.

O'Farrell, T.J. (1993). *Treating Alcohol Problems: Marital and Family Interventions*. New York: Guilford Press.

Pendagast, E.G., and Sherman, C.O. (1977). A guide to the genogram family systems training. *The Family 5*(1), 3–14.

Pokorny, A.D., Miller, B.A., and Kaplan, H.B. (1972). The brief MAST: A shortened version of the Michigan Alcoholism Screening Test. *American Journal of Psychiatry 129*(3), 342–345.

Skinner, H.A. (1982). The drug abuse screening test. *Addiction Behavior 7*(4), 363–371.

Stanton, M.D. (1999). Alcohol use disorders. *AAMFT Clinical Update 1*(3), 1–2.

Stanton, M.D. (1992). The time line and the "Why now?" question: A technique and rationale for therapy, training, organizational consultation and research. *Journal of Marital and Family Therapy 18*(6), 331–343.

Stanton, M.D., and Todd, T.C. (1979). Structural therapy with drug addicts. In E. Kaufman and P. Kaufman (eds.), *Family Therapy of Drug and Alcohol Abuse*. New York: Gardner Press.

Steinglass, P., Bennett, L., Wolin, S., and Reiss, D. (1987). *The Alcoholic Family*. New York: Basic Books.

Substance Abuse and Mental Health Services Administration. (1994). *The Economic Costs of Alcohol and Drug Abuse and Mental Illness*. BKD54. Rockville, MD: Author.

U.S. Department of Health and Human Services (1993). *Prevalence of Substance Abuse Among Racial and Ethnic Subgroups in the United States, 1991–1993*. Rockville, MD: Author.

APPENDIX I

Common Drugs of Abuse

Carolyn E. D'Avanzo, RN, MSN, DNSc
with contributions by David Duncan, DrPh

Classification: Ethyl Alcohol

Alcoholic beverage: liquor, beer, wine
(Slang/street terms: booze, hooch, moonshine, sauce)

HISTORY

Long before references to alcoholism as a disease appeared around 1940, alcohol consumption and drunkenness were described in history and depicted in art. As early as the first century, Seneca observed that while some Romans became drunk by choice, others appeared to be unable to control their consumption. In the fourteenth century, Chaucer made similar observations on individuals' inabilities to control consumption, noting words in Middle English that distinguished excessive drinking from dependence/addiction. Other allusions to the illness of consistent inebriety were noted by Benjamin Rush, the father of American psychiatry (National Council on Alcoholism, 1989) and his British contemporary, Dr. Thomas Trotter (Jellinek, 1960, p. 1). "Alcohol addiction" and "alcoholism" have been listed in the American Standard Classified Nomenclature of Disease since 1933 (Jellinek, 1960; National Council on Alcoholism, 1989). Acceptance by the public of alcoholism as an illness began in the 1940s and is credited to the work of Jellinek in combination with the founding of Alcoholics Anonymous, the first self-help group based on a philosophy of 12 steps to recovery.

Alcohol's use from 8000 B.C.E. to the present time has been evidenced by pots containing wine and beer recovered from the Old Stone Age. Alcohol was used by the Egyptians, Greeks, and Romans, who called alcoholic beverages "elixir vitae," the "elixir of life" (Ray, 1983); the Old and New Testaments contain references to the use of alcoholic beverages in celebrations. The linking of alcohol with life is apparent in the Scandinavian 80-proof beverage Akvavit, which means water of life, and the Gaelic term for whiskey, "usage beath" or "breath of life."

The fermentation of alcoholic beverages probably occurred accidentally as a result of airborne yeast cells combining with the sugar content of fruits (wine), grains (beer), or honey (mead) to produce alcohol. The process of distillation, credited to the Arabian physician

333

Phazes in the tenth century, greatly increases the alcohol content, accounting for the differences in alcohol content of beers, wines, and liquors (Kinney and Leaton, 1995, p. 3).

Alcohol was brought to the United States from the British Isles by the Pilgrims, and wine grapes were planted in California by Spanish missionaries. Rum made in New England from fermented molasses was bartered for slaves in Africa and the West Indies (Roueche, 1960). After the Revolutionary War, grain was converted into whiskey as a less expensive substitute for rum by newly arrived Irish and Scottish immigrants (Hanson and Venturelli, 1995, p. 195). In addition to its mood-lifting euphoria, alcohol was frequently used as an antiseptic and anesthetic. Although drinking was common and alcohol was frequently served with food, strong social sanctions limited drunkenness.

In the early 1800s, heavy drinking was becoming a major problem in the United States; in the 1820s, when the temperance movement began, its leaders urged abstinence from distilled spirits. By the mid-1800s, a resurgence of religious revivals occurred, and total abstinence was called for (Austin, 1978). In 1920, the Eighteenth Amendment to the Constitution was passed making the production, sale, or transport of alcohol illegal; 34 states enacted legislation called prohibition laws. Demands for liquor were met by illegal production called bootlegging. Because of the upswing in organized crime related to illegal activities surrounding liquor, prohibition was repealed by the Twenty-First Amendment in 1933.

SITE OF ACTION/PHARMACOLOGY

Alcohol is absorbed rapidly from the stomach and small intestine, and over 90 percent of alcohol ingested is metabolized by the liver. It directly affects the central nervous system (CNS), and acts as a depressant, which accounts for its being used as an anesthetic in the late nineteenth century. The exact mechanism is unknown, but alcohol apparently disrupts nervous system functioning via brain neurotransmitter systems and the gamma-aminobutyric acid (GABA) receptor complex. When consumption is high, the dissolution of ethanol in the lipid membranes between cells produces the effects consequent to alcohol consumption.

DRUG EFFECTS

Alcohol affects individuals to varying degrees, and can produce relaxation, sedation, lessening of inhibitions, disruptions in judgment, abstract thinking, and lack of motor coordination. Disturbances in memory function are common. There is dilation of peripheral blood vessels, with increased heat loss from the body. The anesthetic qualities of alcohol reduce discomfort or pain.

LENGTH OF EFFECTS

The effects of alcohol are a function of the concentration of alcohol and individual susceptibility to the drug and usually occur within 20 minutes to an hour after ingestion. Alcohol is absorbed more slowly in the presence of water or food, particularly protein. Faster absorption of alcohol occurs in the presence of carbon dioxide, so the effects of carbonated beverages such as champagne or sparkling wine will generally be felt sooner.

SIGNS AND SYMPTOMS

In general, behavioral manifestations of alcohol ingestion increase as the blood alcohol level (BAL) or blood alcohol concentration (BAC) increases. The dependent drinker, however, develops tolerance to ethanol and may not show symptoms even when drinking heavily. Typical signs and symptoms of drinking that may occur are nausea, vomiting, lack of coordination, slurred speech, staggering, disorientation, irritability, short attention span, loud and frequent talking, decreased judgment, decreased inhibitions, interference with memory, unsteady gait, nystagmus, and facial flushing (especially in the case of Orientals). Mood swings, from happy to depressed to violent, link alcohol to homicides and suicides. A dependent drinker may also have blackouts.

SIDE EFFECTS

Individuals who abuse alcohol are prone to numerous physical, social, and psychological problems. Physical complaints include gastrointestinal bleeding, gastritis, pancreatitis, malnutrition, cirrhosis, alcoholic hepatitis, fetal alcohol syndrome and developmental lags in children, and increased rates of cancers of the esophagus and colon. Social problems include violence, high divorce rates, car accidents, and loss of employment. Psychological and mental problems include suicide, blackouts (loss of short-term memory for up to several days), Korsakoff's syndrome (dementia with loss of short-term memory), and Wernicke's encephalopathy (cranial nerve dysfunction and delirium).

After excessive drinking, hangovers result, and the individual may experience malaise, nausea, headache, thirst, and a general feeling of fatigue. Severe overdoses of alcohol, such as those that occur with binge drinking, may result in shallow respirations; cold, clammy skin; and weak, rapid pulse. Symptoms of withdrawal may progress to hallucinations, coma, and death. It is not unusual for alcoholics to drink heavily only on weekends or to have long periods of sobriety followed by binge drinking. If the person is alcohol-dependent, sudden withdrawal may become a life-threatening process with agitation and tremors, increased heart rate and hypertension, hallucinations, delusions and delirium (delirium tremens), and respiratory arrest. Withdrawal is best managed under medical supervision.

PATTERN OF USE

The pattern of use is oral.

Classification: Nicotine

Cigarettes
Smokeless tobacco

HISTORY

The large-leaf variety of tobacco was used by the Aztec Indians of South America for centuries prior to the arrival of the Spaniards. Simultaneously, natives of the North American continent and the West Indies also used a smaller-leaf variety of the tobacco plant. Tobacco was introduced to other parts of the world by Portuguese sailors and was originally hailed as an effective medicine for a variety of illnesses, including boils, headaches, and colds (Schultes, 1978). Nicotine is the active ingredient in tobacco; its psychoactive effects are highly variable, identified as both stimulating and calming. Nicotine is the most rapidly addicting of the drugs of abuse, and abstinence in dependent individuals results in symptoms ranging from irritability to nausea. One early effort to limit its use was Pope Urban VIII's midcentury prohibition of tobacco use in church, followed by another decree in 1650. Neither of these edicts affected the use of either tobacco or snuff. In 1600, smoking was outlawed in China, Russia, and Turkey and was a punishable offense; in the 1600s, laws in Bavaria, Zurich, and Saxony forbade the smoking of tobacco. In 1639, smoking was banned in New Amsterdam (later to become New York City). None of these efforts ever resulted in the elimination of smoking (Siegel, 1989). During the eighteenth century, some reductions in the habit occurred as individuals turned to snuff. Gradually, snuff was partially replaced by chewing tobacco and later, cigars; by the 1920s, use of chewing tobacco and cigarettes achieved relative parity.

Tobacco use resulted in an epidemic of smoking in China, which was later interfaced with smoking opium. Smoking prevalence in the United States kept rising, with 1963 as the peak year for cigarette sales. In 1964, the U.S. Surgeon General's report stated that cigarette smoking was related to lung cancer in men, with the result that the prevalence of smoking decreased. Despite numerous warnings and reports confirming this association and other potentially serious health risks, bans on smoking on commercial airplanes and in public places, and health warnings on cigarettes, millions of Americans continue to smoke. In contrast to other addictive substances, the majority of smokers develop physiologic dependence on nicotine.

SITE OF ACTION/PHARMACOLOGY

Nicotine is absorbed into the blood through the respiratory system (inhaled) or through the mucous membranes (chewed). It directly affects the cardiovascular, endocrine, and central nervous systems.

DRUG EFFECTS

Nicotine causes increased blood pressure and heart rate, affects blood flow to the coronary arteries, and constricts peripheral blood vessels. It is similar to other substances that produce differing levels of euphoria. The individual may experience stimulation, enhanced performance, and hyperalertness. Smokers lose up to 15 percent of the oxygen-carrying capacity of their red blood cells because carbon monoxide in the smoke combines with hemoglobin (Ockene and Kristeller, 1994).

LENGTH OF EFFECTS

The effects of nicotine occur from 30 minutes to about 2 hours depending on the dose, degree of inhalation, and individual characteristics of the smoker.

SIGNS AND SYMPTOMS

Cigarette smokers exhibit a wide range of symptoms such as increased incidence of colds, morning cough with or without sputum production, dyspnea, poor skin color, wrinkles, and stained teeth and skin (Ockene and Kristeller, 1994). Nicotine decreases appetite, which may be perceived as a benefit and a reason to smoke. The relief of anxiety and feelings of relaxation claimed by smokers upon lighting up are actually due to periodic nicotine withdrawal relieved by further nicotine (Frisch and Frisch, 1998). Nicotine appears to improve performance on some motor, but not cognitive, tasks (Edwards, Wesnes, Warburton, and Gale, 1985).

SIDE EFFECTS

Smoking cigarettes is causally linked with the development of coronary heart disease. Toxic gases in cigarette smoke (nitrogen and hydrogen oxides, ammonia, and hydrogen cyanide) are responsible for narrowing the bronchi, paralysis of cilia, thickening of mucus-secreting membranes, and coughs developed by smokers that eventually lead to chronic obstructive pulmonary disease (Ockene and Kristeller, 1994). The tar in "sidestream" smoke contains more cancer-producing substances (aromatic amines) than "mainstream" smoke, which may affect the health of others in the smoker's environment (U.S. Environmental Protection Agency, 1992). Diabetics who smoke risk amputation because of nicotine's vasoconstrictive effects. Smoking cigarettes also accounts for the majority of cases of chronic bronchitis and emphysema. When pregnant women smoke, risks to infants include low birth weight, still-birth, and neonatal death.

Levels of dependence on nicotine are highly idiosyncratic, which is not necessarily true with other addictive drugs. Kicking the nicotine habit may be accomplished either individually or by interventions. Nicotine withdrawal usually occurs 24 hours after the last cigarette and may be characterized by anxiety, irritability, restlessness, dysphoria/depression, problems with concentration, decreased heart rate, and insomnia (American Psychiatric Association, 1994). Recent research suggests that smoking cessation is most successfully achieved through a combination of abstinence/decreased dependence, the use of nicotine patches and gum, and support in the forms of individual counseling and/or social support or psychotherapy groups.

PATTERN OF USE

The pattern of use is oral (it may or may not be inhaled).

Classification: Cannabinoids

Cannabis: marijuana, hashish
(Slang/street terms: grass, joint, pot, ganja, blang, reefer, weed)

HISTORY

Marijuana use has been recorded since 2737 B.C.E. The drug has been used to produce euphoria, to treat a variety of physical complaints such as gout and malaria (Grinspoon and Bakalar, 1995), and as a source of hemp to make rope. The psychoactive compound in marijuana derives from the sticky resin secreted by the tops and leaves of the hemp plant. The word cannabis comes from the Greek word for hemp. Hashish, an even more potent drug, comes from the flower tops of the plant. By 1000 B.C.E., it was being used in India, by the fifth century in Greece, by 1000 A.C.E. in the Eastern Mediterranean and Middle East, and by the fifteenth century in Western Europe. It was brought to North America by English settlers (Pinger, Payne, Hahn, and Hahn, 1995) where in the 1700s it became the source of hemp for rope. In the 1920s, marijuana received considerable criticism for its supposed role in causing violence, which resulted in the Marijuana Tax Act of 1937, when cultivation and distribution were taxed.

In China around 500 B.C., marijuana was banned because it was purported to make youth willful and disrespectful. It was later legalized when use was deemed to be beyond the control of the authorities. The use of marijuana in India has been a part of religious rituals from early history. Missionaries attempted to ban it for centuries, to no avail (Abel, 1982). In the nineteenth century, hashish came to France with Napoleon's soldiers returning from Egypt. Its use spread, as did the use of opium; by the mid-1800s, it became impossible to curb the use of either substance. In the United States, after the Marijuana Tax Act of 1937, many individual states made the use or possession of cannabis illegal (Grinspoon and Bakalar, 1995). Its use increased in the 1960s and 1970s, and it is now the most frequently used illicit substance in the United States, with an estimated 20 million or more current users.

Since 1971, marijuana has been classified as an illicit drug rather than as a narcotic, making possession of a small amount subject to a fine. Its spread as a weed (ditch weed)—especially in the state of Indiana, which produced much of the hemp for rope in World War II—became problematic as use increased. Eradication efforts continue to the present day (Pinger, Payne, Hahn, and Hahn, 1995, p. 306).

SITE OF ACTION/PHARMACOLOGY

The active ingredient in marijuana, delta-6-3,4-tetrahydrocannabinol (THC), is transformed into metabolites when ingested and acts on the cardiovascular and central nervous systems. THC is stored in the fatty tissue of the brain and reproductive systems, in particular. Marijuana acts on many body systems and has been found effective for treatment of a variety of conditions including asthma, glaucoma, epilepsy, hypertension, and the nausea or vomiting that may occur with chemotherapy.

DRUG EFFECTS

The THC content of marijuana determines its potency and therefore, its effects. Physiological symptoms (such as increased heart rate, conjunctival irritation and injection, dilated pupils, nystagmus, cough, decreased coordination, disconnected thoughts, and increased reaction time) may be present. Increased thirst and appetite and a craving for sweets are not uncommon.

LENGTH OF EFFECTS

Effects usually occur in about 20 to 30 minutes and may last for up to 7 hours. THC remains in the body in fatty tissue for long periods of time and has a half-life of about 3 days. Therefore, the effects of marijuana, such as slower reaction time when operating machinery or a motor vehicle, may be sustained for an extended period. Marijuana is detected in urine analysis for about 48 hours after casual use; chronic use may be detected for up to a month after last use.

SIGNS AND SYMPTOMS

The individual may experience mild euphoria, relaxation, lassitude, decreased concentration, lack of motivation, and the sensation of time passing slowly. Short-term memory may be impaired and conversation disjointed. Inhibitions lessen, and both auditory and visual sensations may be enhanced with alterations in the perception of colors and sounds. Some individuals report that they "observe" their own intoxication reactions. Anxiety, hostility, and depression may occur, and adolescents may exhibit personality changes, poor school performance, and social withdrawal.

SIDE EFFECTS

Marijuana is often used with other drugs, for example, to extend a heroin high or to lessen anxiety when snorting cocaine. It is considered to be a gateway drug in that it frequently leads to even more serious drug use, and it may also be the only drug used (the "pothead" who is "stoned" daily). Chronic use may lead to tolerance to the drug, but physiological dependence is not the norm (American Psychiatric Association, 1994). Individuals may have adverse reactions to marijuana such as anxiety or panic attacks, which require professional support in the emergency room (referred to as "talking the person down"). More serious reactions (usually from overdose) are psychotic disorder, when the person suffers from delusions and subsequent anemia, and toxic delirium, which may be characterized by bizarre behavior, paranoia, and hallucinations.

Withdrawal usually produces few symptoms, but chronic users of high doses may exhibit nausea, myalgia, irritability, nervousness, restlessness, insomnia, depression, and increased appetite for high-carbohydrate foods (called the "marijuana munchies") (Millman and Beeder, 1994, p. 102).

PATTERN OF USE

Both marijuana and hashish are smoked. In order to increase the amount of drug effect, the smoke is deeply inhaled and held in the lungs for as long as possible. Marijuana and hashish may be smoked in "joints" or cigarettes, in "bowls" or pipes. Inhaling the smoke through a water-cooled apparatus called a "bong" lessens irritation and aids deeper inhalation. The chronic, high-dose marijuana user is most likely to exhibit withdrawal symptoms when the drug is stopped.

Classification: Stimulants

Amphetamines: Benzedrine (Slang/street terms: black beauties, white crosses)
Caffeine
Cocaine (Slang/street terms: coke, crack [freebase], flake, rock, snow)
Dextroamphetamines: Dexedrine (Slang/street terms: dexies)
Methamphetamines: Desoxyn (Slang/street terms: crank, crystal meth, glass, ice, speed)
Methylphenidates: Ritalin

HISTORY

Stimulant drugs are prescription drugs that are frequently abused and share similar neurochemical and clinical characteristics (Gawin, Khalsa, and Ellinwood, 1994, p. 112).

Amphetamines are synthetic drugs that have been prescribed since the 1930s and were popular in the 1950s and 1960s to treat fatigue, depression, and weight problems. Stimulants were used in World War II to keep soldiers awake, but subsequent oral and intravenous abuse resulted in international efforts to restrict their availability. Amphetamines were initially used medically as bronchial dilators and were available over the counter as benzedrine inhalers. There was an abrupt decline in their use, however, after an American Medical Association (AMA) report of acute paranoid psychotic reaction with hallucinations connected to the use of the inhaler (Monroe and Drell, 1947). Legal restrictions were placed on amphetamine use by the 1980s. However, methamphetamine (crank) and smokable methamphetamine crystals (ice) were produced illegally and gained in popularity: the "poor man's cocaine" (Gawin, Khalsa, and Ellinwood, 1994, p. 111).

Because amphetamines interfere with sleep and decrease appetite, they are presently prescribed for the treatment of narcolepsy and very-short-term weight loss. Methylphenidate (Ritalin), a milder form of amphetamine, is also the drug of choice for attention deficit disorder (ADD) and attention deficit hyperactivity disorder (ADHD). In addition to amphetamines obtained illegally, over-the-counter stimulants are commonly used by individuals attempting to stay awake, such as students cramming for tests, long-distance drivers, and truck drivers. A similar-acting stimulant, phenylpropanolamine (PPA), is also used in most over-the-counter weight control preparations.

The leaves of the coca plant have been chewed by native peoples in the Andes mountains of South America since before the sixteenth century. Earlier use was also a part of religious rituals, and continued use is attributed to the leaf's ability to increase endurance and strength while decreasing hunger. The primary psychoactive substance, cocaine, was isolated in the laboratory in the nineteenth century (*Remmington's Pharmaceutical Sciences,* 1985). Like opium, it was thought to be nonaddictive and was used for pain and anesthesia. It was common in patent medicines, home remedies, and products such as Coca-Cola. Sigmund Freud recommended it as a treatment for depression and morphine addiction, believing it was nonaddictive. Coca leaves were converted to freebase so it could be smoked, and freebase was then mixed with baking soda and water to produce crack cocaine. In recent years, crack (a solid form of cocaine referred to as "rock") has been smoked to produce an almost instantaneous high. The large surface area of the lungs provides rapid absorption and CNS effects, resulting in rapid addiction for some users.

With the realization of cocaine's less benign properties, it was made illegal under the Harrison Narcotic Act of 1914 (Breecher, 1972). Its use, however, increased again in the late 1960s and early 1970s and it remains a popular street drug at present. It is smuggled into the United States, and the supply of cocaine has not decreased appreciably despite strong efforts to prevent its entrance across U.S. borders. Amphetamines and cocaine have alternatively been used since the 1900s, depending on availability and perception of serious side effects.

SITE OF ACTION/PHARMACOLOGY

All stimulants are believed to produce euphoria by activation of mesolimbic or mesocortical dopaminergic pathways in the CNS. Mild stimulants such as caffeine also act on the CNS. Decades of research indicate that dopamine is central to stimulant reward (Gawin, 1991). Although they do not share similar structures, amphetamines, methylphenidates, and cocaine are all alike neuropharmacologically (Gawin, Khalsa, and Ellinwood, 1994).

DRUG EFFECTS

Stimulants produce heightened sensations of well-being, euphoria, energy, and alertness. Pleasures, including sex, seem magnified and more intense; anxiety and depression are reduced. Social inhibitions decrease due to feelings of power, mastery, and self-confidence. High doses of stimulants may cause behavior characterized by heightened sensitivity, compulsions, impairment in decision making, and paranoid psychotic reactions. This may lead to hostile and violent behavior, especially if stimulant use is combined with alcohol. Sustained high doses of stimulants may result in paranoid psychosis with auditory and visual hallucinations. Mild stimulants such as caffeine cause stimulation, restlessness, and anxiety in susceptible individuals.

LENGTH OF EFFECTS

Stimulants taken orally take effect in about 30 minutes and peak about 2 to 3 hours after ingestion. In order to maintain blood levels and the associated euphoria, users may repeat doses at intervals of 4 to 6 hours. The half-life of cocaine is considerably less than that of amphetamines, so that feelings of euphoria may be more intense but short-lived (30 minutes versus 4 hours). Coca leaves deliver cocaine slowly through the mucous membranes, with slow onset of effects and lower blood levels than use of other methods. Injected stimulants produce a rapid orgasmic rush, followed by euphoria and hyperactivity. Along with this rapid effect comes more rapid tolerance to the drug, requiring escalating doses in order to achieve euphoric effects. The effects of caffeine, although a mild stimulant, lasts from 3 to 7 hours.

SIGNS AND SYMPTOMS

Even mild stimulants such as caffeine can raise heart rates and blood pressure temporarily and cause tremors and insomnia. Stronger stimulants greatly increase cardiac and respiratory rates and blood pressure. The individual exhibits dilated pupils, sweating, and agitation, and tremors may progress to seizures. Regular snorting of stimulants irritates the nasal septum, resulting in an inflamed, runny nose. Overdose of stimulants may result in convulsions and cardiac arrest.

SIDE EFFECTS

Psychiatric symptoms may be associated with use during or after the drug use. Chronic abuse results in withdrawal symptoms such as the blues or severe depression as the drug wears off. This crash may initiate depression and lack of energy, and the individual may sleep for prolonged periods. Suicidal ideas during the crash are not uncommon but are usually temporary and should be evaluated in a protective environment such as an emergency room.

PATTERN OF USE

Intranasal or oral stimulant use gives the user the illusion of initial control, while smoking or injection produces rapid and powerful urges for continued use. Regardless of the route of ingestion, the desire for repeated euphoria leads to a compulsion to use.

Classification: Sedative-Hypnotics

Barbiturates: Seconal, Nembutal, Amytal, Tuinal, Phenobarbital
Barbiturate-like: Quaaludes
Benzodiazepines: Valium, Librium, Xanax, Halcion, Ativan
(Slang/street terms: downers, ludes, sopors, trenks, 714s, yellow jackets, reds, blues, rainbow)

HISTORY

Sedative-hypnotics are used to reduce anxiety and treat insomnia. Since 1960, benzodiazepines have largely replaced short-acting barbiturates and other nonbarbiturate sedative-hypnotics (Smith and Wesson, 1994, p. 179). Benzodiazepines, developed as sedative-hypnotics in the 1940s and 1950s, were widely prescribed through the 1970s when their addictive potential was validated. Prescribed for anxiety, these included Valium, Librium, and currently Xanax and Halcion. Large supplies of the drugs have generally been obtained for street sale through fraudulent prescription writing, theft, and/or duping of physicians. They may also be obtained by sharing with persons who have legitimate prescriptions. They are used in combination with alcohol for the sedative effect or to take the edge off withdrawal from cocaine. Barbiturates are preferred as recreational drugs because benzodiazepines generally don't produce euphoric effects unless anxiety is present (Griffiths et al., 1980).

SITE OF ACTION/PHARMACOLOGY

Barbiturates are highly addictive and may cause significant depression of the CNS. They are primary drugs of abuse. Benzodiazepines also act on the CNS, but without significant CNS depression. They are believed to act by altering the balance of the neurotransmitter GABA in the limbic system of the brain, which aids in regulating emotions.

DRUG EFFECTS

Attachment at the benzodiazepine receptor facilitates the effects of GABA and reduces anxiety, provides sedation, and increases the seizure threshold (Smith and Wesson, 1994, p. 180). Individuals may exhibit drowsiness, emotional instability, loss of inhibitions, ataxia, reduction of aggressive and sexual drives, sustained vertical and horizontal nystagmus, and recent memory loss.

LENGTH OF EFFECTS

Onset may occur in 30 to 45 minutes, with effects lasting for 3 to 5 hours.

SIGNS AND SYMPTOMS

The individual appears carefree, happy, and self-confident and may have a sense of grandiosity, while he or she displays poor judgment. Slurred speech, sleepiness, mood swings, and disoriented staggering behavior are not uncommon. Occasionally, a reverse of the drug effect occurs, resulting in anxiety and/or irritability.

SIDE EFFECTS

An overdose of barbiturates is very dangerous. When taken orally, barbiturates are partially metabolized by the liver in stages. The unmetabolized drug is stored in fatty tissue, accumulates, and results in overdose. Symptoms of overdose include weak and rapid pulse, shallow respirations, cold and clammy skin, and possible coma and death. When barbiturates are combined with alcohol, serious overdose can occur rapidly. Doses above the therapeutic range over time cause dependency and can be linked to life-threatening withdrawal, which begins 24 to 72 hours after the last dose, depending on the drug used. Withdrawal symptoms include diaphoresis, marked agitation, insomnia, hallucinations, seizures, and delirium.

With the newer benzodiazepines, death from respiratory depression is rare, even with an overdose of 50 to 100 times the usual therapeutic dose (Smith and Wesson, 1994).

PATTERN OF USE

These drugs are generally taken orally, although it is not uncommon for barbiturates to be used intravenously. Amphetamine abusers may use barbiturates to come down from a high.

Classification: Narcotics/Opioids

Natural opiates: opium, morphine
Semisynthetic narcotic: heroin (Slang/street terms: smack, junk, brown, horse, skunk)
Synthetic opioids: Darvon, Demerol, Dilaudid, Fentanyl (and street fentanyl), methadone, Percodan, Percoset, Talwin

HISTORY

The use of opium and other related narcotics was recorded over 6,000 years ago in Sumerian, Egyptian, and Greek writings. The oriental poppy plant has been grown in the Middle East since that time, and the major source today continues to be the "Golden Triangle" area of Thailand, Laos, and Myanmar (Burma). Narcotics are potent analgesics, and they were commonly used first as treatment for diarrhea and later as sedatives and pain relievers. Opium was used in China, India, and other parts of Asia by the year 1000. By the late 1690s, opium use had moved beyond medicinal use and was outlawed. Opium use was punishable by decapitation or strangulation. When China imposed a ban on opium from India, the British East India Company smuggled opium into China at Canton in ever-increasing amounts until 1838. Conflict between the Chinese and the British governments erupted into the Opium War of 1839–1842. The Chinese were defeated, and opium continued to enter China until 1908 when an agreement between the two countries was reached (Austin, 1978). Opium smoking was brought to the United States when large numbers of Chinese were imported as laborers on the railroads.

Morphine was isolated from opium in 1806. During the Civil War, its use became so prevalent (injected morphine was thought to be nonaddictive) that morphine addiction was called the "soldier's disease" (Hanson and Venturelli, 1995, p. 237). Both opium and morphine were common components of patent medicines after the war. In 1832, a second compound isolated from opium was codeine (Maurer and Vogel, 1967). Morphine was modified to the more potent heroin in 1898. The accessibility of these drugs and their synthetic derivative Demerol has made them the drugs on which health care professionals most often become dependent.

Despite the fact that the Harrison Narcotics Act of 1914 made these drugs illegal in the United States except by prescription (heroin is not legal in the United States, even by prescription), they are easily obtained.

SITE OF ACTION/PHARMACOLOGY

Opiates, whether natural or synthetic, have profound effects on the central nervous system. They appear to be a perfect fit for chemical receptor molecules, called opiate receptors, in the CNS. Opiates also affect nervous tissue in general as well as the respiratory system.

DRUG EFFECTS

Physiological symptoms include constricted pupils, analgesia, psychomotor retardation, hypertension, rhinorrhea, lacrimation, slowed bodily functions, respiratory depression, sedation, and reduction in sexual and aggressive drives.

LENGTH OF EFFECTS

The onset of effects for most opioids is within a half-hour; effects last from 4 to 8 hours, depending on the type of drug used.

SIGNS AND SYMPTOMS

Individuals experience euphoria accompanied by a rush of pleasure (particularly after an intravenous dose), constipation, drowsiness, or relaxation. Speech may be slurred, and individuals may appear lethargic.

SIDE EFFECTS

Both natural opiates and synthetic opioids have great potential for creating physical dependency because tolerance (greater amounts need to be taken in order to produce the same drug effects) occurs quickly. Because Fentanyl is up to 40 times stronger than heroin and up to 100 times stronger than morphine, even the first shot may cause addiction (Gallagher, 1986). Alpha methyl fentanyl (China White) is frequently abused, and overdose is common. Overdose by opioids gives rise to clammy skin, constricted pupils, shallow respirations, coma, and death, if not treated. Poisoning may also be a problem because heroin is frequently "cut" with substances that may contain impurities to increase the quantity for sale. The substitution of methadone for injected opiates, rather than detoxification, is a therapeutic decision made on the basis of individual characteristics. Methadone is addictive (a synthetic narcotic) but does not produce the rush of heroin, and it reduces illegal activities related to drug use. With detoxification, opioids are rapidly metabolized and have shorter but very intense withdrawal symptoms. Symptoms may include muscle aches, backaches, abdominal cramps and diarrhea, watery eyes, running nose, yawning, tremors, panic, chills, sweating, and pupillary dilatation. These symptoms begin to appear after initial symptoms of anxiety and craving about 8 to 10 hours after the last dose, peak within 36 to 48 hours, and tend to be particularly severe in intravenous opioid users. Withdrawal from Demerol (even though a short-acting drug) is usually less intense, but extreme nervousness and muscle twitching may be experienced.

PATTERN OF USE

Opium is taken orally and smoked. Morphine and methadone are taken orally and also injected. Heroin is injected, smoked, and snorted; codeine is taken orally. Regardless of the pattern of use, these are drugs that can induce intense euphoria and may be rapidly addicting.

Classification: Hallucinogens

(by David Duncan, DrPh)

Ketamine (Slang/street terms: green, mauve, L.A. special coke)
Lysergic acid diethylamide (LSD) (Slang/street terms: acid, cid, microdots, windowpane, barrel, blotter, sugar cubes, trips)
MDMA (Slang/street terms: ecstacy, Adam)
Mescaline (Slang/street terms: mesque)
Phencyclidine (Slang/street terms: PCP, angel dust, crystal, hog, tranks, tea)
Psilocybin (Slang/street terms: magic mushrooms, shrooms)

HISTORY

Hallucinogens are classified into two groups: The indoles or indolyalkylamines bear a strong structural resemblance to serotonin; the phenylalkylamines bear a strong resemblance to norepinephrine. Hallucinogens similar to serotonin include lysergic acid diethylamide (LSD), lysergic acid amide (LSA), psilocybin, and psilocin. Those similar to norepinephrine include mescaline and synthetic mescaline-like drugs such as 2,5-dimethoxy-4-methylamphetamine (DOM), 3-4-methylenedioxyamphetamine (MDA), and 3,4-methylenedioxymethamphetamine (MDMA). Other related drugs include phencyclidine and ketamine.

Mescaline, a hallucinogen derived from peyote cactus, has been used since the pre-Colombian period by Native Americans in religious ceremonies (Schultes and Hoffmann, 1973). Although use of mescaline was made illegal by a U.S. Supreme Court ruling in 1990, it continues to be part of Native American religious ceremonies. Peyote is a spineless, carrot-shaped cactus of which only the grayish-green pincushion-like crown containing the mescaline appears above ground. Used for thousands of years by Indians of Mexico and Central America, teonanacatl, or "God's flesh," is a sacramental mushroom. Use of these mushrooms (the source of psilocybin and psilocin) by the Mayan civilization dates back to about 500 B.C.E., despite efforts by the Spanish conquistadors to suppress it. Mushrooms continued to be part of religious ceremonies in Central America as late as the 1950s.

"Organic drugs" such as mescaline and psilocybin were highly valued in the hippie culture of the 1960s and 1970s, but the difficulty of manufacturing them led to the synthesis of a variety of mescaline-like drugs. Most were more powerful than mescaline but less powerful than LSD. The best known of the synthetic mescaline-like drugs is 2,5-dimethoxy-4-methylamphetamine, more widely known as DOM, which appeared on the streets in 1967. Another synthetic that became a black market success was 3,4-methylenedioxyamphetamine or MDA, known as the "love drug." The most controversial synthetic in recent years has been 3,4-methylenedioxymethamphetamine or MDMA, known as "ecstasy" or "Adam." Originally synthesized in 1914, MDMA was never applied to any purpose until it appeared on the black market in the late 1960s. It achieved widespread popularity as a street drug in the 1980s, especially in Western Europe where it was used at mass musical events known as raves.

After exposure to the mind-expanding qualities of psilocybin in Mexico, Dr. Timothy Leary of Harvard became famous for his experimentation with psilocybin and LSD in the 1960s. Leary's research actually focused on positive effects of the hallucinogenic experience, especially spiritual growth (Leary and Clark, 1963). When it was discovered in the 1960s that LSD could induce schizophrenia-like symptoms, it became an illegal substance. LSD is still produced by "garage chemists," however; along with synthetic mushrooms, it is still commonly available on college campuses. Lysergic acid amide (LSA) is the naturally occurring substance in the ergot fungus from which LSD is derived. LSA is in the seeds of several flowering plants like the baby Hawaiian woodrose and morning glory.

Phencyclidine, also known as PCP, is a synthetic drug that was marketed in 1963 as the anesthetic Sernyl. Its effects separate patients in sensory experiences, producing a trancelike state rather than loss of consciousness. Patients, however, began to report that during recovery from the anesthetic they had experienced delirium, disorientation, and agitation. As a result of these reports, Sernyl was withdrawn from the market in 1965. Phencyclidine was first sold in capsules or tablets on the streets in 1965 under the names PCP, crystal, hog, or tranks but did not achieve any great popularity. In the 1970s, however, it became popular as a counterfeit for THC. Since researchers had announced the synthesis of THC (the prime active ingredient in marijuana), street drug users had been eager to obtain it. When THC proved too difficult to make and too unstable to store, drug dealers began selling PCP as THC.

Another drug with effects similar to PCP is ketamine, also known as green, mauve, or L.A. special coke. Originally marketed in 1969 as Ketalar, it is a more potent anesthetic than PCP but with a shorter duration of effects. Ketalar is used primarily as an anesthetic for children. It apparently produces hallucinations less frequently than PCP, and the effects are generally compared to those of cocaine (Duncan and Gold, 1982). Its street reputation is that of an absolutely safe drug that produces cocaine-like stimulation accompanied by giddy laughter (Duncan, 1976). It is in fact probably no safer than PCP, and bad trips and spontaneous occurrence of pain have been reported after ketamine use (Siegel and Jarvik, 1975).

SITE OF ACTION/PHARMACOLOGY

LSD, LSA, psilocybin, and psilocin act on the CNS as partial agonists (Sanders-Bush, Burris, and Knoth, 1988). Mescaline and synthetic mescaline-like drugs such as DOM, MDA, and MDMA also act on the norepinephrine system as partial agonists. Relatively small amounts of these drugs actually reach the brain; much is excreted via the intestinal and urinary systems. PCP is fully metabolized and is excreted in the urine.

DRUG EFFECTS

Individuals who have taken hallucinogens typically describe vivid visual images such as geometric patterns dominated by colors at the red end of the spectrum. The images may take the form of lattices, tunnels, funnels or cones, cobwebs, or spirals. Many report seeing such patterns when they closed their eyes (closed-eye imagery). On opening their eyes, people would often see these images projected on whatever they were looking at and might feel as if they were being swept into the image. Later the images lose the geometric quality and become meaningful images of persons, animals, and objects; nearly three-quarters of the reports are of some kind of religious imagery. Visual phenomena such as afterimages, trails, and halos are reported. An afterimage is an illusion in which a "ghost image" of an object that has been closely observed is projected onto the next thing the subject looks at. Trails are illusions in which a moving object appears to become a series of objects moving one after the other. Lights may seem to be surrounded by a glowing halo or rays of light. Time seems to slow down, and events seem to occur in slow motion. A small number of hallucinogen users experience the phenomenon known as a flashback, in which some of the perceptual effects are experienced without taking another dose of the drug. Most flashbacks consist of very brief experiences of some illusion—usually trails or halo effects. They last for less than 1 minute, very few as long as 5 minutes. Users often experience wandering thoughts and flight of ideas of exceptional speed, diversity, and complexity. New thoughts may be experienced as greatly profound or awe-inspiring, while perceptual illusions may seem incredibly beautiful. On effects of the drug a simple motto may seem to be the essence of all knowledge or the solution to the great problems of the world.

LENGTH OF EFFECTS

Effects of LSD usually occur 30 to 90 minutes after ingestion and last about 8 hours. Because LSD has a half-life of about 110 minutes in humans, much of the drug has left the brain with the onset of effects and is gone before the user has experienced its peak effects. Lysergic acid amide is about one-tenth as potent as LSD. Effects occur about 20 minutes after oral administration of the drug. The effects of psilocybin and psilocin will be felt about 30 minutes after taking an oral dose. Psilocybin is converted into psilocin in the body, and it appears that psilocin is the active agent. Effects of mescaline-like drugs such as DOM may last for 16 to 24 hours. PCP is known for its rapid onset of 2 to 3 minutes, with effects lasting up to 4 to 6 hours, sometimes followed by a period of depression that lasts 24 hours to a week.

SIGNS AND SYMPTOMS

LSD users show signs of dizziness, restlessness, inability to concentrate, visual disturbances, and uncontrollable laughter. At small doses, LSA produces a languid, dreamy state while thought processes remain alert. At higher doses, this state is intensified, with the user falling into a deep sleep after about an hour. Visual hallucinations or illusions are uncommon except at extremely high doses of LSA. Taken by mouth or snorting, mescaline may initially produce nausea and often vomiting. Muscle tremors and difficulty in speaking coherently soon follow. The hallucinogenic dose of mescaline is about 200 mg, about 4,000 times as much as the dose for LSD.

Small doses of DOM produce feelings of euphoria, distortions of body image, and closed-eye imagery. Larger doses produce a full range of LSD-like effects. MDA induces feelings of serenity, joy, and insightfulness without either perceptual changes or depersonalization. Large doses of MDA produce a full range of hallucinogenic effects lasting for 8 to 12 hours, with the most intense effects during the first 2 hours. MDMA taken orally induces a state of relaxed euphoria similar to that produced by marijuana or a very low dose of LSD. In small doses, PCP produces relaxation, euphoria, "spaciness," numbness, tingling sensations, muscular weakness, problems with perception and coordination, elevated blood pressure, bloodshot eyes, and slurred speech.

Side Effects

At moderate doses, PCP produces indifference to pain, sweating and flushing, drooling, distorted vision, bulging eyeballs, rigid muscles, difficulty in speaking, slowed mental processes, slowed movements, and inability to comprehend time and space. At larger doses, mental processes become labored and almost impossible. Large-enough doses will produce coma and can result in death. PCP users are more likely to die of accidents while under the influence, however, than of overdoses. At any of these dosage levels, reaction time is impaired, and users may experience sudden swings in mood—laughing one moment and crying the next—behaviors that range from manic excitation to catatonia-like withdrawal. The state of disorientation and delirium resulting from PCP use can be very marked and may include violence. There is no clear evidence, however, that PCP causes users to become violent or to be impervious to pain and possessed of superhuman strength. Concentration is often difficult, short-term memory is impaired, and users forget what they were just doing, but other memory functions are generally undisturbed. Problem solving is likely to be impaired as are such cognitive functions as mathematical calculations and color naming.

Tolerance to LSD and the other hallucinogens is striking for the rapidity with which it develops. If LSD is taken daily, its effects on perception, cognition, and emotion (but not on autonomic arousal) disappear completely over the course of just 2 or 3 days. No amount of the drug taken thereafter will produce effects. Tolerance for the hallucinogens dissipates almost as rapidly as it develops. Full sensitivity returns within a week of nonuse. There is cross-tolerance among LSD, psilocybin, and mescaline, and probably with the other hallucinogens as well. None of the hallucinogens have ever been shown to produce physical dependence and withdrawal symptoms.

As with hallucinogen users, PCP users have typically used the drug only sporadically. Instances of daily use, however, seem to be becoming increasingly common. With such daily use, tolerance develops, and there is some evidence of dependence and of withdrawal symptoms (Grinspoon and Bakalar, 1979). These withdrawal symptoms include tooth grinding, diarrhea, tremors, and difficulty staying awake.

Despite media reports, there has never been a case of human death as a result of an overdose of any hallucinogen. Overdoses of MDMA, however, are reported to cause arrhythmias, hyperthermia with seizures, and intracerebral hemorrhage. A lethal dose of LSD could cost $100,000 to $250,000 at typical street prices. There are also a variety of urban legends about people jumping off buildings in the belief that they could fly, assaulting someone seen as a monster, or engaging in other dangerous behavior as a result of hallucinations. There is no evidence that any of these things have ever actually happened. Unlike users of psychotics, hallucinogen users are usually fully aware that their hallucinations are hallucinations. Some observations indicate that some patients use hallucinogens and other drugs for self-control of their prepsychotic and psychotic symptoms, however. When self-control fails or is interrupted, a psychotic break may occur, but the psychosis cannot be said to have been caused or precipitated by the drugs.

Psychotic behavior lasting up to several months may be precipitated by heavy PCP use, even in individuals without any prior psychotic tendencies. Although this is a transient condition and not a true chronic psychosis, retrospective studies of patients hospitalized for PCP use show that PCP-intoxicated patients could not be distinguished from schizophrenics based on presenting symptoms (Erard, Luisada, and Peele, 1980; Yesavage and Freeman, 1978). Follow-up studies of patients who have undergone LSD therapy have not shown any ill effects in terms of mental, physical, or social health.

PATTERN OF USE

LSD is usually taken orally as a pressed tablet, a square of gelatinous material, or a piece of blotter paper on which liquid LSD has been dropped. It can also be injected or absorbed through the mucous membranes. Current users prefer smaller doses than those used in the 1960s so that the effect is more like the euphoria produced by marijuana than the hallucinogenic experience sought by earlier users.

Mescaline is taken orally or snorted. Typical hallucinogenic effects of mescaline begin about an hour after ingesting the drug and continue for 3 to 4 hours.

PCP sold in the form of saltlike crystals is snorted into the nostrils or sprinkled onto marijuana, tobacco, or mint leaves and then smoked. In the first instance, it was commonly called tea; in the second instance, it was usually called angel dust.

Classification: Anabolic Steroids

Brand names: Anadrol, Anavar, Dianobol, Durabolin, Equipose, Finajet, Halotestin, Maxibolin, Winstrol

HISTORY

Manipulation of hormones is not new. In ancient times, athletes used stimulants like cocaine and strychnine to reduce fatigue and improve performance, male hormones were manipulated through castration to produce desired effects, and various plants and aphrodisiacs were ingested to influence gender-related sexual performance (Ray and Ksir, 1993). Although there is little research documenting the prevalence of steroid abuse, it is known that these drugs are abused singly and in combination. Negative effects on health have been clearly substantiated, and withdrawal is characterized by uncomfortable symptoms of depression, fatigue, restlessness, anorexia, and insomnia. Steroid abuse is especially prevalent among prepubertal and pubertal youth who take the drugs to improve athletic performance, muscular development, and self-image, as well as to increase libido, euphoria, and well-being (Cicero and O'Connor, 1990).

Therapeutic steroids were used under medical supervision after World War II to help emaciated individuals gain weight. In recent years, however, the taking of anabolic-androgenic steroids, self-administered, has become an increasingly visible problem in professional and amateur competitive sports. The 1997 Monitoring the Future (MTF) study, for example, reported that steroid use in high school seniors almost doubled between 1996 and 1997 (Johnston, O'Malley, and Bachman, 1998). Whether bought legally through mail orders or health food stores or obtained illegally, the use of steroids to maximize athletic performance has been ignored as a health risk. Efforts are now being made to educate health care professionals, national governments, and sports organizations about steroid dependence and negative health effects related to their use. Because steroid use is often denied, the detection of use in order to prevent fatal consequences is of particular importance. Health care practitioners must be able to identify symptoms of steroid use and the clinical indications for urine testing.

SITE OF ACTION/PHARMACOLOGY

Anabolic steroids are converted to testosterone in the body, with growth that increases the size of muscle mass and internal organs. It maximizes calcium uptake in the bones, increases synthesis of proteins, and affects the control and distribution of body fat. In addition, there may be CNS effects: users report an increase in energy and less fatigue and a stimulant-like high (Ray and Ksir, 1993).

DRUG EFFECTS

A serious effect of steroids is the possible premature closing of the growth plates of the long bones, resulting in shorter stature. Increases in blood pressure and blood lipids, heart disease, liver tumors, jaundice, fluid retention, baldness, acne, and increased breast size may occur. Women using anabolic steroids may build muscle, grow facial hair, develop a deeper voice, and have increased clitoral size even with small amounts of additional testosterone.

LENGTH OF EFFECTS

Effects are particularly noticeable during use, with some residual effects.

SIGNS AND SYMPTOMS

These preparations are called ergogenic agents, agents that enhance performance. Although difficult to entirely substantiate through research, there are masculinizing effects, increases in muscle tissue, increased muscle mass and strength, and increased aerobic capacity and endurance.

SIDE EFFECTS

Feelings of invincibility and aggression are commonly reported side effects of steroid use and may result in violent behaviors. Pronounced mood swings and manic-like episodes, called "roid rage," are also reported.

PATTERN OF USE

Steroids are taken orally or by intramuscular injection. To avoid developing a tolerance to the drug, users generally administer them in cycles of weeks or months, called "cycling," rather than continuously.

Classification: Inhalants

Benzene (paint thinner, cleaning fluids)
Freon
Gasoline/lighter fluid
Nitrous oxide
Shoe polish
Toluene (airplane glue)
Typewriter correction fluid

HISTORY

Inhalation is the major route of ingestion for a number of common household and industrial products. These are ingested through sniffing, huffing, bagging, and spraying. Such substances have been used at various times throughout history to experience temporary stimulation, to achieve euphoria, and to reduce inhibitions. In recent years, the use of inhalants has doubled among preadolescents and early adolescents. These products are accessible to these groups in and around their households, while other drugs may be more difficult to obtain.

SITE OF ACTION/PHARMACOLOGY

Inhalants affect the CNS and are also extremely damaging to the cardiovascular and respiratory systems of the user.

DRUG EFFECTS

Inhalants have profound effects on the heart and may cause permanent damage. Elevated heart rates, arrhythmias, ventricular fibrillation, and decreased cardiac output may occur. Irreversible damage also may be done to other body systems such as the liver, brain, bone marrow, and kidneys.

LENGTH OF EFFECTS

The absorption of inhalants is rapid: Euphoria can occur within 15 minutes.

SIGNS AND SYMPTOMS

Considerable variations in signs and symptoms occur, depending on the substance inhaled. The user may be euphoric, giddy, and excited or may complain of fatigue, drowsiness, headache, and visual hallucinations. Irritated conjunctiva, anemia, cough, and pulsing headache are common symptoms. Users frequently have poor academic performance as a result of intoxication or physiological damage. "Glue sniffer's rash," a contact dermatitis, may be seen on the hands, on the nose, and around the mouth.

SIDE EFFECTS

Those who abuse inhalants may show signs of peripheral neuropathies and exhibit tremors and weakness. Protein in the urine and symptoms of myocardial ischemia are evidence of serious physiological damage. The user may collapse suddenly due to cardiovascular effects and require immediate emergency medical treatment. Sudden death is one terrible consequence of inhalant abuse.

PATTERN OF USE

Inhalants are taken directly (as from gas tanks) or from rags soaked with the substance and put into plastic bags. Liquids that produce fumes to inhale are frequently put into soda cans to escape the detection of family members or school officials.

Classification: Laxative Abuse

HISTORY

With the desire of adolescents in recent years to achieve fashion-model thinness, and the increase in eating disorders in this group in general, misuse of over-the-counter laxatives has increased in popularity among high school and college students. It is frequently a component of the purging behaviors of bulimia and anorexia nervosa. Laxatives also are abused by the elderly, with about 30 percent of individuals age 60 or older being regular users (Lee and Bennett, 1991). Laxative abuse is estimated to occur ten times more frequently in women than in men (Kokke, Saidi, Watson, and Donowitz, 1996).

SITE OF ACTION/PHARMACOLOGY

Laxatives act in the gastrointestinal system.

DRUG EFFECTS

These drugs increase peristalsis, irritate the intestinal mucosa, and increase the amount of water in the intestines.

LENGTH OF EFFECTS

The effects of various laxatives depend on the qualities and dosage of the drug used.

SIGNS AND SYMPTOMS

Individuals who abuse laxatives frequently have chronic bloating, pain and cramping, weakness, and frequent bowel movements or diarrhea.

SIDE EFFECTS

As part of the syndrome of bulimia nervosa, laxative abuse signals a psychological problem in need of professional assistance. Inadequately digested food accompanied by malabsorption of important nutrients leads to hypocalcemia and hypokalemia. Weight loss coupled with protracted diarrhea may result in life-threatening electrolyte disturbances and dangerous or fatal heart arrhythmias (Roseborough and Felix, 1994). Dependence on laxatives to have bowel movements can result in alterations in colonic function.

PATTERN OF USE

Laxatives are used by adolescents and young adults to increase intestinal motility, reduce food absorption, and therefore decrease the intake of calories. Older adults may use laxatives habitually in place of fiber-rich foods, fluids, and a program of regular exercise.

REFERENCES

Abel, E.A. (1982). *Marihuana: The First Twelve Hundred Years*. New York: McGraw-Hill.

American Psychiatric Association. (1994). *Diagnostic and Statistical Manual of Mental Disorders* (4th ed.). Washington, DC: American Psychiatric Association.

Austin, G. (1978). Perspectives on the history of psychoactive substance abuse. *National Institute on Drug Abuse Research Issues 23*. Washington, DC: U.S. Department of Health, Education, and Welfare.

Breecher, E.M. (1972). *Licit and Illicit Drugs*. Boston: Little, Brown.

Cicero, T.J., and O'Connor, L.H. (1990). Abuse liability of anabolic steroids and their possible role in the abuse of alcohol, morphine, and other substances. *NIDA Research Monograph 102*, 1–28.

Duncan, D.F., and Gold, R.S. (1982). *Drugs and the Whole Person*. New York: Macmillan

Edwards, J.A., Wesnes, K., Warburton, D.M., and Gale, A. (1985). Evidence of more rapid stimulus evaluation following cigarette smoking. *Addictive Behaviors 10*, 113–126.

Erard, R., Luisada, P.V., and Peele, R. (1980). The PCP psychosis: Prolonged intoxication or drug-precipitated functional illness. *Journal of Psychedelic Drugs 12*, 235–245.

Frisch, N.C., and Frisch, L.E. (1998). The client who abuses chemical substances. In N.C. Frisch and L.E. Frisch (eds.), *Psychiatric Mental Health Nursing*. New York: Delmar Publishers.

Gallagher, W. (1986). Pandora's pharmacy. *This World*, August 31, 7–9.

Gawin, F.H. (1991). Cocaine addiction: Psychology and neurophysiology [published erratum appears in *Science 253*, 494, 1991]. *Science 251*, 1580–1586.

Gawin, F., Khalsa, M.E., and Ellinwood, E. (1994). Stimulants. In M. Galanter and H. Kleber (eds.), *Textbook of Substance Abuse Treatment*. New York: American Psychiatric Press.

Griffiths, R.R., Bigelow, G.E., Liebson, I., et al. (1980). Drug preference in humans: Double-blinded choice comparison of pentobarbital, diazepam, and placebo. *Journal of Pharmacology and Experimental Therapy 215*, 649–661.

Grinspoon, L., and Bakalar, J.B. (1995). *Marijuana: The Forbidden Medicine*. New Haven: Yale University Press.

Hanson, G., and Venturelli, P.J. (1995). *Drugs and Society*. Boston: Jones and Bartlett Publishers.

Jellinek, E.M. (1960). *The Disease Concept of Alcoholism*. New Brunswick, NJ: Hillhouse Press.

Johnston, L.D., O'Malley, P.M., and Bachman, J.G. (1998). *National Survey Results on Drug Use from The Monitoring The Future Study, 1975–1997*. NIH Pub. No. 98-4345. Rockville, MD: U.S. Department of Health and Human Services, National Institute on Drug Abuse.

Kinney, J., and Leaton, G. (1995). *Loosening the Grip: A Handbook of Alcohol Information*. St Louis: Mosby-YearBook.

Kokke, F.T., Saidi, R.F., Watson, A.J.M., and Donowitz, M. (1996). In J.D. Stobo, D.B. Hellmann, P.W. Ladenson, B.G. Petty, and T.A. Traill (eds.), *The Principles and Practice of Medicine* (23rd ed.). Stamford, CT: Appleton and Lange.

Leary, T., and Clark, W.H. (1963). Religious implications of consciousness expanding drugs. *Religious Education 58*, 251–256.

Lee, J.H., and Bennett, G. (1991). Substance abuse in adulthood. In E.G. Bennett and D. Woolf (eds.), *Substance Abuse: Pharmacologic, Developmental and Clinical Perspectives* (2nd ed.). Albany, NY: Delmar Publishers.

Maurer, D., and Vogel, V. (1967). *Narcotics and Narcotic Addiction*. Springfield, IL: Thomas Publishers.

Millman, R.B., and Beeder, A.B. (1994). Cannabis. In M. Galanter and H.D. Kleber (eds.), *Textbook of Substance Abuse Treatment*. Washington, DC: American Psychiatric Press.

Monroe, R.R., and Drell, H.J. (1947). Oral use of amphetamines obtained from inhalers. *Journal of the American Medical Association 135*, 909–915.

National Council on Alcoholism. (1989). *Who Says Alcoholism Is a Disease?* (Brochure), New York.

Ockene, J.K., and Kristeller, J.L. (1994). Tobacco. In M. Galanter and H.D. Kleber (eds.), *Textbook of Substance Abuse Treatment*. Washington, DC: American Psychiatric Press.

Pinger, R.R., Payne, W.A., Hahn, D.B., and Hahn, E.J. (1995). *Drugs: Issues for Today* (2nd ed.). St. Louis, MO: Mosby-YearBook.

Ray, O.S. (1983). *Drugs, Society and Human Behavior*. St. Louis, MO: CV Mosby.

Ray, O.S., and Ksir, C. (1993). *Drugs, Society and Human Behavior* (6th ed.). St. Louis, MO: CV Mosby.

Remmington's Pharmaceutical Sciences (17th ed.). (1985). Easton, PA: Mack Publishing.

Roseborough, G.S., and Felix, W.A. (1994). Disseminated intravascular coagulation complicating gastric perforation in a bulimic woman. *Canadian Journal of Surgery 37*, 55–58.

Roueche, B. (1960). *The Neutral Spirit: A Portrait of Alcohol*. Boston: Little, Brown.

Sanders-Bush, E., Burris, J.K., and Knoth, K. (1988). Lysergic acid diethylamide and 2,5-dimethoxy-4-methylamphetamine are partial agonists at serotonin receptors linked to phosphoinositide hydrolysis. *Journal of Pharmacology and Experimental Therapeutics 246*, 924–928.

Schultes, R.E. (1978). Ethnopharmacological significance of psychotropic drugs of vegetable origin. In W.G. Clark and J. del Giudice (eds.), *Principles of Pharmacology* (2nd ed.). New York: Academic Press.

Schultes, R.E., and Hoffmann, A. (1973). *The Botany and Chemistry of the Hallucinogens*. Springfield, IL: Charles C. Thomas Publishers.

Siegel, R.K. (1989). *Intoxication*. New York: E.P. Dutton.

Siegel, R.K., and Jarvik, M.E. (1975). Drug-induced hallucinations in animals and man. In R.K. Siegal and L.J. West (eds.), *Hallucinations*. New York: Wiley.

Smith, D., and Wesson, D.R. (1994). Benzodiazepines and other sedative-hypnotics. In M. Galanter and H.D. Kleber (eds.), *Textbook of Substance Abuse Treatment*. Washington, DC: American Psychiatric Association Press.

U.S. Environmental Protection Agency. (1992). *Respiratory Health Effects of Passive Smoking: Lung Cancer and Other Disorders* (Review Draft). Washington, DC: Office of Research and Development.

Yesavage, J.A., and Freeman, A.M. III. (1978). Acute phencyclidine (PCP) intoxication. *Journal of Clinical Psychiatry 44*, 664–665.

APPENDIX II

National Health Promotion and Disease Prevention Objectives

Goals to Be Achieved by the Year 2000

Source: Healthy People 2000: National Health Promotion and Disease Prevention Objectives. (U.S. Department of Health and Human Services, Public Health Service, 1991)

Health Status Objective 3: Tobacco

3.1 Reduce coronary heart disease deaths to no more than 100 per 100,000 people.

3.2 Slow the rise in lung cancer deaths to achieve a rate of no more than 42 per 100,000 people.

3.3 Slow the rise in deaths from chronic obstructive pulmonary disease to achieve a rate of no more than 25 per 100,000 people.

Risk Reduction Objective 3: Tobacco

3.4 Reduce cigarette smoking to a prevalence of no more than 15 percent among people age 20 and older.

3.5 Reduce the initiation of cigarette smoking by children and youth so that no more than 15 percent have become regular cigarette smokers by age 20.

3.6 Increase to at least 50 percent the proportion of cigarette smokers age 18 and older who stopped smoking cigarettes for at least 1 day during the preceding year.

3.7 Increase smoking cessation during pregnancy so that at least 60 percent of women who are cigarette smokers at the time they become pregnant quit smoking early in pregnancy and maintain abstinence for the remainder of their pregnancy.

3.8 Reduce to no more than 20 percent the proportion of children age 6 and younger who are regularly exposed to tobacco smoke in the home.

3.9 Reduce smokeless tobacco use by males ages 12 through 24 to a prevalence of no more than 4 percent.

Health Status Objective 4: Alcohol and Other Drugs

4.1 Reduce deaths caused by alcohol-related motor vehicle crashes to no more than 8.5 per 100,000 people.

4.2 Reduce cirrhosis deaths to no more than 6 per 100,000 people.

4.3 Reduce drug-related deaths to no more than 3 per 100,000 people.

4.4 Reduce drug abuse–related hospital emergency department visits by at least 20 percent.

Risk Reduction Objective 4: Alcohol and Other Drugs

4.5 Increase by at least 1 year the average age of first use of cigarettes, alcohol, and marijuana by adolescents ages 12 through 17.

4.6 Reduce the proportion of young people who have used alcohol, marijuana, and cocaine in the past month.

4.7 Reduce the proportion of high school seniors and college students engaging in recent occasions of heavy drinking of alcoholic beverages to no more than 28 percent of high school seniors and 32 percent of college students.

4.8 Reduce alcohol consumption by people age 14 and older to an annual average of no more than 2 gallons of ethanol per person.

4.9 Increase the proportion of high school seniors who perceive social disapproval associated with the heavy use of alcohol, occasional use of marijuana, and experimentation with cocaine.

4.10 Increase the proportion of high school seniors who associate risk of physical or psychological harm with the heavy use of alcohol, regular use of marijuana, and experimentation with cocaine.

4.11 Reduce to no more than 3 percent the proportion of male high school seniors who use anabolic steroids.

Theoretical Models of Addiction: An Overview

Carolyn E. D'Avanzo, RN, MSN, DNSc
Madeline Naegle, RN, CS, PhD, FAAN

George Jellinek's Early Contributions

The interrelationships among alcohol addiction and various genetic, physical, environmental, and social factors have been difficult to determine. Jellinek (1960) noted the interaction of these many factors and stated that "there is not one alcoholism but a whole variety" (p. 10). In Jellinek's (1960) view, alcoholism was "any use of alcoholic beverages that causes any damage to the individual, society or both" (p. 35). Using this broad definition, he singled out what he called "species" of alcoholism, arbitrarily using letters of the Greek alphabet such as alpha and gamma (Jellinek, 1960). The types of alcoholism described were differentiated by patterns of onset, loss of control, and rates of progression. Each species differed somewhat from the others; in combination, they contained the symptoms now considered indicators of alcoholism, although all need not be present for an accurate diagnosis.

Jellinek actually described patterns of alcohol abuse and dependence and included such symptoms as psychological dependence; consumption of alcohol at the expense of adequate nutrition, leading to physical ills such as gastritis, cirrhosis of the liver, and polyneuropathy; tolerance to alcohol at a cellular level; craving (an overpowering desire to drink); inability to control the time or amount of one's drinking; withdrawal symptoms; periodic binge drinking such as on weekends; and marked behavioral changes even after moderate drinking.

Valliant's Model of Alcoholism in Men

The understanding of the multidetermined nature of alcoholism was further advanced by the longitudinal studies of George Valliant (1983). He acknowledged major questions on the etiology of alcoholism, such as whether alcoholism is caused by heredity or environment, whether it is the cause or the result of mental illness, and whether it is a sin or a sickness. He sought accurate information in long-term prospective studies and selected subjects before signs of disease existed, following them for decades and recording their subsequent problems with alcohol (or lack thereof).

Valliant's study, one of the first to examine the development of alcohol abuse, was a prospective, epidemiological study at the Harvard Medical School's Study of Adult Development. Valliant followed 660 men from adolescence to late middle life from 1940 to 1980. The sample consisted of 204 men who were upper-middle-class sophomores and 456 inner-city boys of junior high school age. In addition, information was elicited from 100 alcohol-dependent women and men admitted to a detoxification unit who were followed for 8 years.

More recent study results suggest that alcoholism may simultaneously manifest a conditioned habit and a disease, and that the disease of alcoholism can be defined by medical or sociological models; some types of alcoholism are more under genetic control and some are more under environmental control. Findings suggest that, once developed, alcoholism is chronic. Valliant describes common phases as insidious, fulminating, and intermittent, as well as acknowledging recovery achieved with or without treatment. Quantities cited are based on the male sample. He describes the course of alcoholism in three stages (1983, pp. 309–310):

> Stage I: Heavy "social" drinking is characterized by ingestion of three to five drinks daily for up to a lifetime. The individual may reverse to more moderate levels of consumption, may continue this pattern without apparent symptoms, or may progress to the next stage.
>
> Stage II: The individual encounters medical, social, occupational, and legal difficulties associated with drinking. Consumption is at the level of about eight drinks daily. In this group, about half become abstinent or return to controlled drinking.
>
> Stage III: About 3 percent to 5 percent of American adults (men outnumber women 3 or 4 to 1) will progress to this stage of physical dependence/addiction. Once addiction has occurred, the individual progresses to social incapacity or death. Spontaneous recovery is generally uncommon. Sobriety may be reached, however, by detoxification and treatment, including the use of support groups like Alcoholics Anonymous.

Contemporary Disease Model

Although illness and disease are often used interchangeably today, the word illness was more frequently used to describe alcoholism by physicians who believed it to be less frightening to the public (Jellinek, 1960). The correspondence between alcoholism and criteria for disease can be explained as follows. The American Medical Association (1963, p. 506) defined disease as "any deviation from a state of health; an illness or sickness; more specifically, a definite marked process having a characteristic train of symptoms. It may affect the whole body or any of its parts, and its etiology, pathology, and prognosis may be known or unknown." The marked psychological and physical effects of alcohol addiction over time engender little disagreement over the concept among health care providers today, although disputes about the etiology of alcoholism and other substance misuse continue. The current disease model, revised from Jellinek, acknowledges the heterogeneity of patterns in abuse and addiction described by Valliant and incorporates the following five points:

1. There is a unique entity that can be identified as alcoholism; this occurs in heterogeneous types.
2. Alcoholics and prealcoholics are essentially different from nonalcoholics.
3. Alcoholics may experience an irresistible physical craving for alcohol and/or a psychological compulsion to drink.
4. Alcoholics gradually develop loss of control over drinking and possibly the inability to stop drinking.
5. Alcoholism is a progressive disease that follows an inexorable development through a distinct series of phases as long as the person continues to ingest alcohol.

The disease concept of alcoholism is endorsed by a number of groups including the American Medical Association, the American Nurses Association, the American Heart Association, the American Psychiatric Association, and the World Health Organization.

Research findings that support the biologic etiology of at least some manifestations of alcoholism continue to mount. Findings of studies of twins and half-siblings raised apart from alcoholic parents, dating from the 1970s (Cloninger, Sigvardsson, and Bohman, 1988; Goodwin et al., 1973), suggest that genetic factors have at least a modest influence on the development of alcoholism. The observation that children of alcoholics have high rates of alcoholism even when raised by adoptive parents whose drinking was light to moderate supports the view that a susceptibility to alcoholism is inborn and determined biologically. A recent study of fraternal and identical male and female twins found that the relationship between parental alcoholism and twin concordance for alcohol abuse varied according to the type of twin and sex (Pickens et al., 1991). Nongenetic familial factors were supported by observations of Worobec and others (1990) that alcoholics with alcoholic parents are at increased risk for severe alcoholism because they are more reliant on ethanol to manage moods, and they are less able to recognize the negative effects of drinking. Even abstinence does not remove the neurophysiological response that some individuals have to alcohol, which may lead to its abuse. Research further indicates that an inborn lack of sensitivity to the effects of alcohol may lead to heavy drinking (Schuckit, 1991). This lack of sensitivity results in habitual ingestion of large amounts of alcohol in order to achieve euphoric or relaxing effects.

Social Learning Models

Sociological models of addiction link the cause of substance abuse to factors external to the individual. These factors include families, peer groups, neighborhoods, or communities. Drug use is learned in contacts with other individuals who teach or model drug use behaviors. Initiation into cocaine use, for example, might entail where to obtain it, how to snort it or use drug apparatus, and what is felt in a high. It is clear that many adolescents often begin experimentation with alcohol and other drugs in response to social/peer pressure, particularly if they bond with a drug-using group. The work of Kandel (1982) supports the notion that the use of alcohol by adolescents is frequently a gateway to the use of marijuana and then to harder drugs such as cocaine and heroin.

The presence of positive role models and one's confidence in reaching goals influence the individual's ability to achieve such goals (Bandura, 1977). Goals set by adolescents are frequently congruent with those of their families and/or peer groups. Factors that appear to increase an adolescent's risk for substance abuse include poverty, sexual and/or physical abuse (Boyd, 1993), dysfunctional families, low self-esteem and poor psychological functioning (Dembo, Williams, Schmeidler, and Wothke, 1993), limited coping skills, and lack of positive role models. Interventions directed at modifying these social factors and based on the social learning model have been incorporated into many prevention programs for school-age children and youth.

Social concerns about alcoholism supported the temperance movement of the early 1800s, founded on the premise that drunkenness was evil and a moral failing rather than a biological or psychological disease. The Women's Christian Temperance Union advocated abstinence, religion, prayer, and reformation as antidotes to drunkenness. Additional social action in 1920 led to the passage of the Eighteenth Amendment, which prohibited the manufacture and sale of liquor. While it failed, it remains a significant first social effort acknowledging the negative effects of substance use on health. For some health care providers and the public, the identification of alcoholism as a disease is objectionable. Some believe that the illness/disease concept absolves the individual of personal responsibility in the development and continuation of addiction. Valliant (1983) noted that, in this view, calling alcoholism a disease is a semantic trick because, for some, excessive drinking can be overcome by willpower. Viewing alcoholism and drug dependence as "moral weaknesses" implies that abusers use substances not because they are biologically susceptible, but because they make a personal choice to do so. This view leads to various forms of punishment as intervention strategies. Incarceration, job loss, fines, revocation of motor vehicle and professional licenses, and mandatory alcohol or driving education courses are social actions implemented as deterrents to drinking (Nusbaumer, 1994).

Psychological Perspectives

Psychological models addressing the development and treatment of addiction emerged in early psychoanalytic writings and were based on the notion that alcoholism is rooted in the individual's personality characteristics and signifies the presence of unresolved, unconscious conflicts, including self-destructive and oral-dependent psychodynamics. In this view, existing psychopathology predisposed certain individuals to become addicts, and treatment was directed at the underlying psychodynamic cause (Levin, 1990). Personality characteristics were linked with the notion of a prealcoholic or alcoholic personality and included depression and antisocial characteristics such as aloofness, dependency, and difficulty with social relationships. Linkages between one particular personality type and the development of addiction, however, have not been supported by research.

Early psychoanalytic approaches were notably unsuccessful in the treatment of alcoholism and other addictions, resulting in continued skepticism about their relevance. Because such treatment failed to adequately acknowledge the biological determinants and social factors that support addiction, considerable negativity about the ability of physicians and nurses to treat addiction was generated. Modified psychotherapeutic approaches to alcoholism treatment emerged in the 1960s (Fox, 1965; Tiebout, 1961), and others have continued to refine models of treatment that address psychological issues in the development of addiction: those that accompany the course of the illness, and those that must be addressed in ongoing recovery. Newer models include abstinence as a goal and the need for involvement in self-help programs as developed in the 12-step Alcoholics Anonymous model (Kaufman, 1989; Zimberg, 1985). In the early 1980s, addictions were classified as diseases akin to medical conditions, and the popularity of psychological perspectives waned.

It is now generally accepted that addiction has psychological as well as physical components and affects social function as well. Psychiatrists, psychiatric nurses, and other mental health specialists are expected to be knowledgeable about identifying and treating addiction. In addition, they bring expert knowledge to the assessment and treatment of dual diagnosis. In dual diagnosis, addiction cooccurs with a major psychiatric disorder, and the client requires both substance abuse and psychiatric intervention. Because abuse and dependence on drugs are so prevalent in Western society, persons with these problems are seen in every health care setting. Most individuals with drug problems do not seek treatment for them. Of those who do, some are legally mandated to treatment, some are referred by employers, some are treated because their addictions cause long-term medical problems, and some seek treatment in response to family, legal, or social problems. Since the early 1980s, the federal government, addiction treatment groups, and professional organizations have sought to increase addictions education among social workers, physicians, and nurses in general practice. The most recent initiatives are directed at increasing the detection and referral of persons with drug problems seen in primary care settings to specialty treatment.

Multifactorial Models: Alcoholism as a Biopsychosocial Phenomenon

Multifactorial models consider the many possible factors that may contribute to substance-using patterns: genetics, beliefs/attitudes, personality and developmental traits, social and cultural factors, and coping/interpersonal skills. Biological research now provides strong support for the existence of genetic and neurophysiological traits that contribute to an individual's response to the pharmacological effects of drugs. Cultural, social, and learning factors often determine whether a person experiments with drugs at all and/or experiments and continues to use to degrees of abuse or dependence. Models acknowledging these many factors are known as biopsychosocial models.

Heterogeneity in humans invalidates the use of unidimensional causality for an understanding of substance use behaviors. Similarly, research and experience have proved that the cookie-cutter approach to treatment is unpredictable in outcome and lacks strong evidence of success. Increasingly, providers are recognizing that assessment and treatment must be individualized, and newer multifactorial models, which acknowledge many variables, are gaining acceptance. These include Cloninger's (1987) model of neurogenic learning, von Knorring and associates' (1985) early and late-onset subtyping, and Zucker's (1987) developmental sequencing model. These theories incorporate a multidimensional view of substance use disorders and evaluate genetic factors, personality, and psychopathology with patterns of drinking (Galanter and Kleber, 1994, p. 15). The biopsychosocial model is the most comprehensive model of causality applied to addictive disorders. It includes genetic predisposition in interaction with psychological and sociocultural factors that result in patterns of abuse or dependence on alcohol, tobacco, and/or other drugs in combination. This model acknowledges the roles of genetic and familial predispositions, the importance of pharmacology in initial and continued drug use, learning as a factor in experimentation and positive reinforcement, and the psychological conflicts that predispose one to use and continue problematic use. This model proposes that drug users are not a homogeneous population and that subpopulations within this group share characteristics, patterns, and consequences of use.

The multitude of clinical problems faced by clients with addictions appears to be best served when the biopsychosocial model serves as the basis for clinical approaches. Because addiction has multiple origins and affects all spheres of one's life, care providers from many disciplines contribute to the comprehensive treatment of the drug-dependent individual and his or her family. The multifactorial model facilitates comprehensive assessment and treatment that use a range of modalities.

REFERENCES

American Medical Association. (1963). *Narcotics Addiction: Official Actions of the AMA.* Chicago: American Medical Association.

Bandura, A. (1977). *Social Learning Theory.* Englewood Cliffs, NJ: Prentice-Hall.

Bohn, M.J., and Meyer, R.E. (1994). Typologies of addiction. In M. Galanter and H.D. Kleber (eds.), *The American Psychiatric Press Textbook of Substance Abuse Treatment.* Washington, DC: American Psychiatric Press.

Boyd, C.J. (1993). Antecedents of women's crack cocaine abuse. *Journal of Substance Abuse Treatment 10,* 433–438.

Cloninger, C.R. (1987). Neurogenic adaptive mechanisms in alcoholism. *Science 236,* 410–416.

Cloninger, C.R., Sigvardsson, S., and Bohman, M. (1988). Childhood personality predicts alcohol abuse in young adults. *Alcohol Clinical Experimental Research 12,* 494–505.

Dembo, R., Williams, L., Schmeidler, J., and Wothke, W. (1993). A longitudinal study of predictors of the adverse effects of alcohol and marijuana/hashish use among a cohort of high risk youths. *International Journal of the Addictions 28*(11), 1045–1083.

Fox, R. (1965). Psychiatric aspects of alcoholism. *American Journal of Psychotherapy 19,* 408–416.

Goodwin, D.W., Schulsinger, F., Hermansen, L., Guze, S.B., and Winokur, G. (1973). Alcohol problems in adoptees raised apart from alcoholic biological parents. *Archives General Psychiatry, 28,* 238–242.

Jellinek, E.M. (1960). *The Disease Concept of Alcoholism.* New Brunswick, NJ: Hillhouse Press.

Kandel, D. (1982). Epidemiologic and psychosocial perspectives on adolescent drug use. *Journal of American Academy of Child Psychiatry 21*(4), 328–347.

Kaufman, E. (1989). Psychotherapy of dually diagnosed patients. *Journal of Substance Abuse Treatment 6,* 9–18.

Levin, J.D. (1990). *Alcoholism: A Bio-Psychological Approach.* New York: Hemisphere.

Nusbaumer, M.R. (1994). Governmental control of deviant drinking: The manipulation of morals in medicine. In P.J. Venturelli (ed.), *Drug Use in America: Social, Cultural and Political Perspectives.* Boston: Jones and Bartlett.

Pickens, R.W., Svikis, D.S., McGue, M., Lykken, D.T., Heston, L.L., and Clayton, P.J. (1991). Heterogeneity in the inheritance of alcoholism: A study of male and female twins. *Archives of General Psychiatry 48,* 19–28.

Schuckit, M.A. (1991). A clinical model of genetic influence in alcohol dependence. *Journal of Studies on Alcohol 55,* 5–17.

Tiebout, H.M. (1961). Alcoholics Anonymous: An experiment in nature. *Quarterly Journal of Studies on Alcohol 22,* 62–68.

Valliant, G. (1983). *The Nature of Alcoholism.* Cambridge, MA: Harvard University Press.

von Knorring, L., Palm, V., and Andersson, H.E. (1985). Relationship between treatment outcome and subtype of alcoholism in men. *Journal of Studies in Alcohol 46,* 388–391.

Worobec, T.G., Turner, W.M., O'Farrell, T.J., Cuttee, H.S., Bayog, R.D., Tsuang, M.T. (1990). Alcohol use by alcoholics with and without a history of parental alcoholism. *Alcoholism, Clinical and Experimental Research 14*(6), 887–892.

Zimberg, S. (1985). Principles of alcoholism psychotherapy. In S. Zimberg, J. Wallace, and S. Blume (eds.), *Practical Approaches to Alcoholism Psychotherapy* (2nd ed.). New York: Plenum Press.

Zucker, R.A. (1987). The four alcoholisms: A developmental account of the etiologic process. In P.C. Rivers (ed.), *Alcohol and Addictive Behavior.* Lincoln, NE: University of Nebraska Press.

APPENDIX IV

Self-Help Programs for the Addictions

Alcoholics Anonymous (AA) is the best-known and most successful self-help program. In 1935 in Ohio. an alcoholic now known as Bill W. had a spiritual experience that prompted him to stop drinking. After a year of abstinence from alcohol, rather than giving in to an urge to begin drinking again, he sought out another alcoholic for support. He remained sober, recognized the need for peer support, and began the AA organization. There were no dues, and the only requirement for membership was a sincere desire for sobriety—a full life without the abuse of alcohol. Independent from religious, social, or political organizations, AA members were alcoholics helping other alcoholics by means of meetings, peer support, sharing of stories, and reliance on a "higher power." Total abstinence was stressed. These components—spirituality, emotional and social engagement, and commitment to getting sober—remain central to the organization as it exists today.

In 1939, about 100 members of the fledgling organization published "The Big Book," (Alcoholics Anonymous, 1939) a collection of their experiences along the path to sobriety. By 1983, there were an estimated 1 million members worldwide and by 1992, there were well over 2 million members (Alcoholics Anonymous World Services, 1992).

A survey of its members by the General Service Office of AA in 1992 showed that men outnumbered women members about 2 to 1. Multisubstance use was reported by 79 percent of its members under age of 21 and by 60 percent under age 31. Of its membership in 1992, 31 percent were new members who had been sober less than a year, 34 percent had been sober from 1 to 5 years, and 35 percent had been sober for more than 5 years (Kinney and Leaton, 1995).

AA meetings are available 7 days a week in larger metropolitan areas throughout the world and may run 24 hours a day during holiday seasons when members feel more vulnerable to "slipping." Nurses and nursing students can gain invaluable information about self-help programs by attending these meetings. Meetings that are designated as open may be attended by any interested person as well as spouses or significant others. Often there are several more experienced members who speak about their experiences, including what brought them to AA and how their lives have been changed by sobriety. These meetings have many elements of group therapy, such as development of a cohesive group, a sense of universality of shared experiences, and altruism toward others, which partially explains their effectiveness. There is a strong sense of service in AA; a sponsor acts as a friend and mentor to new AA members and is available in the community as well as at meetings.

Alcoholics Anonymous has become the model for numerous self-help groups founded in the same 12-step model. These include Narcotics Anonymous, Overeaters Anonymous, Survivors of Incest, Gamblers Anonymous, and others. The expectation that regular meeting attendance will assist in attaining and maintaining sobriety makes these groups helpful adjuncts to professional focused treatment. In addition, the availability of meetings, comradeship, and 24-hour sponsorship provide support not generally available in the professional community. Although research on the effectiveness of AA alone is limited, many people attribute their sobriety and the preservation of their lives to involvement with the fellowship. Self-help is based in a philosophy that emphasizes the potential inner strength of the individual, the group, and the community—it means help built around an inner core rather than help offered from outside. The early work of AA has been followed by various self-help and advocacy groups.

Additional groups for addiction have developed using different treatment philosophies or psychological models and include Rational Recovery (based on the rational emotive therapy approach), Women for Sobriety, secular organizations for sobriety, and groups directed at the needs of dually diagnosed individuals. Groups based on the 12-step model are utilized for all phases of treatment including in-patient treatment, aftercare, relapse prevention, and ongoing recovery. It is important to note that in one study only a small percentage of former problem drinkers in the United States sought help from professionals, Alcoholics Anonymous, or informal helping networks. Individuals who had sought help reported that they had done so in response to social pressures or a compulsion to drink (Hasin and Grant, 1995). This observation, as well as reports of others who stopped drinking or using drugs without treatment, suggests that social norms that stigmatize heavy drinking and illicit drug use may be increasingly prevalent in the United States.

REFERENCES

Alcoholics Anonymous. (1939). *Alcoholics Anonymous.* New York: Alcoholics Anonymous World Services.

Alcoholics Anonymous. (1992). *This is AA: An introduction to the AA recovery program* (Brochure). Alcoholics Anonymous World Services.

Hasin, D.S., and Grant, B.F. (1995). AA and other helpseeking for alcohol problems: Former drinkers in the U.S. general population. *Journal of Substance Abuse 7*(3), 281–292.

Kinney, J., and Leaton, G. (1995). *Loosening the Grip: A Handbook of Alcohol Information.* St. Louis, MO: Mosby-YearBook.

Resources and Programs on Alcohol, Tobacco, and Other Drug Abuse

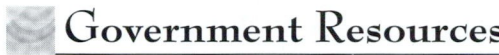 Government Resources

Center for Substance Abuse Treatment (CSAT) Hot Line
Phone: 800-662-4357

National Clearinghouse for Alcohol and Drug Information (NCADI)
P.O. Box 2345, Rockville, Maryland 20847-2345
Phone: 800-729-6686

National Association of State Alcohol and Drug Abuse Directors (NASADAD)
444 North Capitol Street, NW, Suite 642, Washington, DC, 20001
Phone: 202-783-6868

National Institute on Drug Abuse
National Institutes of Health
6001 Executive Boulevard, Room 5213, Bethesda, Maryland 20892-9561
Phone: 301-443-6245

Office of Minority Health Resource Center (OMHRC)
U.S. Department of Health and Human Services
P.O. Box 37337, Washington, DC 20013-7337
Phone: 800-444-6472, TDD: 301-230-7199, Fax: 301-230-7198, Email: info@omhrc.gov
http://www.omhrc.gov

Resources/Programs for Alcohol and Drug Abuse

Adult Children of Alcoholics (ACA/AcoA)
P.O. Box 3216, Torrance, California 90510
Phone: 310-534-1815

Alcoholics Anonymous World Service Office (AA)
P.O. Box 459, Grand Central Station, New York, New York 10163
Phone: 212-870-3400

Cocaine Anonymous World Service Office (CAWS)
P.O. Box 2000, Los Angeles, California 90049-8000
Phone: 310-559-5833, Fax: 310-559-2554

Jews in Recovery from Alcoholism and Drug Abuse
426 West 58th Street, New York, New York 10019
Phone: 212-397-4197, Fax: 212-489-6229, Email: jacs@jacsweb.org

Nar-Anon Family Groups
P.O. Box 2562, Palos Verdes Peninsula, California 90274
Phone: 213-547-5800

Narcotics Anonymous (NA)
P.O. Box 9999, Van Nuys, California 91409
Phone: 818-780-3951

National Families in Action
2296 Henderson Mill Road, Suite 300, Atlanta, Georgia 30345
Phone: 770-934-6364, Fax: 770-934-7137, Email: nfia@web.cc.emory.edu

National Resource Center for Prevention of Perinatal Abuse of Alcohol and Other Drugs
515 King Street, Suite 410, Alexandria, Virginia 22314
Phone: 703-836-8761 or 703-684-6048

Rational Recovery Systems
Box 800, Lotus, California 95651
Phone: 916-621-2667

Secular Organizations for Sobriety (SOS)
P.O. Box 5, Buffalo, New York 14215
Phone: 716-834-2922

Women for Sobriety
P.O. Box 618, Quakertown, Pennsylvania 18951
Phone: 800-333-1606

Other National Organizations

Latino Council on Alcohol and Tobacco (LCAT)
UMDNJ-Robert Wood Johnson Medical School
675 Hoes Lane, Room N110, Piscataway, New Jersey 08854
Phone: 908-235-5041

National Association for Children of Alcoholics (NACoA)
11426 Rockville Pike, Suite 100, Rockville, Maryland 20852
Phone: 301-468-0985

National Association for Native American Children of Alcoholics (NANACoA)
1402 Third Avenue, Suite 1110, Seattle, Washington 98101
Phone: 206-467-7686 or 800-322-5601, Fax: 206-467-7689, Email: nanacoa@ao!.com

National Black Alcoholism Addictions Council (NBAC)
1629 K. Street, NW, Suite 802, Washington, DC 20006
Phone: 202-296-2696

National Council on Alcoholism and Drug Dependence (NCADD)
12 West 21st Street, New York, New York 10010
Phone: 212-206-6770, 800-622-2255, Fax: 212-645-169O

National Rural Institute on Alcohol and Drug Abuse
c/o Arts and Sciences Outreach, University of Wisconsin, Eau Claire, Wisconsin 54702-4004
Phone: 715-836-2031

 # Resources for Women

Mothers Against Drunk Driving (MADD)
511 East John Carpenter Freeway, Suite 700, Irving, Texas 75062
Phone: 214-744-6233 or 800-GET-MADD

Women for Sobriety
P.O. Box 618, Quakertown, Pennsylvania 18951
Phone: 800-333-1606

Women's Health Network
1325 G Street, NW, Washington, DC 20005
Phone: 202-347-1140

 # Resources for Youth

American Youth Work Center
1200 17th Street, NW, 4th floor, Washington, DC 20036
Phone: 202-785-0764

Boys Clubs of America
771 First Avenue, New York, New York 10017
Phone: 212-351-5906

Camp Fire, Inc.
4601 Madison Avenue, Kansas City, Missouri 64112
Phone: 816-756-1950

Center for Science in the Public Interest
1875 Connecticut Avenue, NW, Suite 300, Washington, DC 20009-5728
Phone: 202-332-9110

Girls Clubs of America, Inc.
30 East 33rd Street, 7th floor, New York, New York 10016
Phone: 212-689-3700

International Institute for Inhalant Abuse
450 W. Jefferson, Englewood, Colorado 80110
Phone: 303-788-1951

"Just Say No" International
2101 Webster Street, Suite 1300, Oakland, California 94612
Phone: 800-258-2766

March of Dimes
1275 Mamaroneck Avenue, White Plains, New York 10605
Phone: 914-428-7100

National Agriculture Library
Youth Development Education Center
Room 304, 10301 Baltimore Boulevard, Beltsville, Maryland 20705-2351
Phone: 301-504-6400

National Association of Teen Institutes
87909 Manchester Road, St. Louis, Missouri 63144
Phone: 314-962-3456

National Black Child Development Institute (NBCDI)
463 Rhode Island Avenue, NW, Washington, DC 20005
Phone: 202-387-1281

National Collaboration for Youth
1319 F Street, NW, Suite 601, Washington, DC 20004
Phone: 202-347-2080

National Family Partnership
11159-B South Towne Square, St. Louis, Missouri 63123-7824
Phone: 314-845-1933

National 4-H Council
7100 Connecticut Avenue, Chevy Chase, Maryland 20815-4999
Phone: 301-961-2800

National Head Start Association
201 N. Union Street, Suite 320, Alexandria, Virginia 22314
Phone: 703-739-0875

National Network of Runaway and Youth Services, Inc.
1400 Eye Street, NW, Suite 330, Washington, DC 20004
Phone: 202-783-7949

YMCA of the USA
101 North Wacker Drive, Chicago, Illinois 60606
Phone: 312-977-0031
726 Broadway, New York, New York 10003
Phone: 212-614-2700

Internet Resources for Youth

Girl Power! Campaign
http://www. health.org/gpower/index.htm

Kids Campaign Site
http://www.kidscampaign.org

Youth Info Department of Health and Human Services
http://youth.os.dhhs.gov/

Resources for People with Disabilities

Center for Empowerment of Deaf Alcoholics in Recovery (CEDAR)
3041 University Avenue, San Diego, California 92104
Phone: 619-293-3820, TDD: 619-293-3746

Clearinghouse on Disability Information
OSERS/Department of Education
Switzer Building, Room 3132, 400 Maryland Avenue, SW, Washington, DC 20202-2524
Phone: 202-205-8412, Fax: 202-732-1252

Congress on Chemical Dependency and Disability (CCDD)
15519 Crenshaw Boulevard, Gardenia, California 90249
Phone: 310-679-9126

Institute on Alcohol, Drugs and Disability
P.O. Box 7044, San Mateo, California 94403
Phone: 707-644-2677, TDD: 707-664-2958

Minnesota Chemical Dependency Program for Deaf and Hard of Hearing Individuals
2450 Riverside Avenue, Minneapolis, Minnesota 55454
Phone: 612-337-4114, TDD: 612-337-4114, Voice and TDD: 800-282-DEAF

National Information Center for Children and Youth with Disabilities (NICHCY)
P.O. Box 1492, Washington, DC 20013
Phone: 800-695-0285, 202-884-8200, Fax: 202-884-8441, http://www.nichcy.org/

Resource Center on Substance Abuse Prevention and Disability
1331 F Street, NW, Suite 800, Washington, DC 20004
Phone: 202-783-2900, TDD: 202-737-0645

Substance Abuse Resources
1806 Highway 35, Oakhurst, New Jersey 07755
Phone: 732-663-1800, Email: ncadd@monmouth.com, http://www.subabuseresources.com

Substance Abuse Resources and Disability
Wright State University School of Medicine, SARDI, Dayton, Ohio 45435
Phone: 513-873-3588, TDD: 513-873-3579
http://www.med.wright.edu/SOM/academic/SubAbuse/SAIP.HTML

Internet Resources for People with Disabilities

National Association on Alcohol, Drugs and Disability, Inc. (NAADD)
http://www.health.org/

National Center for the Dissemination of Disability Research (NCDDR)
http://www.ncddr.org/

National Clearinghouse of Rehabilitation Training Materials (NCRTM)
http://www.nchrtm.okstate.edu/

National Rehabilitation Information Center (NARIC)
http://www.cais.com/naric/

Resources for Elders

Administration on Aging
330 Independence Avenue, SW, Washington, DC 20201
Phone: 800-677-1116 (Eldercare Locator), 202-619-0724 (public inquiries), 202-401-4541 (Office of Assistant Secretary for Aging), 202-619-7501 (AoA's National Aging Information Center for technical information), TDD: 202-401-7575, Fax: 202-260-1012
http://www.aoa.dhhs.gov, Email: esec@ban-gate.aoa.dhhs.gov

National Institute on Aging Information Center
P.O. Box 8057, Gaithersburg, Maryland 20898-8057
Phone: 800-222-2225, TTY: 800-222-4225, Fax: 301-589-3014
Email: niainfo@lkacc.com, http://www.nih.gov/nia

National Resource Center on Minority Aging Populations (NRC-MAP)
University Center on Aging, San Diego State University, College of Human Services, San Diego, California 92182-0273
Phone: 619-594-675, Fax: 619-594-2811

Resources for the Workplace

Drug-Free Workplace Helpline
M-F 9 am to 8 pm EST
Phone: 800-WORKPLACE

Employee Assistance Professional Association (EAPA)
4601 North Fairfax Drive, Suite 1001, Arlington, Virginia 22203
M-F 8 am to 6 pm EST
Phone: 703-522-6272

Employee Assistance Society of North America
P.O. Box 3909, Oak Park, Illinois 60303
Phone: 708-383-6668

North America Congress on Employee Assistance Programs
1863 Technology Drive, Suite 200, Troy, Michigan 48083
Phone: 313-588-7733

Resources for Gays/Lesbians/Bisexuals

National Resources

Al-Anon Family Groups
1600 Corporate Landing Parkway, Virginia Beach, Virginia 23454-5617
Phone: 800-344-2666, http://www.al-anon.alateen.org

Gay and Lesbian Medical Association (GLMA)
459 Fulton Street, Suite 107, San Francisco, California 94102
Phone: 415-255-4547

International Advisory Council for Homosexual Men and Women
in Alcoholics Anonymous (IAC)
P.O. Box 18212, Washington, DC 20036-8212

National Association of Lesbian & Gay Addiction Professionals (NALGAP) c/o PRTA
440 Grand Avenue, Suite 401, Oakland, California 94610-5012
Phone: 510-465-0547, TDD: 510-465-2888, Fax: 510-465-0505, Email: kfolger@flash.net

National Youth Advocacy Coalition
1711 Connecticut Avenue, NW, Suite 206, Washington, DC 20009-1139
Phone: 202-319-7596

Parents, Families and Friends of Lesbians and Gays (PFLAG)
1726 M Street NW, Suite 400, Washington, DC 20036
Phone: 202-638-4200, Fax: 202-467-8194, Email: info@pflag.org, http://www.pflag.org

Project Connect
Lesbian and Gay Community Services Center
208 West 13th Street, New York, New York 10011
Phone: 212-620-7310, http://www.gaycenter.org/index.html

Regional/State/Community Resources

Addiction Recovery Services
Los Angeles Gay & Lesbian Center
1625 N. Schrader Boulevard, Los Angeles, California 90028-9998
Phone: 213-993-7655

Alcoholism Center for Women
1147 S. Alvarado Street, Los Angeles, California 90006
Phone: 213-381-8500

Coalition of Lavender Americans on Smoking and Health (CLASH)
170 Columbus Avenue, Suite 200, San Francisco, California 94133
Phone: 415-956-1811

Fenway Community Health Center
7 Haviland Street, Boston, Massachusetts 02115
Phone: 617-267-0900

Gay Men's Health Crisis
129 West 20th Street, New York, New York 10011-3629
Phone: 212-337-1228

Hetrick-Martin Institute
2 Astor Place, New York, New York 10003
Phone: 212-674-2400

Lambda Program
Livengrin Foundation
4833 Hulmeville Road, Salem, Pennsylvania 19020
Phone: 215-638-5200

Lyon-Martin Women's Health Services
1741 Market Street, Suite 201, San Francisco, California 94102
Phone: 415-565-7667

New Leaf Services for Our Community
1853 Market Street, San Francisco, California 94103
Phone: 415-626-7000

Pacific Research and Training Alliance
440 Grand Street, Suite 401, Oakland, California 94610-5012
Phone: 510-465-0547

Pride Institute
14400 Martin Drive, Eden Prairie, Minnesota 55344
Phone: 612-934-7554

The Stepping Stone
3425 Fifth Avenue, San Diego, California 92103
Phone: 619-295-3995

Stonewall Recovery Series
430 Broadway Avenue East, Seattle, Washington 98102
Phone: 206-461-4546

Triangle Treatment Program
Robinson Institute
1841 Broadway, Suite 201, New York, New York 10023

Van Ness Recovery House
1919 North Beachwood Drive, Hollywood, California 90068
Phone: 213-463-4266

Whitman Walker Clinic
1407 S. Street, NW, Washington, DC 20009
Phone: 202-797-3500

Resources for African Americans

African American Parents for Drug Prevention
4025 Red Bud Avenue, Cincinnati, Ohio 45229
Phone: 513-961-4158, Fax: 513-961-6719

Institute on Black Chemical Abuse Resource Center
2616 Nicollet Avenue, South, Minneapolis, Minnesota 55407
Phone: 612-872-7878

National Association of African Americans for Positive Imagery
3536 North 16th Street, Philadelphia, Pennsylvania 19140
Phone: 215-225-5232

National Black Alcoholism and Addictions Council (NBAC)
1629 K Street, NW, Suite 802, Washington, DC 20006
Send correspondence to: 285 Jenesee Street, Upica, New York 103501
Phone: 202-296-2696, Fax: 202-775-7465

National Black Child Development Institute, Inc.
1023 15th Street, NW, Suite 600, Washington, DC 20005
Phone: 202-387-1281, Fax: 202-734-1738

Resources for Hispanics/Latinos

For Kids Only (English and Spanish versions)
National Clearinghouse for Alcohol and Drug Information (NCADI)
P.O. Box 2345, Rockville, Maryland 20847-2345
Phone: 800-729-6686, http://www.health.org/kidsarea/index.htm

Latino Caucus of the American Public Health Association
P.O. Box 92198, Long Beach, California 90809
Phone: 310-570-4016

National Coalition of Hispanic Health and Human Services Organization (COSSMHO)
1501 16th Street, NW, Washington, DC 20036
Phone: 202-387-5000, Fax: 202-797-4353, http://www.cossmho.org

National Council of La Raza
1111 19th Street NW, Suite 1000, Washington, DC 20036
Phone: 202-785-1670, http://www.nclr.org/

National Hispanic Education and Communications Projects
1000 16th Street, NW, Suite 603, Washington, DC 20036
Phone: 202-452-8750

National Hispano/Latino Community Prevention Network
Route 1, Box 204, Espanola, New Mexico 87532
Phone: 505-747-1889, Fax: 505-747-1623, Email: hmontoya@aol.com

Sue~os Publications
15865-B Gale Avenue, #1004
Hacienda Heights, California 91745
Phone: 310-693-9373

U.S.-Mexico Border Health Association
6006 N. Mesa, Suite 600, El Paso, Texas 79912
Phone: 915-581-6645

Internet Resources for Hispanics/Latinos

Instituto para el Estudio de las Adicciones
http://www.arrakis.es/iea/

Latin American Network Information Center (UT-LANIC)
telnet://lanic.utexas.edu, login=lanic
gopher://lanic.utexas.edu
http://lanic utexas.edu/

Latin American Youth Center
http://www.youthlink.net/layc/index.htm

MANA: A National Latina Organization
http://www.hermana.org/

National Hispano/Latino Community Prevention Network
http://www.emory.edu/NFIA/CONNECTIONS/NHLCPN/

The National Latino/A Research Center
http://www.rohan.sdsu.edu/dept/nlrc/

Prevention Program: Mothers and Daughters
http://www.health.org/gpower/AdultsWhoCare/walkn2wrlds.htm

WHEEL Council
http://home.fia.net/~wheel

Resources for Asian Pacific Islanders

Asian American Drug Abuse Program
5318 South Crenshaw Boulevard, Los Angeles, California 90043
Phone: 213-293-6284

Asian American Recovery Services, Inc.
785 Market Street, 10th Floor, San Francisco, California 94103
Phone: 415-541-9285

Asian & Pacific Islander American Health Forum
942 Market Street, Suite 200, San Francisco, California 94102
Phone: 415-954-9959, Fax: 415-954-9999
Washington, DC Area
Phone: 703-841-9128, Fax: 703-841-9017, Email: marnelle@apiahf.org

Chinatown Youth Center
1693 Polk Street, San Francisco, California 94109
Phone: 415-775-2636

Japanese Community Youth Council
2012 Pine Street, San Francisco, California 94115
Phone: 415-563-8052

Lao Family Community of Minnesota, Inc.
320 West University, St. Paul, Minnesota 55103
Phone: 612-221-0069

Midwest Regional Center for Drug Free Schools and Communities
1900 Spring Road, Suite 300, Oakbrook, Illinois 60521
Phone: 708-571-4710

National Asian Pacific American Families Against Substance Abuse (NAPAFASA)
1887 Maplegate Street, Monterey Park, California 91755-6536
Phone: 213-725-1311 or 213-278-0031, Fax: 213-278-9078,
Email: fkuramoto@prevline.health.org

National Development and Research Institutes, Inc.
Two World Trade Center, 16th Floor, New York, New York 10048
Phone: 212-845-4414

Northeast Regional Center for Drug Free Schools and Communities
12 Overton Avenue, Sayville, New York 11782
Phone: 516-589-7022

Office of Minority Health Resource Center
P.O. Box 37337, Washington, DC 20013
Phone: 800-444-6472

Santa Clara Valley Health and Hospital System
Department of Alcohol and Drug Services Prevention Division
595 Millich Drive, Campbell, California 95008
Phone: 408-378-6805

Southeast Asian Prevention and Intervention Network (SEAPIN) Resource Center
c/o United Cambodian Association of Minnesota
1821 University Avenue, Suite 319 South, St. Paul, Minnesota 55104
Phone: 612-645-7841

Southeast Regional Center for Drug Free Schools and Communities
Spencerian Office Plaza, Suite 350, University of Louisville, Louisville, Kentucky 40292
Phone: 502-852-0052
University of Oklahoma, 555 Constitution Avenue, Suite 138, Norman, Oklahoma 73072
Phone: 405-325-1454

Western Regional Asian Pacific Agency
8616 La Tijera Boulevard, Suite 200, Los Angeles, California 90045
Phone: 310-337-1550

Western Regional Center for Drug Free Schools and Communities
Northwest Regional Education Laboratory
101 SW Main Street, Suite 500, Portland, Oregon 97204
Phone: 503-275-9486

Internet Resources for Asian Pacific Islanders

Asian and Pacific Islander American Health Forum
http://www.igc.apc.org/apiahf/index.html

Countries of Asia
http://webhead.com/~sergio/asiacountries.html

Hmong Homepage
http://www.stolaf.edu/people/cdr/hmong/

Singapore Online Guide
http://www.travel.com.sg/sog

Viet-Net Web
http://www.vnet.org/

Resources for American Indians/Alaskan Natives

Department of Health and Human Services Administration for Native Americans
200 Independence Avenue, SW, Room 348F, Washington, DC 20201
Phone: 202-690-7776

Department of the Interior
Bureau of Indian Affairs, Office of Substance Abuse Prevention
1818 C Street, NW, Washington, DC 20240-0001
Phone: 202-208-2654, http://www.doi.gov/bia/

Indian Health Service (IHS)
Alcoholism and Substance Abuse Program
Room 5A-25, 5600 Fishers Lane, Rockville, Maryland 20857
Phone: 301-443-4297, http://www.ihs.gov

National Association for Native American Children of Alcoholics (NANACoA)
1402 Third Avenue, Suite 1110, Seattle, Washington 98101-2118
Phone: 206-467-7686, 800-322-5601, Fax: 206-467-7689, http://www.nanacoa.org/

Northern Plains Native American Chemical Dependency Association (NPNACDA)
P.O. Box 1153, Rapid City, South Dakota 57709
Phone: 605-341-5360, Email: npna@rapidnet.com,
http://www.rapidnet.com/npna/welcome.htm

Southwest Regional Center for Drug Free Schools and Communities
555 Constitution Avenue, Suite 138, Norman, Oklahoma 73072-7820
Phone: 800-234-SWRC

Internet Resources for American Indians/Alaskan Natives

Aboriginal Youth Net Solvent Abuse Module
http://www.ayn.ca/modules/solvent/index.html

AIDS Prevention and Education Network Contacts for Native American
and Aboriginal Populations
http://www.health.org/na.htm

Native American Voices
http://www.umc.org/naco/

Naturally Native Production
http://www.umc.org/naco/redhorse.htm

PowWows and Festivals by Lisa Mitten at the University of Pittsburgh
http://www.pitt.edu/~lmitten/powwows.html

Internet Resources and Referral Guide

Federal Resources

Centers for Disease Control and Prevention
http://www.cdc.gov/cdc.htm

**National Clearinghouse for Alcohol and Drug Information (NCADI)
and PREVline**
http://www.health.org

National Health Information Center
http://nhic-nt.health.org/

National Institutes of Health
http://www.nih.gov/

Office of Minority Health
http://www.os.dhhs.gov/progorg/ophs/omh/

Office of National Drug Control Policy
http://www.whitehouse.gov/WH/EOP/ondcp/html/ondcp.html

Online Drug Policy Library
http://www.druglibrary.org/

Partnership Against Violence Network (PAVnet)
gopher://cyfer.esusda.gov:70/11/violence
http://www.usdoj.gov/pavnet.htm

Substance Abuse and Mental Health Services Administration
http://www.samhsa.gov/

U.S. Department of Health and Human Services
http://www.os.dhhs.gov/

Additional Resources

Al-Anon/Alateen
http://www.al-anon.alateen.org

Alcoholics Anonymous
http://www.aa.org

American Council for Drug Education
http://www.acde.org

American Lung Association—Smoking and Pregnancy
http://www.lungusa.org/noframes/global/news/report/smking/smksmprefac.html

American Lung Association—Women and Smoking
http://www.lungusa.org/noframes/global/news/report/smking/smkwomenfac.html

American Society of Addiction Medicine
http://www.asam.org

Betty Ford Center
http://www.bettyfordcenter.com

Brink's Place
http://www.brinksplacetv.com

Bureau of Alcohol, Tobacco and Firearms
http://www.atf.treas.gov

Canadian Center on Substance Abuse
http://www.ccsa.ca

Center for Alcohol and Addiction Studies at Brown University
http://caas.caas.biomed.brown.edu

Center for Science in the Public Interest
http://www.cspinet.org

Center for Substance Abuse Prevention
http://www.samhsa.gov

Center for Substance Abuse Research
http://www.bsos.umd.edu/cesar/cesar.html

Christopher D. Smithers Foundation
http://www.com/smithers

Cocaine Anonymous
http://www.ca.org

Community Anti-Drug Coalitions of America
http://www.cadca.org

Drug Strategies
http://www.drugstrategies.org

Employee Assistance Professionals Association
http://www.EAP-Association.com

Employee Assistance Programs
http://www.healthtouch.com

Entertainment Industries Council
http://eiconline.org

Facing Alcohol Concerns Through Education (FACE Initiative)
http://faceproject.org

Fighting Back
http://www.mc.vanderbilt.edu/vumc/centers/varc/fightback/fight_back.html

Hazelden Foundation
http://www.hazelden.org

Jewish Alcoholics, Chemically Dependent Persons and Significant Others
http://www.jacsweb.org/

Johnson Institute
http://www.johnsoninstitute.com

Join Together
http://www.jointogether.org

Just Say No International
http://www.justsayno.org

Krooz Controlled
http://www.tiac.net/users/krooznet

McGovern Family Foundation
http://www.mcgovernfamily.org

The Marin Institute
http://www.marininstitute.org

Monitoring the Future Study: A Continuing Study of American Youth
http://www.isr.umich.edu/src/mtf/

Mothers Against Drunk Driving (MADD)
http://www.madd.org

Moyers on Addiction: Close to Home
http://www.wnet.org/closetohome/

Narcotics Anonymous
http://www.wsoinc.com

National Association for Children of Alcoholics (NACoA)
http://www.health.org/nacoa

National Association of Alcoholism and Drug Abuse Counselors (NAADAC)
http://www.naadac.org

National Association of State Alcohol and Drug Abuse Directors (NASADAD)
http://www.nasadad.org

National Association on Alcohol, Drugs and Disability, Inc. (NAADD)
http://www.naadd.org

National Center on Addiction and Substance Abuse at Columbia University
http://www.casacolumbia.org

National Clearinghouse for Alcohol and Drug Information
http://www.health.org

National Coalition of Hispanic Health and Service Organizations
http://www.cossmho.org

National Families in Action
http://www. emory.edu/NFIA

National Highway Traffic Safety Administration
http://www.nhtsa.dot.gov

National Inhalant Prevention Coalition
http://www.inhalants.org

National Institute on Alcohol Abuse and Alcoholism
http://www.niaaa.nih.gov

National Institute on Drug Abuse
http://www.nida.nih.gov

National Organization on Fetal Alcohol Syndrome
http://www.nofas.org

National PTA
http://www.pta.org/commonsense

National Women's Resource Center
http://www.nwrc.org

New York State Addiction Technology Transfer Center
http://www.albany.edu/pdp/attc/

New York State Office of Alcoholism and Substance Abuse Services
http://www.oasas.state.ny.us/

New York University Interdisciplinary Consortium on Substance Abuse—Resource Center
http://www.nyu.edu/education/icsa/resources/centers.html

Office of Minority Health Resource Center
http://www.omhrc.gov

Office of National Drug Control Policy
http://www.whitehousedrugpolicy. gov

Oxford House
http://www.oxfordhouse.org

Parents Resource for Drug Education
http://www.prideusa.org

Partnership for a Drug-Free America
http://www.drugfreeamerica.org

Phoenix House
http://www.phoenixhouse.org

Resources for Diversity
http://www.nova.edu/Inter-Links/diversity.html

Robert Wood Johnson Foundation
http://www.rwjf.org

Rutgers University Center of Alcohol Studies Library
http://www.rci.rutgers.edu/~cas2

Secular Organizations for Sobriety
http://www.codesh.org/sos

SMART Recovery
http://www.smartrecovery.org

Therapeutic Communities of America
http://www.tcanet.org

The Trauma Foundation
http://www.traumafdn.org

United Methodists in Recovery
Email: umrlist@aol.com

Women for Sobriety
http://www.mediapulse.com/wfs

Substances and Pregnancy: Audiovisual Resources and Publications

Audiovisual Resources

Addiction Research Foundation
33 Russell Street, Toronto, Canada M5S 251
Fetal Alcohol Syndrome discusses effects of alcohol on the fetus and fetal alcohol syndrome. Reviews techniques for diagnosis, detection, and prevention.

American Journal of Nursing Company
Educational Services Division
555 West 57th Street, New York, New York 10019-2961
Phone: 800-223-2282 or 212-582-8820
Death of the High Risk Infant outlines stages of grieving and provides guidelines for assisting parents in their grief. 30 minutes. Videocassette rental ($60) or sale ($250).

Harvard Medical School
Mental Health Training Film Program
58 Fenwood Road, Boston, Massachusetts 02115
Born with a Habit describes the pregnant addict, prenatal care, delivery problems, and treatment of the addicted neonate. For rental or sale.

March of Dimes
Supply Division
1275 Mamaroneck Avenue, White Plains, New York 10605
Born Hooked views complex medical, social, and ethical problems related to the pregnant drug addict and to the newborn suffering from narcotic withdrawal. 13:30 minutes. Videocassette or 16mm film.

Vida Health Communications
6 Bigelow Street, Cambridge, Massachusetts 02139
A Challenge to Care examines all aspects of chemical dependency and pregnancy. This film provides specific strategies for the comfort and care of the drug-exposed newborn.

National Publications

National Association for Perinatal Addiction Research and Education (NAPARE)
11 East Hubbard Street, Suite 200, Chicago, Illinois 60611
Phone: 302-329-2512

National Clearinghouse for Alcohol and Drug Information
Information Services
P.O. Box 2345, Rockville, Maryland 20852
Phone: 301-468-2600
Publications catalogue with material on alcohol and drug abuse for educators, health care providers, and clients.

National Council on Alcoholism and Drug Dependence, Inc.
12 West 21st Street, Eighth Floor, New York, New York 10010
Phone: 800-NCA-CALL or 212-206-6770
Materials on alcoholism, FAS, and FAE.

National Head Start Association
1220 King Street, Suite 200, Alexandria, Virginia 22314
Phone: 703-739-0875
Materials and support for preschool education and parenting.

National Sudden Infant Death Syndrome Clearinghouse
8201 Greensboro Drive, Suite 600, McLean, Virginia 22102
Phone: 703-821-8955
Materials to explain this serious risk associated with drug use during pregnancy.

Teratology Society
9650 Rockville Pike, Bethesda, Maryland 20814
Phone: 301-571-1841
Information on specific teratogenic agents.

Publications: Drugs and Pregnancy

March of Dimes Birth Defects Foundation
1275 Mamaroneck Avenue, White Plains, New York 10605
Phone: 914-428-7100
Drugs, Alcohol, and Tobacco Abuse During Pregnancy (1987). A 2-page booklet with basic facts about the effects on the fetus and newborn of exposure to tobacco, alcohol, prescription drugs, antacids, aspirin, laxatives, vitamins, caffeine, uppers, downers, and street drugs. Single copies are free and can be duplicated.

Trish Magyari
Georgetown University Child Development Center
3800 Reservoir Road, NW, Washington, DC 20008
Phone: 202-687-8635
I Want to Have a Healthy, Happy Baby (1988). A 6-page pamphlet describing the dangers of alcohol, cigarettes, and other drugs during pregnancy. It also discusses risks for AIDS. It is developed for a primarily black, inner-city audience in the District of Columbia. Single copies are free and can be duplicated.

Publications: Tobacco and Pregnancy

American Lung Association
1740 Broadway, New York, New York 10019
Phone: 212-315-8700
Freedom from Smoking for You and Your Baby (1986). A 10-day self-help guide for mothers to stop smoking. It includes a progress record. Copies are $1.40 each.

March of Dimes Birth Defects Foundation
1275 Mamaroneck Avenue, White Plains, New York 10605
Phone: 914-428-7100
Babies Don't Thrive in Smoke-Filled Rooms (1986). A 4-page pamphlet that highlights risks of smoking during pregnancy.

National Institute of Health
NHLBI Smoking Educational Program Information Center
4733 Bethesda Avenue, Suite 530, Bethesda, Maryland 20814
Phone: 301-951-3260
Pregnant? That's Two Good Reasons to Quit Smoking (1983). An 8-page booklet that describes risks and encourages mothers to quit smoking. There is an accompanying poster. Single copies are free.

Index